Clinical Pharmacology of Gastrointestinal and Liver Disease

Guest Editor

RICHARD H. HUNT, FRCP, FRCPEd, FRCPC, FACG, AGAF

GASTROENTEROLOGY CLINICS OF NORTH AMERICA

www.gastro.theclinics.com

September 2010 • Volume 39 • Number 3

SAUNDERS an imprint of ELSEVIER, Inc.

W.B. SAUNDERS COMPANY

A Division of Elsevier Inc.

Elsevier Inc. • 1600 John F. Kennedy Blvd., Suite 1800 • Philadelphia, Pennsylvania 19103-2899

http://www.theclinics.com

GASTROENTEROLOGY CLINICS OF NORTH AMERICA Volume 39, Number 3
September 2010 ISSN 0889-8553, ISBN-13: 978-1-4377-2524-7

Editor: Kerry Holland

Gastroenterology Clinics of North America (ISSN 0889-8553) is published quarterly by Elsevier Inc., 360 Park Avenue South, New York, NY 10010-1710. Months of issue are March, June, September, and December. Business and Editorial Offices: 1600 John F. Kennedy Blvd., Suite 1800, Philadelphia, PA 19103-2899. Customer Service Office: 6277 Sea Harbor Drive, Orlando, FL 32887-4800. Periodicals postage paid at New York, NY and additional mailing offices. Subscription prices are $264.00 per year (US individuals), $135.00 per year (US students), $416.00 per year (US institutions), $290.00 per year (Canadian individuals), $507.00 per year (Canadian institutions), $366.00 per year (international individuals), $186.00 per year (international students), and $507.00 per year (international institutions). Foreign air speed delivery is included in all *Clinics* subscription prices. All prices are subject to change without notice. **POSTMASTER**: Send address changes to *Gastroenterology Clinics of North America*, Elsevier Health Sciences Division, Subscription Customer Service, 3251 Riverport Lane, Maryland Heights, MO 63043. Telephone: 1-800-654-2452 (U.S. and Canada); 314-447-8871 (outside U.S. and Canada). Fax: 314-447-8029. E-mail: journalscustomerservice-usa@elsevier.com (for print support); journalsonlinesupport-usa@elsevier.com (for online support).

Reprints. For copies of 100 or more, of articles in this publication, please contact the Commercial Reprints Department, Elsevier Inc., 360 Part Avenue South, New York, New York 10010-1710. Tel. (212) 633-3813, Fax: (212) 462-1935, E-mail: reprints@elsevier.com.

Gastroenterology Clinics of North America is also published in Italian by Il Pensiero Scientifico Editore, Rome, Italy; and in Portuguese by Interlivros Edicoes Ltda., Rua Commandante Coelho 1085, 21250 Cordovil, Rio de Janeiro, Brazil.

Gastroenterology Clinics of North America is covered in *MEDLINE/PubMed (Index Medicus)*, *Excerpta Medica*, *Current Contents/Clinical Medicine*, *Science Citation Index*, *ISI/BIOMED*, and *BIOSIS*.

Printed and bound by CPI Group (UK) Ltd, Croydon, CR0 4YY
Transferred to Digital Print 2011

Contributors

GUEST EDITOR

RICHARD H. HUNT, FRCP, FRCPEd, FRCPC, FACG, AGAF
Professor, Division of Gastroenterology and Farncombe Family Digestive Disease
Research Institute, McMaster University Health Science Centre, Hamilton, Ontario,
Canada

AUTHORS

DAVID ARMSTRONG, MA, MB BChir, FRCP(UK), FACG, AGAF, FRCPC
Associate Professor, Division of Gastroenterology, McMaster University, Hamilton,
Ontario, Canada

MATTHEW R. BANKS, BSc, MB BS, PhD, FRCP
Consultant Gastroenterologist, Department of Gastroenterology, University College
Hospital; Honorary Senior Lecturer, University College London, London, United Kingdom

ALAN BARKUN, MD, CM, MSc (Clinical Epidemiology)
Research Scholar (Chercheur National), Fonds de la Recherche en Santé du Québec,
Division of Gastroenterology, Montreal General Hospital, The McGill University Health
Center, Montréal, Canada

WOJCIECH BLONSKI, MD, PhD
Division of Gastroenterology, University of Pennsylvania, Philadelphia, Pennsylvania;
Department of Gastroenterology, Medical University, Wroclaw, Poland

ROBERT S. BRESALIER, MD
Professor of Medicine, Resoft Distinguished Professor of GI Oncology, Department
of Gastroenterology, Hepatology and Nutrition, The University of Texas, MD Anderson
Cancer Center, Houston, Texas

MICHAEL CAMILLERI, MD
Clinical Enteric Neuroscience Translational and Epidemiological Research (CENTER),
Mayo Clinic College of Medicine, Rochester, Minnesota

CHENG E. CHEE, MD
Hematology/Oncology Fellow, Department of Oncology, Mayo Clinic, Rochester,
Minnesota

STEPHEN M. COLLINS, MD
Farncombe Family Digestive Health Institute, McMaster University Medical Centre,
Hamilton, Ontario, Canada

RAYMOND N. DUBOIS, MD, PhD
Provost and Executive Vice President of MD Anderson Cancer Center and Professor,
Department of Gastrointestinal Medical Oncology and Cancer Biology, The University
of Texas MD Anderson Cancer Center, Houston, Texas

RICHARD N. FEDORAK, MD, FRCPC
Professor of Medicine, Division of Gastroenterology; and Associate Vice-President, Research, University of Alberta, Edmonton, Alberta, Canada

JOSE G.P. FERRAZ, MD, PhD
Clinical Associate Professor, Inflammation Research Network, University of Calgary, Calgary, Alberta, Canada

TAKAHISA FURUTA, MD, PhD
Associate Professor, Center for Clinical Research, Hamamatsu University School of Medicine, Higashi-Ku, Hamamatsu, Japan

GUADALUPE GARCIA-TSAO, MD
Professor of Medicine, Section of Digestive Diseases, Yale University School of Medicine, New Haven, Connecticut

MARC G. GHANY, MD, MHSc
Liver Diseases Branch, National Institute of Diabetes and Digestive and Kidney Diseases, National Institutes of Health, Bethesda, Maryland

DAVID Y. GRAHAM, MD, PhD
Professor of Medicine, Molecular Virology and Microbiology, Michael E. DeBakey Veterans Affairs Medical Center, Baylor College of Medicine, Houston, Texas

JOSHUA GREENSPOON
Division of Gastroenterology, Montreal General Hospital, The McGill University Health Center, Montreal, Canada

BJORN I. GUSTAFSSON, MD, PhD
Senior Research Scientist, Department of Gastroenterology, Institute for Cancer Research and Molecular Medicine, NTNU, Trondheim; Senior Gastroenterology Consultant, Department of Gastroenterology, St Olavs University Hospital, Trondheim, Norway

CHANUNTA HONGTHANAKORN, MD
Research Fellow, Division of Gastroenterology, University of Michigan, Ann Arbor, Michigan

COLIN W. HOWDEN, MD
Professor of Medicine, Division of Gastroenterology, Northwestern University Feinberg School of Medicine, Chicago, Illinois

RICHARD H. HUNT, FRCP, FRCPEd, FRCPC, FACG, AGAF
Professor, Division of Gastroenterology and Farncombe Family Digestive Disease Research Institute, McMaster University Health Science Centre, Hamilton, Ontario, Canada

ALEXANDRA J. KENT, MBChB
Research Fellow, Department of Gastroenterology, John Radcliffe Hospital, Oxford, United Kingdom

MARK KIDD, PhD
Research Scientist, Gastrointestinal Pathobiology Research Group, Yale University School of Medicine, New Haven, Connecticut

BEN LAWRENCE, MBChB, MSc
Medical Oncology Registrar, Department of Medical Oncology, Auckland City Hospital, Auckland, New Zealand; Postdoctoral Associate, Gastrointestinal Pathobiology Research Group, Yale University School of Medicine, New Haven, Connecticut

THOMAS W. LEE, MBBS, FRACP
Inflammatory Bowel Disease Fellow, University of Alberta, Edmonton, Alberta, Canada

GARY R. LICHTENSTEIN, MD
Professor of Medicine, Division of Gastroenterology, University of Pennsylvania, Philadelphia, Pennsylvania

MING VALERIE LIN, MD
Department of Internal Medicine, Pennsylvania Hospital, University of Pennsylvania Health System, Philadelphia, Pennsylvania

ANNA S.F. LOK, MD
Professor of Medicine, Division of Gastroenterology, University of Michigan, Ann Arbor, Michigan

CECILIA MIÑANO, MD, MPH
Gastroenterology Fellow, Section of Digestive Diseases, Yale University School of Medicine, New Haven, Connecticut

IRVIN MODLIN, MD, PhD, DSc, FRCS (Eng & Ed)
Professor, Gastrointestinal Pathobiology Research Group, Yale University School of Medicine, New Haven, Connecticut

MAZEN NOUREDDIN, MD
Liver Diseases Branch, National Institute of Diabetes and Digestive and Kidney Diseases, National Institutes of Health, Bethesda, Maryland

NEEHAR PARIKH, MD
Fellow, Division of Gastroenterology, Northwestern University Feinberg School of Medicine, Chicago, Illinois

SATISH S.C. RAO, MD, PhD, FRCP (Lon)
Division of Gastroenterology/Hepatology, Department of Internal Medicine, University of Iowa Carver College of Medicine, University of Iowa Hospitals and Clinics, Iowa City, Iowa

CARMELO SCARPIGNATO, MD, DSc (Hons), PharmD (h.c.), FRCP (Lond), FCP, FACG
Professor, Division of Gastroenterology, Department of Clinical Sciences; Laboratory of Clinical Pharmacology, School of Medicine and Dentistry, University of Parma, Italy

MEHNAZ A. SHAFI, MD
Associate Professor of Medicine, Department of Gastroenterology, Hepatology and Nutrition, The University of Texas, MD Anderson Cancer Center, Houston, Texas

FERGUS SHANAHAN, MD
Professor and Chair, Department of Medicine, and Director, Alimentary Pharmabiotic Centre, University College Cork, National University of Ireland, Ireland

DANIEL SIFRIM, MD, PhD
Professor of GI Physiology, Director of Upper GI Physiology Unit, Barts and The London School of Medicine and Dentistry, Wingate Institute of Neurogastroenterology, London, United Kingdom

FRANK A. SINICROPE, MD
Professor of Oncology and Medicine, Department of Oncology and Division of Gastroenterology, Mayo Clinic, Rochester, Minnesota

SIDDHARTH SINGH, MD
Division of Gastroenterology/Hepatology, Department of Internal Medicine, University of Iowa Carver College of Medicine, University of Iowa Hospitals and Clinics, Iowa City, Iowa

IRENE SONU, MD
University of Pennsylvania School of Medicine, Philadelphia, Pennsylvania

JAN F. TACK, MD
Department of Gastroenterology, University Hospitals Leuven, Leuven, Belgium

JOHN L. WALLACE, PhD, MBA
Professor of Medicine, Farncombe Family Digestive Health Research Institute, McMaster University, Hamilton, Ontario, Canada

DINGZHI WANG, PhD
Professor, Department of Cancer Biology, The University of Texas MD Anderson Cancer Center, Houston, Texas

Contents

Preface   xv

Richard H. Hunt

CLINICAL PHARMACOLOGY OF THE GASTROINTESTINAL TRACT AND PANCREAS

New Pharmacologic Approaches in Gastroesophageal Reflux Disease   393

David Armstrong and Daniel Sifrim

This article highlights current and emerging pharmacological treatments for gastroesophageal reflux disease (GERD), opportunities for improving medical treatment, the extent to which improvements may be achieved with current therapy, and where new therapies may be required. These issues are discussed in the context of current thinking on the pathogenesis of GERD and its various manifestations and on the pharmacologic basis of current treatments.

The Pharmacological Therapy of Non-Variceal Upper Gastrointestinal Bleeding   419

Joshua Greenspoon and Alan Barkun

The modern management of patients with upper gastrointestinal bleeding includes, in selected patients, the performance of timely multimodal endoscopic hemostasis followed by profound acid suppression. This article discusses the available data on the use of antisecretory regimens in the management of patients with bleeding peptic ulcers, which are a major cause of non-variceal upper gastrointestinal bleeding, and briefly addresses other medications used in this acute setting. The most important clinically relevant data are presented, favoring fully published articles.

Nonsteroidal Antiinflammatory Drug-Related Injury to the Gastrointestinal
Tract: Clinical Picture, Pathogenesis, and Prevention   433

Carmelo Scarpignato and Richard H. Hunt

Increasing life expectancy in developed countries has led to a growing prevalence of arthritic disorders, which has been accompanied by increasing prescriptions for nonsteroidal antiinflammatory drugs (NSAIDs). These are the most widely used agents for musculoskeletal and arthritic conditions. Although NSAIDs are effective, their use is associated with a broad spectrum of adverse reactions in the liver, kidney, cardiovascular system, skin, and gut. Gastrointestinal (GI) side effects are the most common. The dilemma for the physician prescribing NSAIDs is, therefore, to maintain the antiinflammatory and analgesic benefits, while reducing or preventing GI side effects. The challenge is to develop safer NSAIDs by shifting from a focus on GI toxicity to the increasingly more appreciated cardiovascular toxicity.

Pharmacologic Aspects of Eradication Therapy for *Helicobacter pylori* Infection   465

Takahisa Furuta and David Y. Graham

The commonly used regimens for the eradication of *Helicobacter pylori* infection consist of administration of proton pump inhibitors (PPIs) and 1 to 3 antimicrobial agents, such as amoxicillin, clarithromycin, metronidazole, fluoroquinolone, or tetracycline. Each agent has its own pharmacologic characteristics. PPIs are metabolized by cytochrome P450 2C19 (CYP2C19), which is polymorphic. CYP2C19 genotypic differences in the pharmacokinetics and pharmacodynamics of PPIs influence the eradication rates of *H pylori* infection by PPI-containing regimens. Amoxicillin is a time-dependent antibiotic, whereas clarithromycin, metronidazole, tetracycline, and fluoroquinolone are not. The plasma half-life of antimicrobial agents also differs among these antibiotics. To achieve consistently high eradication rates, the eradication regimens must be designed based on a good understanding of the resistance patterns of the bacteria and the pharmacologic characteristics of the agents used for *H pylori* eradication therapy.

Current Medical Treatments of Dyspepsia and Irritable Bowel Syndrome   481

Michael Camilleri and Jan F. Tack

Dyspepsia is a highly prevalent condition characterized by symptoms originating in the gastroduodenal region without underlying organic disorder. Treatment modalities include acid-suppressive drugs, gastroprokinetic drugs, *Helicobacter pylori* eradication therapy, tricyclic antidepressants, and psychological therapies. Irritable bowel syndrome is a multifactorial, lower functional gastrointestinal disorder involving disturbances of the brain-gut axis. The pathophysiology provides the basis for pharmacotherapy: abnormal gastrointestinal motor functions, visceral hypersensitivity, psychosocial factors, intraluminal changes, and mucosal immune activation. Medications targeting chronic constipation or diarrhea may also relieve irritable bowel syndrome. Novel approaches to treatment require approval, and promising agents are guanylate cyclase cagonists, atypical benzodiazepines, antibiotics, immune modulators, and probiotics.

Pharmacological Management of Diarrhea   495

Alexandra J. Kent and Matthew R. Banks

According to the World Health Organization, there are approximately 2 billion annual cases of diarrhea worldwide. Diarrhea is the leading cause of death in children younger than 5 years and kills 1.5 million children each year. It is especially prevalent in the developing world, where mortality is related to dehydration, electrolyte disturbance, and the resultant acidosis, and in 2001, it accounted for 1.78 million deaths (3.7% of total deaths) in low- and middle-income countries. However, diarrhea is also a common problem in the developed world, with 211 million to 375 million episodes of infectious diarrheal illnesses in the United States annually, resulting in 73 million physician consultations, 1.8 million hospitalizations, and 3100 deaths. Furthermore, 4% to 5% of the Western population suffers from chronic diarrhea. Given the high prevalence of diarrhea, research has been directed at learning more about the cellular mechanisms underlying diarrheal illnesses in order to develop new medications directed at novel cellular targets. These cellular mechanisms and targets are discussed in this article.

Pharmacologic Management of Chronic Constipation   509

Siddharth Singh and Satish S.C. Rao

Chronic constipation is a common digestive problem in North America, with significant psychosocioeconomic implications. Dietary and lifestyle measures and low-cost traditional over-the-counter laxatives are usually the first line of therapy but help only half of the patients. Several newer agents that act by increasing colonic peristalsis, altering colonic secretion, and/or antagonizing enteric opioid receptors have been developed that are effective in treating constipation and its related symptoms as well as improving quality of life. This article focuses on the pharmacology of traditional and newer agents for the treatment of constipation.

The Safety of Drugs Used in Acid-related Disorders and Functional Gastrointestinal Disorders   529

Neehar Parikh and Colin W. Howden

Medicines are frequently used in the management of acid-related disorders and functional gastrointestinal disorders. With the exception of complicated peptic ulcer disease, these disorders are not associated with appreciable mortality. Drug treatments have consequently been held to the highest standards of safety. Some medicines have been withdrawn or restricted based on assessments and perceptions of risk. However, the risk of serious toxicity is low for most of the agents discussed in this article. Assessments are made of the safety and adverse-event profiles of certain drug classes and, where appropriate, individual medicines. For conditions with a low risk of mortality or serious morbidity, clinicians need to balance the risks of potential adverse events with the anticipated benefits of a successful outcome of specific drug treatment.

Tumor Necrosis Factor-α Monoclonal Antibodies in the Treatment of Inflammatory Bowel Disease: Clinical Practice Pharmacology   543

Thomas W. Lee and Richard N. Fedorak

In the last 10 years, anti-tumor necrosis factor (TNF)-α therapy has become a cornerstone in the management of autoimmune diseases. Clinical trial data have consistently found that infliximab, adalimumab, and recently certolizumab pegol offer therapeutic benefits to patients with inflammatory bowel diseases (Crohn's disease and ulcerative colitis). Recent understanding on how these monoclonal antibodies evoke changes at the physiological and molecular levels have provided insights into disease pathogenesis and helped to identify new targets for future drug therapy. With increased experience in the use of these anti-TNF-α antibodies the long-term safety data, use in pregnancy have become available. This article provides an overview of the current knowledge regarding anti-TNF-α therapies for clinicians caring for patients with Crohn's disease and ulcerative colitis.

Clinical Pharmacology of 5-ASA Compounds in Inflammatory Bowel Disease   559

Irene Sonu, Ming Valerie Lin, Wojciech Blonski, and Gary R. Lichtenstein

Mesalamine has been the first-line of therapy in patients with inflammatory bowel disease (IBD) since the 1960s. This article serves as a review of the different 5-aminosalicylic acid compounds, release formulations, use and dosing in the treatment of IBD, in particular ulcerative colitis.

Targeted Therapeutic Agents for Colorectal Cancer   601

Cheng E. Chee and Frank A. Sinicrope

The treatment of colorectal cancer (CRC) has evolved substantially during the past decade with the advent of molecular targeted therapies. Inhibitors to the vascular endothelial growth factor and epidermal growth factor receptor (EGFR) pathways have been shown to enhance the efficacy of cytotoxic chemotherapy in patients with advanced CRC, and anti-EGFR antibodies demonstrate modest activity as monotherapeutic agents. These biologic agents have improved patient outcomes and survival and have been incorporated into routine clinical practice establishing a new standard of care. Molecular markers have recently been adopted into clinical practice with the finding that the *KRAS* oncogene is a predictive biomarker for anti-EGFR therapy, whereby the therapeutic benefit of anti-EGFR treatment is restricted to tumors with wild-type *KRAS*. The use of molecular targeted agents has fewer yet more specific toxicities compared with conventional cytotoxic drugs and enables a more personalized approach to cancer therapy. In contrast to the results for advanced CRC, targeted therapies have not shown a benefit in the adjuvant setting for patients with resected colon cancer. The goal of this review is to provide an update on the medical management of CRC, with a focus on the use of targeted therapy.

New Pharmacologic Therapies for Gastroenteropancreatic Neuroendocrine Tumors   615

Ben Lawrence, Bjorn I. Gustafsson, Mark Kidd, and Irvin Modlin

Successful treatment of unresectable and metastatic gastroenteropancreatic neuroendocrine tumors (GEP-NETs) requires the thoughtful choice of systemic therapy as a component of a multidisciplinary therapeutic approach. The role of somatostatin analogues is established in symptom relief, but the efficacy of interferon and radiopeptide targeted therapy is not clear. The utility of a variety of tyrosine kinase and antiangiogenic agents is variable and under investigation, whereas the role of cytotoxic chemotherapy in poorly differentiated GEP-NETs is accepted. Overall, the ideal treatment of more indolent tumors is less certain. Reassessments of the GEP-NET pathology classification has provided improved logic for the role of a variety of agents, whereas the precise positioning of many new agents that target molecular pathways of angiogenesis and proliferation is under examination. This article describes the current options for systemic therapy for GEP-NETs within the framework of the current World Health Organization classification system.

The Gastrointestinal Complications of Oncologic Therapy   629

Mehnaz A. Shafi and Robert S. Bresalier

A spectrum of oncologic treatments including chemotherapy, radiotherapy, and molecular targeted therapies is available to combat cancer. These treatments are associated with adverse effects in several organ systems including the gastrointestinal (GI) tract. The immunocompromised state induced by oncologic therapy is also an important contributing factor underlying GI complications. This review discusses common GI complications that can result from cancer therapy. The pathologic mechanisms underlying each complication and the pharmacology of the agents used to treat these complications are discussed.

CLINICAL PHARMACOLOGY OF THE LIVER

Pharmacokinetics and Pharmacodynamics of Peginterferon and Ribavirin: Implications for Clinical Efficacy in the Treatment of Chronic Hepatitis C   649

Mazen Noureddin and Marc G. Ghany

The pharmacokinetics and pharmacodynamics of standard interferon alfa-2a and interferon alfa-2b are substantially altered by pegylation. The size, geometry, and site of attachment of the PEG moiety affect the pharmacokinetics and pharmacodynamics as evidenced by the different absorption, volume of distribution, and clearance of the linear 12-kDa peginterferon alfa-2b and the branched 40-kDa peginterferon alfa-2a. Despite these differences, the clinical efficacy, safety, and tolerability of the 2 peginterferons are similar. However, evidence exists that peginterferon alfa-2 plus ribavirin is associated with small but significantly higher sustained virological response rates compared with peginterferon alfa-2b. This article discusses the pharmacokinetics and pharmacodynamics of the 2 peginterferons and their combination with ribavirin.

New Pharmacologic Therapies in Chronic Hepatitis B   659

Chanunta Hongthanakorn and Anna S.F. Lok

Approximately 350 million persons worldwide are chronically infected with hepatitis B, which can result in cirrhosis, liver failure, and hepatocellular carcinoma. Currently, 2 interferons and 5 nucleos(t)ide analogues have been approved for the treatment of chronic hepatitis B (CHB). This article discusses the mechanisms of action, pharmacokinetics, optimal dose, clinical efficacy, and side effects of medications used for the treatment of CHB.

Clinical Pharmacology of Portal Hypertension   681

Cecilia Miñano and Guadalupe Garcia-Tsao

Portal hypertension is an increase in pressure in the portal vein and its tributaries. It is defined as a portal pressure gradient (the difference in pressure between the portal vein and the hepatic veins) greater than 5 mm Hg. Although this gradient defines portal hypertension, a gradient of 10 mm Hg or greater defines clinically significant portal hypertension, because this pressure gradient predicts the development of varices, decompensation of cirrhosis, and hepatocellular carcinoma. The most direct consequence of portal hypertension is the development of gastroesophageal varices that may rupture and lead to the development of variceal hemorrhage. This article reviews the pathophysiologic bases of the different pharmacologic treatments for portal hypertension in patients with cirrhosis and places them in the context of the natural history of varices and variceal hemorrhage.

NEW DIRECTIONS IN CLINICAL PHARMACOLOGY OF GI DISEASES

Therapeutic Potential of Peroxisome Proliferator-Activated Receptors in Chronic Inflammation and Colorectal Cancer   697

Dingzhi Wang and Raymond N. DuBois

Peroxisome proliferatoreactivated receptors (PPARs) are members of the nuclear hormone receptor superfamily and have been implicated in a variety of physiologic and pathologic processes, such as nutrient metabolism, energy homeostasis, inflammation, and cancer. This article highlights breakthroughs in our understanding of the potential roles of PPARs in inflammatory bowel disease and colorectal cancer. PPARs might hold the key to some of the questions that are pertinent to the pathophysiology of inflammatory diseases and colorectal cancer and could possibly serve as drug targets for new antiinflammatory therapeutic and anticancer agents.

New Pharmacologic Therapies in Gastrointestinal Disease   709

John L. Wallace and Jose G.P. Ferraz

Many gastrointestinal diseases remain poorly responsive to therapies, and even in the cases of conditions for which there are many effective drugs, there is still considerable room for improvement. This article is focused on drugs for digestive disorders that have entered the marketplace recently, or are expected to reach the marketplace within the next 1 to 2 years. Although advances have been made in understanding gastrointestinal motility, visceral pain, mucosal inflammation, and tissue repair, the major gastrointestinal diseases remain as significant therapeutic challenges.

Pharmabiotic Manipulation of the Microbiota in Gastrointestinal Disorders, from Rationale to Reality   721

Fergus Shanahan and Stephen M. Collins

The viewpoints of enthusiasts and skeptics in relation to the role of probiotics should not be allowed to distract clinicians from the bigger issue, which is the pivotal role of the microbiota in the protection against many disorders and in the pathogenesis of others. However, all probiotics, like all bacteria, are not created equal, and therapeutic deployment in a generic sense is as absurd as the administration of pills or tablets without regard for the nature of the active ingredient and the intended effect. The rationale for therapeutic manipulation or supplementation of the microbiota is sound in conditions where the intestinal ecosystem is poorly developed, such as in low birth weight neonates, or where it is profoundly disturbed, such as after broad-spectrum antibiotics. In other conditions, such as irritable bowel disorder (IBD), the efficacy of some, but not all, probiotics has been a welcome surprise. However, the impact of probiotics is likely to be modest and is probably more complicated in IBD. In choosing a probiotic strategy, clinicians should adhere to the principles of evidence-based therapeutics. These include: selection from a reputable supplier, with appropriate documentation of contents and shelf life; anticipation of strain-specific effects; avoidance of cocktails without documentation of the activities of each ingredient with absence of interstrain antagonism; and published evidence of efficacy from clinical trials.

Index   727

FORTHCOMING ISSUES

December 2010
Advanced Imaging in Gastroenterology
Ralf Kiesslich, MD,
Guest Editor

March 2011
Irritable Bowel Syndrome
William D. Chey, MD,
Guest Editor

June 2011
Women's Issues in Gastroenterology
Barbara B. Frank, MD, and
Asyia Ahmad, MD,
Guest Editors

RECENT ISSUES

June 2010
Gallbladder Disease
Cynthia W. Ko, MD, MS,
Guest Editor

March 2010
Gastroenterologic Issues in the Obese Patient
David A. Johnson, MD,
Guest Editor

December 2009
Challenges in Inflammatory Bowel Disease
Miguel Regueiro, MD, and
Arthur M. Barrie III, MD, PhD,
Guest Editors

THE CLINICS ARE NOW AVAILABLE ONLINE!

Access your subscription at:
www.theclinics.com

FORTHCOMING ISSUES

December 2010
Advanced Imaging in Gastroenterology
Asif Khalfeh, MD
Guest Editor

March 2011
Irritable Bowel Syndrome
William D. Chey, MD,
Guest Editor

June 2011
Women's Issues in Gastroenterology
Barbara B. Blanc, MD, and
Asyia Ahmad, MD
Guest Editors

RECENT ISSUES

June 2010
Gallbladder Disease
Cynthia W. Ko, MD, MS
Guest Editor

March 2010
Gastroenterologic Issues in the
Cancer Patient
David A. Johnson, MD
Guest Editor

December 2009
Challenges in Inflammatory Bowel Disease
Miguel Regueiro, MD, and
Arthur M. Barrie III, MD, PhD
Guest Editors

Preface

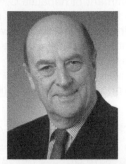

Richard H. Hunt, FRCP, FRCPEd, FRCPC, FACG, AGAF
Guest Editor

The evolution of drug therapy moves rapidly and it is often difficult for the practitioner to keep up with the introduction of new drugs or the subtle changes in regimen or dose to optimize clinical outcomes. This is especially true for diseases managed by gastroenterologists, who often look after the full spectrum of cases ranging from upper GI disorders to inflammatory bowel disease, GI bleeding, those with hepatobiliary and pancreatic disease, and increasingly, patients with GI oncology diagnoses. Regrettably, there is less emphasis in the current curricula of many medical schools on clinical pharmacology and the teaching of therapeutics or *materia medica*, as it was often called. Thus, many busy clinicians find that managing optimal treatments for such a wide range of GI problems is very challenging. This volume of *Gastroenterology Clinics of North America* sets out to address some of these issues.

I should like to acknowledge the distinguished authors whose contributions are assembled here. They have provided an informative background to the therapeutic choices in a range of commonly encountered conditions and they highlight current best clinical practice based on the available evidence.

The topics range in order of presentation from GERD, NSAIDs, and the GI tract, eradication of H pylori infection, upper GI nonvariceal bleeding, and the functional GI disorders including management of diarrhea and constipation. There is also an article on the safety of drugs used in these disease areas. There are contributions in IBD on the commonly used 5-ASA drugs and the anti-TNFα biological agents. There is a section on oncology focused on the medical management of colorectal cancer, on new approaches to GI tumors, and on new treatments for gastroenteropancreatic neuroendocrine tumors, and it ends with the adverse effects seen in the GI tract from oncological treatment protocols in general. In the section on liver disease, articles cover treatment of hepatitis B and C and the management of portal hypertension.

The contributions have been chosen to clarify areas where there is evidence of confusion about the clinical pharmacology, to update our knowledge in fast-moving therapeutic areas, or to highlight new approaches. Examples of the former are the

Gastroenterol Clin N Am 39 (2010) xv–xvi
doi:10.1016/j.gtc.2010.08.016
0889-8553/10/$ – see front matter © 2010 Elsevier Inc. All rights reserved.

use of PPIs in patients with GERD, eradication of *H pylori* infection, and UGI bleeding or the use of 5-ASA drugs in IBD. Examples of fast-moving therapeutic areas include the management of colorectal cancer and the treatment of hepatitis C. Highlighting new approaches are the new medical treatments for GI tumors and for neuroendocrine tumors. The volume ends with 2 glimpses to the future including new pharmacological treatments for GI disease and the second more provocative on the potential to manipulate the gastrointestinal microbiota for therapeutic benefit.

Both the authors and I hope that you will find their contributions to be of help and value in your practice and as stimulating education about those therapeutic areas that you do not typically cover in your daily practice.

Richard H. Hunt, FRCP, FRCPEd, FRCPC, FACG, AGAF
Division of Gastroenterology and
Farncombe Family Digestive Disease Research Institute
McMaster University Health Science Centre
Room 4W8A, 1200 Main Street West
Hamilton, ON L8N 3Z5, Canada

E-mail address:
huntr@mcmaster.ca

New Pharmacologic Approaches in Gastroesophageal Reflux Disease

David Armstrong, MA, MB BChir, FRCP(UK), AGAF, FRCPC[a],
Daniel Sifrim, MD, PhD[b],*

KEYWORDS

- Gastroesophageal reflux disease • GERD
- Pharmacologic therapies • Heartburn

Gastroesophageal reflux disease (GERD) has come to be regarded as a simple condition that is easy to treat; proton pump inhibitors (PPIs) are generally considered the most effective medical treatment of GERD. Patients with mild or infrequent symptoms often do not require PPI therapy but those with more severe or frequent symptoms may benefit significantly from regular PPI therapy.

One of the major challenges in GERD management is the persistence of symptoms despite regular, once-daily therapy, considered by some as PPI failure. However, this is not necessarily a failure of acid suppression therapy. Current, first-generation PPIs have a short plasma half-life and cannot provide day-long acid suppression; thus, there are opportunities for improved outcomes with (1) more frequent dosing using current PPIs, (2) longer-acting PPIs or potassium-competitive acid blockers (P-CABs), (3) antireflux agents, (4) visceral pain modulators, or (5) mucosal protectants. In the short-term, improved outcomes can be achieved by fine-tuning treatment using currently available medications, based on their pharmacology and the patient's disease manifestations; a careful consideration of the choice of drug, dose, and treatment regimen is crucial in the day-to-day management of GERD. For the future, an improved understanding of GERD and the pharmacology of available medications is essential for improving symptoms and quality of life.

BACKGROUND

The prevalence of GERD is increasing worldwide and it has become the most prevalent gastrointestinal disorder. It is responsible for a substantial proportion of health

[a] Division of Gastroenterology, HSC-4W8F, McMaster University Medical Centre, 1200 Main Street West, Hamilton, ON L8N 3Z5, Canada
[b] Barts and The London School of Medicine and Dentistry, Wingate Institute of Neurogastroenterology, 26 Ashfield Street, London E12AJ, UK
* Corresponding author.
E-mail address: d.sifrim@qmul.ac.uk

Gastroenterol Clin N Am 39 (2010) 393–418
doi:10.1016/j.gtc.2010.08.019
0889-8553/10/$ – see front matter © 2010 Elsevier Inc. All rights reserved.

care expenditure in the developed world.[1] In the last 3 decades, the development of increasingly potent acid suppressants has revolutionized the medical management of GERD. Initially, histamine H_2-receptor antagonists (H_2-RAs) supplanted antacids for the healing of erosive esophagitis (EE); H_2-RAs were, in turn, supplanted, to a large extent, by PPIs, which provided healing and symptom relief in a significantly greater proportion of patients than H_2-RAs.[2,3] Despite the success of acid suppression, GERD is not primarily a disorder of acid secretion and there have been many attempts to develop pharmacologic, endoscopic, and surgical treatments to increase basal lower esophageal sphincter (LES) pressure, reduce the frequency and duration of inappropriate transient LES relaxations (TLESRs), improve esophageal clearance, and accelerate gastric emptying. The attractions of targeting the pathophysiologic basis of GERD rather than acid suppression have not yielded new medications that produce healing and symptom relief comparable with those reported for PPIs.

Documented costs for managing GERD are attributable predominantly to the costs of pharmacotherapy,[4,5] although surgical therapy is also associated with substantial costs, as are over-the-counter remedies.[6-9] The costs of treating GERD and its complications have prompted close scrutiny of prescribing habits with the expectation that management guidelines and consequent constraints on pharmacotherapy will reduce expenditure.[9,10] Reports that antireflux therapy may be provided without documentation of a diagnostic indication, in up to one-third of patients,[11,12] suggest a significant opportunity to reduce the costs of GERD treatments. However, GERD is associated with an increased risk of esophageal adenocarcinoma and other complications[13,14] and with substantial impairment of patients' sleep, work productivity, and quality of life that warrant therapy.[13] Furthermore, despite apparently optimal therapy, many patients continue to experience symptoms attributable to GERD, suggesting that there are still unmet needs.

The aim of this article to is to highlight current and emerging treatments for GERD, opportunities for improving medical treatment, the extent to which improvements may be achieved with current therapy, and where new therapies may be required. These issues are discussed in the context of current thinking on the pathogenesis of GERD and its various manifestations and on the pharmacologic basis of current treatments.

PATHOPHYSIOLOGY OF GERD

The Montreal definition of GERD as "a condition which develops when the reflux of stomach contents causes troublesome symptoms and/or complications",[13] is widely accepted; however, this definition does not specify how and why reflux occurs, which organs are affected by the reflux, or what symptoms and complications may be associated with the reflux of gastric contents.

Gastroesophageal reflux (GER) occurs in healthy individuals without any obvious sequelae; it is generally considered normal for the esophagus to be exposed to gastric acid (pH < 4) for up to 3% to 4% of the day (approximately 45–60 minutes a day). Similarly, TLESRs are normal events that occur in response to physiologic gastric distension. The duration of esophageal acid exposure, documented at one point, 5 cm above the LES, is often termed the reflux time; this implies that it is gastric acid or, more precisely, esophageal luminal fluid with a pH less than 4.0, that causes GERD. However, in an unknown proportion of patients, GERD symptoms seem to be associated with the presence of weakly acidic or alkaline conditions in the esophagus, suggesting that factors other than gastric acid and pepsin may be responsible for GERD.

Thus, excessive GER can occur for several reasons (**Box 1**), which may be amenable to pharmacologic therapy; however, the range of causes is such that not

---

Box 1
Potential mechanisms underlying symptoms or signs of GERD

Excessive GER

- Delayed gastric emptying with retention of gastric contents

  Gastroparesis

  Gastric outlet obstruction

  Small bowel dysmotility (carbohydrate, gluten intolerance)

- Hiatus hernia

- Reduced basal LES pressure

- Excessive TLESRs

- Increased gastric acid secretion

  Zollinger-Ellison syndrome

  Rebound hypersecretion after withdrawal of acid suppression therapy

  Helicobacter pylori-negative status

  Increased duodenogastroesophageal reflux

  Bile acids

  Pancreatic secretions

Excessive esophageal exposure to noxious agents

- Impaired esophageal clearance

  Disordered esophageal body motility

  Impaired salivary secretion

- Hiatus hernia

- Luminal agents

  Acidic foods

  Alcohol

  Medications (eg, bisphosphonates, antibiotics)

Excessive esophageal sensitivity

- Functional esophageal disease (Rome)

- Esophageal hyperalgesia

- Central hyperalgesia

  Depression

  Irritable bowel syndrome

- Concurrent inflammation

  Eosinophilic esophagitis

---

all of these causes could be responsive to the same medication or to a single, standard treatment regimen. Depending on the causes of an individual's GERD, it may be appropriate to target dietary factors, motility factors, concurrent therapy, meal-related factors, daytime or night-time acid secretion, structural factors (eg, hiatal hernia), or psychological factors.

MANIFESTATIONS OF GERD

GERD is remarkable for the variety of possible causes and for its protean manifestations (**Box 2**). Although it is generally accepted that heartburn and regurgitation are diagnostic of GERD,[13] these typical symptoms may occur in the absence of GERD (so-called functional heartburn).[15] Moreover, GERD may present with other atypical symptoms referable to the esophagus or to other organs.[13] Although GER and GERD symptoms are common postprandially, recent studies highlight the association between GERD and sleep disturbances and the observation that sleep disturbances may improve with effective antireflux therapy.[13] The diurnal patterns of GER that lead to typical symptoms may therefore be different from those associated with sleep

---

Box 2
Potential manifestations of GERD

- Symptomatic: esophageal

  Typical symptoms

    Heartburn, regurgitation

    Chest pain

    Dysphagia

  Atypical symptoms

    Abdominal pain or burning

    Nausea, vomiting

- Symptomatic: nonesophageal

  Cough

  Wheeze

  Hoarseness

  Shortness of breath

  Sleep disturbance

  Earache

  Dysphagia/globus symptoms

  Glossitis

  Toothache

- Complications

  Esophageal mucosal breaks (erosions/ulcers)

  Esophageal stricture

  Barrett esophagus

  Esophageal adenocarcinoma

  Reflux laryngopharyngitis

  Bronchitis

  Pneumonia

  Otitis media

  Dental erosions

disturbance or noncardiac chest pain; similarly, the timing and duration of reflux episodes documented in patients with nonerosive reflux disease (NERD) are different from those observed in patients with EE or Barrett esophagus.[16] Data are limited with respect to the characteristics of reflux in patients with laryngopharyngitis, asthma, otitis media, or dental erosions attributed to GERD. However, it would not be surprising if, for example, the diurnal reflux patterns in patients with presumed reflux laryngopharyngitis differed from those in patients with EE. Thus, even if the causes of the reflux episodes were similar in patients with different manifestations of GER, one might expect differing therapeutic requirements for different presentations.

ACID SUPPRESSION THERAPY

For a variety of reasons, including patient adherence and commercial considerations, emphasis has been placed on developing antireflux therapies that need to be taken only once daily. Although this strategy is associated with greater adherence than multiple daily doses,[17,18] it is appropriate only if the pharmacologic profile is consistent with therapeutic goals. Prompt acid neutralization by antacids is associated with rapid relief of reflux symptoms but the effect is short-lived with no prospect of antacids being used as a once-daily therapy. Histamine H_2-RAs have a significantly longer duration of action, offset by the fact that their effect is not immediate. In the treatment of GERD, H_2-RAs were evaluated twice daily; although H_2-RAs are more effective than placebo for healing EE, their long-term effectiveness is compromised by tachyphylaxis[19–23] and there is little, if any, benefit from using doses up to twice the standard healing dose.[24] The short duration of effect and tachyphylaxis of H_2-RAs limits their benefit when used once daily.

PPIs have proved significantly more effective than antacids or H_2-RAs for healing and maintaining remission in EE and for maintaining symptom relief.[2,3] Studies documented more prolonged acid suppression with PPIs than with H_2-RAs and the degree of acid suppression, because the proportion of the 24-hour period during which gastric pH exceeded 4.0 correlated with the proportion of patients with healing of their EE over 8 weeks.[25] Gastric pH studies confirmed that, although currently available PPIs have their C_{max} (maximum concentration) at 90 to 120 minutes after administration, they produce more prolonged acid suppression (gastric pH ≥ 4.0) because they are covalently bound to the proton pumps; this suppression is overcome only when new proton pumps are inserted into the secretory membrane of the parietal cell canaliculus. As a result, current PPIs, taken once daily, can produce sufficient gastric acid suppression to achieve healing and symptom relief in many patients with GERD. Despite this situation, currently available PPIs have identifiable limitations related to their mechanism of action.[26] Conventional PPIs do not have a rapid onset of action because they are prodrugs, administered in an enteric, acid-resistant formulation, to prevent premature inactivation by gastric acid; after dissolution of the enteric coating, the prodrug is absorbed in the small intestine. Because PPIs are weak bases, they are concentrated in the highly acidic, secretory canaliculus; activation of the prodrug to its sulphenamide form occurs only in the acidic secretory canaliculus of an actively secreting parietal cell, when the activated sulphenamide produces irreversible inhibition of those proton pumps (H+-K+ ATPase) that are actively inserted in the secretory canalicular membrane. These events occur only if circulating blood levels are high enough to allow sufficient PPI prodrug to concentrate in active parietal cells; however, because conventional PPIs have a t_{max} (time of maximum concentration) of about 1 to 6 hours and a half-life of about 60 to 130 minutes, the PPI plasma residence time is less than 12 hours (**Fig. 1**), such that plasma levels decrease below the therapeutic

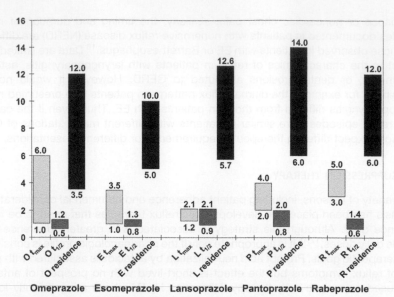

Omeprazole Esomeprazole Lansoprazole Pantoprazole Rabeprazole

Fig. 1. Pharmacokinetic data for 5 PPIs that are widely available; t_{max} and $t_{1/2}$ vary for each drug, with t_{max} ranging overall from 1.0 hours to 6.0 hours and $t_{1/2}$ ranging overall from 0.5 hours to 3.5 hours; the calculated residence time (the time, after ingestion, during which the plasma concentrations remain greater than 3% of the C_{max}) does not exceed 14.0 hours for any PPI. (*Data from* Klotz U. Pharmacokinetic considerations in the eradication of *Helicobacter pylori*. Clin Pharmacokinet 2000;38:243–70; Shi S, Klotz U. Proton pump inhibitors: an update of their clinical use and pharmacokinetics. Eur J Clin Pharmacol 2008;64:935–51.)

threshold within 4 to 10 hours of drug ingestion.[27,28] Parietal cells that become active more than 4 to 10 hours after drug ingestion remain uninhibited because plasma PPI levels have fallen below the therapeutic threshold (**Fig. 2**); as a result, gastric acidity steadily recovers over the 16 to 18 hours that remain until the next single daily dose. Because blocked proton pumps are not replaced for 3 to 4 days, PPIs have a progressively greater effect in reducing gastric acidity over the first 3 to 5 days of administration but, despite this, their effect diminishes over the 24-hour period between doses as new proton pumps are synthesized and acid secretion gradually increases.[29] This situation may not be a problem for many patients with GERD whose symptoms occur predominantly during the daytime but, for other patients, the loss of PPI effect may permit nocturnal return of acid secretion (**Fig. 3**A) and nocturnal acid reflux (see **Fig. 3**B), leading to persistent night-time symptoms on once-daily PPI therapy. For some patients, the PPI effect is influenced by differences in PPI pharmacokinetics; variability in blood PPI levels, and hence in gastric acidity, and may be to the result of differences in absorption or differences in PPI metabolism related, for example, to CYP2C19 polymorphisms.[30,31] As a result, 24-hour gastric acidity can vary by as much as 3 to 4 log units between individuals (**Fig. 4**); furthermore, this interindividual variability does not seem to disappear after 3 days of once-daily oral dosing.[32]

Pure PPI isomers, such as esomeprazole, dexlansoprazole, and TU-199 (an isomer of tenatoprazole), generally produce higher blood levels than the racemic mixtures, leading to an increase in gastric acid suppression; in early studies with esomeprazole, the increase in gastric acid suppression was attributed to an increased area under the

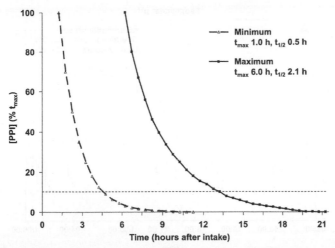

Fig. 2. Simulated plasma concentration curves for 2 theoretic PPIs that have the shortest t_{max} and $t_{1/2}$ (minimum) and longest t_{max} and $t_{1/2}$ (maximum) reported for the 5 PPIs that are, currently, most widely available; even under the latter conditions (maximum), plasma concentrations decrease to less than 10% off the C_{max} by 13 to 14 hours after PPI ingestion. Thus, minimal PPI is available to inhibit proton pump function for the last 8 to 11 hours of the day in patients receiving once-daily PPI. (*Data from* Klotz U. Pharmacokinetic considerations in the eradication of *Helicobacter pylori*. Clin Pharmacokinet 2000;38:243–70; Shi S, Klotz U. Proton pump inhibitors: an update of their clinical use and pharmacokinetics. Eur J Clin Pharmacol 2008;64:935–51.)

curve (AUC) for the concentration-time curve[33,34] but more recent studies with dexlansoprazole[35] and other PPIs suggest that there is a threshold effect; that is, regardless of the peak concentration or AUC, acid suppression is achieved as long as blood levels exceed a threshold level.[35–37] In clinical practice, threshold blood levels can be maintained by multiple daily oral dosing[38,39] or by continuous infusion as in the management of upper gastrointestinal bleeding.[39–41] Multiple daily dosing regimens raise concerns about patient adherence, and concerns remain that first-generation PPIs are slow to achieve an effective reduction in gastric acidity.

Recognition that current PPIs do not address all clinical needs has led to new antisecretory agents that offer more rapid onset and a more prolonged duration of action.[42,43] Speed of onset has been addressed by an immediate-release (IR) omeprazole formulation that contains uncoated omeprazole powder (20 mg or 40 mg) plus sodium bicarbonate (1680 mg)[44]; the sodium bicarbonate neutralizes gastric acid, protecting the acid-labile omeprazole from degradation and, in addition, stimulating gastrin release by increasing gastric pH; the latter effect stimulates insertion of acid pumps, analogous to food-stimulated acid secretion, such that the parietal cells are activated and, hence, susceptible to omeprazole. The antisecretory effect of IR omeprazole is evident more quickly than that of classic delayed-release PPIs.[45–47] Esomeprazole, the first pure isomer PPI, produces a greater AUC than racemic omeprazole, and the associated increase in acid suppression is associated with a small, but significant increase in healing rates for EE.[48–53] Another approach to prolonged acid suppression is to extend the period during which blood levels of the PPI exceed the threshold level needed to achieve therapeutic levels of the PPI in the secretory canaliculus of the parietal cell. Dexlansoprazole, the R-isomer of lansoprazole, is metabolized more slowly than the S-isomer; it is now approved in the United States as

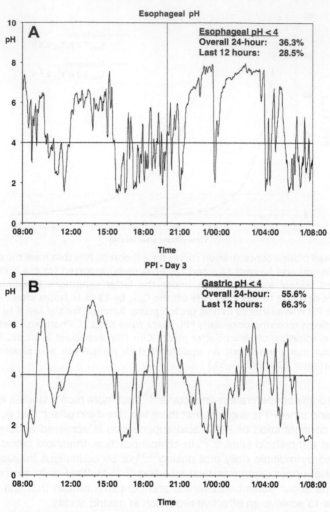

Fig. 3. Luminal pH recordings from (A) the esophagus and (B) the stomach. (A) A 24-hour esophageal pH recording, off therapy, from a patient who has severe LA grade C EE; there is significant esophageal acid exposure through the day but, importantly, there is prolonged acid exposure during the latter half of the recording (pH < 4.0 for 28.5% of the recording). (B) A 24-hour gastric pH recording in a healthy, H pylori-negative patient after 3 days of rabeprazole, 20 mg daily; during the latter half of the recording, the gastric pH is acidic (<4.0) for 66.3% of the time.

a modified, dual-release formulation in which some of the R-isomer has a standard enteric coating and some a modified coating that releases the PPI at a higher pH; as a result, there is a second peak in blood levels and a more prolonged increase of dexlansoprazole levels above threshold levels. Clinically, dual-release dexlansoprazole (60 mg and 90 mg daily) healed EE after 8 weeks in 92.7% and 93.3% of patients, respectively, whereas standard lansoprazole, 30 mg daily, produced healing in 88.9% of patients (P<.01).[54] Although differences for healing, symptom relief, and maintenance of remission[55–57] are comparable with the differences between esomeprazole 40 mg daily and omeprazole 20 mg daily,[49,50] it is not clear how much of the effect

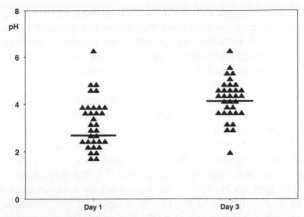

Fig. 4. Median 24-hour gastric pH values from 33 healthy, *H pylori*-negative patients on the first (day 1) and third (day 3) days during which they received rabeprazole 20 mg daily. The group median pH values were 3.1 (day 1) and 4.3 (day 3) but there was marked, interpatient variability with respect to the individual median 24-hour gastric pH values. (*Data from* Armstrong D, James C, Camacho F, et al. Oral rabeprazole vs. intravenous pantoprazole: a comparison of the effect on intragastric pH in healthy subjects. Aliment Pharmacol Ther 2007;25:185–96.)

is because of the change in formulation and how much to the absolute increase in dosage. Neither of the other isomeric PPIs, S-pantoprazole[58] or dexrabeprazole,[59] is available clinically and their benefit in clinical practice remains uncertain.[60]

Other PPIs, still in development, include AGN 201,904-Z,[37] ilaprazole (IY-81,149),[61] and tenatoprazole (TU-199).[36,62–66] AGN 201,904-Z, the sodium salt of an acid stable omeprazole prodrug, is designed to provide continued metered absorption throughout the gut and, thus, prolong the plasma PPI residence time; the prodrug is converted rapidly to omeprazole in the systemic circulation, producing faster and greater acid suppression than esomeprazole 40 mg daily in healthy, *H pylori*-negative male volunteers.[37] Ilaprazole is a benzimidazole derivative that has a longer half-life and greater acid suppression than omeprazole.[42] Racemic tenatoprazole, an imidazo-pyridine derivative, has a longer half-life ($t_{1/2} \sim$ 8–9 hours) than first-generation benzimidazole-derived PPIs, with the result that it produces a significantly higher median 24-hour pH than esomeprazole, 40 mg daily, after 7 days' administration.[62–64] A crossover study comparing isomeric S-tenatoprazole sodium, 30 mg, 60 mg, and 90 mg daily, with esomeprazole, 40 mg daily, showed that the higher doses produced significantly greater and more prolonged dose-dependent 24-hour and nocturnal acid suppression than esomeprazole.[66] A meta-analysis of individual subject data from 4 pharmacodynamic studies has shown, also, that S-tenatoprazole sodium, 60 mg daily, produces greater acid suppression than esomeprazole, 40 mg daily, and is comparable with esomeprazole, 40 mg twice daily,[67] although there are no clinical trial data in patients.

In the last few years, another class of acid suppressants has been developed; the P-CABs also inhibit the H^+-K^+ ATPase but, unlike PPIs, they target the potassium-binding region of the proton pump. P-CABs are lipophilic weak bases with a high pKa and are stable at low pH. They are absorbed rapidly and are concentrated, up to 100,000-fold, in the secretory canaliculus; the protonated form then binds ionically, but reversibly to the proton pump,[68] producing rapid and profound acid suppression.[69,70] Initial studies with P-CABs such as linaprazan (AZD-0865), revaprazan (YH1885), and soraprazan indicated that these compounds have a more rapid onset of action and the potential for greater acid suppression than conventional PPIs.[71–74] Linaprazan (AZD-0865) given once daily was not superior to esomeprazole, 40 mg daily, in the treatment of EE and NERD,[75,76] and the development program for this compound has been halted.

Although antacids and H_2-RAs are less effective than PPIs, they still have a role in management of patients with GERD, particularly as over-the-counter medications.[77] As prescription medications, H_2-RAs alone are not, generally, effective for more severe grades of GERD; however, they are still recommended and used widely for patients with mild or infrequent symptoms[78,79] and also, in combination with PPIs, for patients with persistent nocturnal symptoms.[80] Initial enthusiasm for combined therapy with a PPI and an H_2-RA[81] was tempered by a diminution in benefit that was observed as tachyphylaxis to the H_2-RA developed[19,82]; however, more recent data, and studies with combinations of a PPI and an H_2-RA, suggest that there is still a role for combination acid suppression therapy in some patients with GERD.[42,79–81,83]

NONACID SUPPRESSION THERAPY

Acid suppression therapy remains the mainstay of medical management for GERD, and PPIs provide the most effective acid suppression therapy. Despite this, PPIs are less effective for complete symptom relief and, furthermore, relapse of symptoms and complications such as erosions, strictures, and hemorrhage can occur, even with maintenance PPI therapy. There are good pharmacologic reasons why some patients might not respond to standard, once-daily therapy with a PPI and, although there is good reason to assume that increased acid suppression improves response rates, there are several other mechanisms that might underlie PPI failure in GERD, including the presence of esophagitis or other esophageal diseases, persistent weakly acidic reflux or duodenogastroesophageal reflux, delayed gastric emptying, esophageal hypersensitivity, concomitant functional bowel disorders, and psychological comorbidity. Identification of the individual underlying mechanisms for persistent symptoms, where possible, might be relevant for the management of refractory GERD. Several agents under development may have a role in selected refractory reflux patients. They include motility agents to accelerate gastric emptying and improve esophageal clearance, antireflux agents that reduce the frequency of TLESRs and thereby the number of acid and nonacid reflux episodes, visceral pain modulators to reduce visceral hypersensitivity, and mucosal protection agents. None of these agents, on its own, is likely to be as effective as a PPI in so many patients but there may be a role for these medications in combination with acid suppression therapy.

MOTILITY AGENTS

A significant factor in the pathophysiology of GERD is disordered gastroesophageal motility,[84] including one or more of these abnormalities: delayed gastric emptying, reduced LES pressure, increased incidence of reflux during TLESRs, and ineffective esophageal clearance. Together with a hiatal hernia, disordered gastroesophageal motility may favor GER and/or determine the volume, proximal extent, and composition of the refluxates. Gastroesophageal hypomotility might be a cofactor involved in refractoriness to PPI treatment.[85] Several prokinetic agents can stimulate gastrointestinal motility and many of these agents have been used, either alone or in combination with a PPI or H_2-RA, for the treatment of GERD. Bethanechol, metoclopramide, domperidone, cisapride, and macrolides, such as erythromycin or ABT-229, have all been used in patients with GERD.[86-97] Although these drugs are believed predominantly to impart their effect by enhancing esophageal motility, reflux clearance, basal LES pressure, reducing TLESRs, and by accelerating gastric emptying, many of these compounds are not highly selective and have off-target effects. This situation means that the mechanism of action responsible for their therapeutic effects often remains controversial, and undesirable side effects are often encountered. For example, cisapride, a 5-HT$_4$ agonist that was approved for use in GERD before subsequently being withdrawn for safety reasons, not only increased the rate of gastric emptying but also modified saliva secretion and bicarbonate content and gastric acid secretion, believed to occur via potassium channels,[92,98] which also mediated the adverse cardiac effects of cisapride. Although cisapride was more effective than placebo in symptom relief and healing esophagitis, studies indicated that cisapride has little effect on esophageal motility and, notably, no effect on TLESRs after 4 weeks of oral (20 mg twice daily) administration.[89] Tegaserod, another partially selective 5-HT$_4$ agonist, also showed some efficacy in small GERD trials. Tegaserod (1 and 4 mg/d) reduced postprandial reflux and TLESRs but did not alter LES tone.[93] However, as with cisapride, it is uncertain whether the beneficial effects of tegaserod were because of the effect on motor function or other recently documented effects on salivary flow rate, salivary bicarbonate and epidermal growth factor secretion, and bicarbonate secretion from esophageal submucosal glands.[99,100] Tegaserod has also been withdrawn from the market for safety issues.

Motilin is a peptide found in specific endocrine cells in the epithelia of the upper small intestine.[101,102] Motilin receptor agonists can increase gastric emptying after ingestion of a meal; this action is mediated via the cholinergic system of the stomach.[103] Much of this evidence is derived from the use of erythromycin, a macrolide antibiotic that also acts as a motilin receptor agonist.[95] Erythromycin, given at low doses, which have no antibiotic effect, was the first motilin agonist used in several clinical situations, particularly in severe gastroparesis. Early studies found erythromycin to be of no value in the control of reflux.[86] ABT-229, an erythromycin derivative devoid of antibiotic activity, accelerates gastric emptying and increases LES pressure[103] in healthy persons; however, the therapeutic effect of ABT-229 in patients with GERD was limited in terms of modulation of both esophageal motility (LES pressure and TLESRs) and acid exposure.[104,105] The development of ABT-229 has been discontinued because of a rapid onset of tachyphylaxis and worsening of symptoms in dyspeptic patients. In a recent study in patients after lung transplantation, another macrolide antibiotic, azithromycin, reduced the number of reflux events and total esophageal acid exposure and also reduced the proximal extent to which reflux regurgitated.[94]

There are several limitations when using macrolides as prokinetics in GERD. The most consistent data supporting their role as prokinetics in reflux disease come from studies in which the drug was administered intravenously[86,88,106]; this would not be suitable for a broader GERD population. In addition, repeat administration of macrolides induces desensitization of the motilin receptor, reducing their efficacy over time.[102,107] Macrolides also induce side effects, including nausea and abdominal cramping, which are believed to be caused by direct activation of motilin receptors on gastric smooth muscle, which occurs at higher doses[102] and which makes macrolides difficult to tolerate for many patients. A more selective motilin agonist, which could be taken orally, would be highly desirable to test in patients with GERD with compromised gastroesophageal motor function.

Few studies have assessed the value of the current therapeutic approach to delayed gastric emptying in patients with GERD, who failed PPI therapy. However, it is likely that these patients also complain about other dyspeptic symptoms related to slow gastric motor activity. There are no data about the value of adding a promotility drug in patients who have failed PPI therapy, given once or twice per day. However, in patients with delayed gastric emptying and persistent GERD symptoms on PPI therapy, the use of a promotility agent remains an attractive option.

ANTIREFLUX AGENTS

Prevention of GER, either acidic or nonacidic, should be the ultimate goal of GERD treatment. As reflux mainly occurs during TLESRs,[108,109] drugs targeting this motor pattern may be useful to reduce GERD symptoms.[110,111] Although most studies show no difference in the number of TLESRs, between healthy individuals and patients with GERD, patients with GERD have acid reflux twice as often during a TLESR compared with healthy individuals.[112,113] A recent study described a possible reason for this difference. The position of a proximal gastric acid pocket is largely determined by the presence of a hiatal hernia. Entrapment of the pocket above the diaphragm, especially in patients with hiatal hernia, is a major risk factor underlying the increased occurrence of acidic reflux during a TLESR in patients with GERD.[114] The importance of hiatal hernia and other reflux mechanisms, such as straining, absent LES pressure, and reflux induced by swallowing, should also be emphasized when considering the efficacy of drugs aimed at reducing the occurrence of TLESRs.

Several pharmacologic agents, including γ-aminobutyric acid-B (GABA$_B$[115–123]) and GABA$_A$ receptor agonists,[124] cholecystokinin A antagonists,[125] morphine,[126] glutamate antagonists,[127] cannabinoids,[128,129] metabotropic glutamate receptor agonists and antagonists,[129–131] and nitric oxide synthase inhibitors,[132] all reduce the triggering of TLESRs. These drugs have not reached clinical development, mainly owing to their undesirable pharmacologic profile and/or side effects.

GABA$_B$RECEPTOR AGONISTS

Baclofen, a GABA$_B$receptor agonist, used in the clinical management of spasticity, reduces TLESRs in animals[133] and healthy volunteers.[118] The maximal inhibition of TLESRs provoked by baclofen in humans varies between 40% and 60%.[118,121] Administration of baclofen also increases basal LES pressure and reduces the number of reflux episodes in patients with GERD.[115–117,119–121,134] One study evaluated the effect of baclofen (4–10 mg daily) for 4 weeks in patients with GERD[116] and showed a significant reduction in acid exposure and symptoms. These results reinforce the point that reflux inhibition is a valid concept in treating GERD, because the inhibition of TLESRs seems to be associated with a reduction in acid exposure. Furthermore, they show that humans do not become tolerant of baclofen when it is taken for a longer period. Short-term studies showed that baclofen was also effective in patients with hiatal hernia.[135] However, because baclofen increases basal LES pressure it is possible that this effect adds to the effect on TLESRs in patients with hiatal hernia.

Baclofen not only reduces acid reflux but also has a similar inhibitory effect on nonacid reflux and duodenal reflux. Vela and colleagues[120] showed that 40 mg of baclofen reduced both postprandial acid and nonacid reflux measured with impedance-pH monitoring and decreased associated symptoms in healthy individuals and patients with heartburn. Similarly, Koek and colleagues[117] showed that baclofen (5 mg, 3 times daily) effectively reduced duodenal reflux (measured by Bilitec) and associated PPI-resistant symptoms.

Arbaclofen placarbil is a prodrug of R-baclofen, the active stereoisomer of baclofen. A recent trial in 50 patients with GERD revealed that it is well tolerated and reduced the number of reflux episodes and associated heartburn.[136] However, the effect was marginal and larger studies are required.

Baclofen has effects on the central nervous system (CNS) that limit its value for treating GERD. As the drug crosses the blood-brain barrier, a variety of CNS-related side effects may occur, including somnolence, confusion, dizziness, lightheadedness, drowsiness, weakness, and trembling. Baclofen has a short pharmacologic half-life (3–4 hours), which necessitates dosing 3 or more times per day.

Attention is focusing on the development of new GABA$_B$ receptor agonists that act primarily at peripheral sites and therefore have better tolerability. For example, lesogaberan[137] has a similar pharmacodynamic effect on reflux parameters to baclofen, resulting in almost complete inhibition of TLESRs in dogs, and a similar degree of inhibition as baclofen in healthy individuals.[122] However, in contrast to baclofen, this agent seems to act in the periphery, with a low incidence of CNS-related adverse effects, making it more interesting as an add-on therapy for the treatment of patients with GERD with an incomplete response to PPI therapy. A recent randomized trial with 232 patients has shown a significant difference in symptom response with lesogaberan compared with placebo.[138]

GLUTAMATE RECEPTOR ANTAGONISTS

Glutamate is involved in the vagovagal reflex, triggering TLESRs. Glutamate binds to metabotropic glutamate receptors (mGluRs) structurally related to GABA$_B$ receptors. A recent study showed that riluzole (a benzothiazole inhibiting the release of excitatory amino acids such as glutamate and aspartate) attenuated the rate of TLESRs triggered by isovolumetric distention in healthy volunteers.[127]

More selective mGluR5 antagonists potently inhibit TLESRs and reflux in ferrets and dogs.[130,139] Recent studies showed that ADX10059, a potent, selective, negative allosteric modulator of mGluR5, improved esophageal pH-metry and clinical symptoms in patients with GERD.[131,140] Further development of this drug for chronic use in reflux disease was canceled because of liver toxicity.

CANNABINOID RECEPTOR AGONISTS

Cannabinoid CB$_1$ receptors have been localized in brain areas involved in the triggering of TLESRs. A study in dogs showed that the CB receptor agonist WIN 55,212-2 reduced the occurrence of TLESRs in response to gastric distension by 80%.[128] A study in ferrets confirmed involvement of CB$_1$ receptors in the central regulation of LES relaxation and showed the presence of CB$_1$ receptors in the brain centers involved in the triggering of TLESRs.[141] These data indicate that CB$_1$ agonists may be clinically useful to reduce TLESRs in humans but, like baclofen, central side effects were reported and so more specific CB$_1$ agonists devoid of central side effects need to be further investigated.

PPI treatment does not abolish nonacid reflux[142] and the esophagus continues to be exposed to gastric contents with mild ongoing mucosal irritation and possible persistence of symptoms. Patients with GERD who failed PPI therapy may show an association between their symptoms and 3 different types of GER: weak acidic/alkaline reflux, acidic reflux, and duodenal GER. Drugs targeting the mechanisms underlying GER or TLESRs could also reduce nonacid and DGER. Patients with NERD or low-grade esophagitis mainly reflux during TLESRs. This subgroup should benefit most from drugs that reduce TLESRs. More probably, the best indication for reflux inhibitors in GERD is to improve PPI-resistant symptoms by reducing persistent nonacid and acid reflux. This strategy implies that reflux inhibitors are prescribed as add-on treatment in this subgroup of patients.

VISCERAL PAIN MODULATORS

There are no studies specifically evaluating the value of visceral pain modulators in patients with GERD with persistent heartburn despite PPI treatment. However, given that most patients who fail PPI treatment originate from the NERD group, and that up to 40% of PPI failures show a lack of either weak or acidic reflux during intraesophageal impedance assessment, the use of these agents is highly attractive. Pain modulators such as tricyclic antidepressants, trazodone, and selective serotonin reuptake inhibitors (SSRIs) all improve esophageal pain in patients with noncardiac chest pain.[143–145] It is thought that these agents confer their visceral analgesic effect by acting on the CNS and/or sensory afferents. The pain modulators are used in non-mood-altering doses, and provide a therapeutic alternative until more novel and esophageal-specific compounds become available.

Human studies supporting a spinal mechanism in the development of visceral hypersensitivity are limited; however, using a model of acid-induced esophageal pain hypersensitivity, the development of secondary allodynia in the nonacid-exposed proximal esophagus after a distal esophageal acid infusion has been shown.[146] This secondary allodynia is believed to occur through sensitization of spinal neurons, and can be attenuated by both the prostaglandin E_2 receptor-1[147] and N-methyl-D-aspartate receptor antagonist, ketamine.[148] These studies suggest that spinal neurons can induce visceral hypersensitivity and may also be treated using specific therapies.

MUCOSAL PROTECTION

The human esophagus contains esophageal submucosal glands (SMGs), which secrete bicarbonate, mucin, and other products. Esophageal SMG secretions are likely to serve a protective effect against injury to the mucosa by refluxed gastric acid either by direct buffering of luminal acid or by creating a preepithelial defense and buffer zone close to the mucosal surface. Given these observations, drugs that stimulate SMG secretion may have beneficial effects in patients with GERD.

Sucralfate is protective against acid or acid-pepsin injury to rabbit and cat esophagus. Its beneficial action is due, in part, to enhanced mucosal defense (cytoprotection) because it can occur in the absence of luminal buffering of hydrogen ion.[149]

Tegaserod is a secretogogue that increases duodenal bicarbonate secretion; the presence of serotonin receptors in the esophagus may explain the finding that tegaserod stimulates esophageal SMG bicarbonate secretion, an effect that likely accounts for the observed protection against acid-pepsin injury to pig, but not rabbit, esophagus.[99]

Exposure of esophageal epithelial cells to unconjugated bile acids increases intracellular reactive oxygen species, and this effect is blocked by antioxidants. Recent preliminary studies showed that changes in esophageal mucosal integrity induced by weakly acidic solutions with unconjugated bile acids, similar to reflux in patients with GERD on PPI, can be prevented with antioxidants.[150]

IMPLICATIONS FOR CURRENT CLINICAL PRACTICE

Current PPIs, given once daily, achieve healing in more than 90% of patients with mild EE (Los Angeles [LA] grade A).[2,48–52] Although healing rates are markedly lower for more severe EE (LA grades C and D),[53] and 6-month remission rates on maintenance therapy are generally less than 75% to 85%,[151,152] it has been proposed that increased acid suppression produces little improvement in outcomes.[153,154] This proposition, along with reports linking acid suppression therapy to gastrointestinal infections, fractures, vitamin B_{12} deficiency and respiratory infections,[1,43] has triggered considerable interest in alternative antireflux therapies to address the substantial impairment in quality of life and a risk of complications associated with GERD.[14,155]

Box 3
Therapeutic options for persistent GERD symptoms

- Optimization of once-daily PPI therapy

  Ensure adherence

  Take before breakfast

  Switch to different PPI

  　PPI with slower metabolism

  　Pure isomeric PPI

  　IR PPI for rapid onset

  Modify diet: avoid foods that delay gastric emptying or promote reflux

- Supplementation of once-daily PPI therapy

  Antacids for acute, infrequent exacerbations

  　Intermittent

  Bicarbonate, with PPI, to accelerate PPI absorption

  H_2-RA therapy (nocturnal)

  　Intermittent

  Prokinetic therapy

  　Domperidone

  　Metoclopramide

  Reflux inhibitory therapy

  　Baclofen

  Epithelial protection

  　Sulcrate

- Increase of PPI therapy

  Twice-daily therapy

  Multiple daily dose therapy

- Use of sensory modulator (with or without acid suppression)

  Tricyclic antidepressant

  SSRI antidepressant therapy

  Antispasmodic for reflux-induced spasm

  　Nitrates

  　Anticholinergic

  　Botulinal toxin (endoscopic)

However, there is no direct alternative to PPI therapy. Although GERD symptoms may persist, despite healing of EE,[49–52] in up to 40% of patients with GERD taking once-daily PPI therapy,[131,153,154,156] there are no data to indicate that other agents are more effective for healing or symptom resolution. Similarly, persistent symptoms in patients diagnosed with NERD may indicate that they have functional heartburn rather than true GERD[157,158] but, in most trials, patients with NERD have received lower-dose PPIs for a shorter period than EE patients and there are no data to indicate that other agents would be more effective. Complete absence of a response to once-daily PPI therapy may suggest PPI failure[154,159] but an incomplete response does not necessarily indicate PPI failure.[154] There are few clinical data on multiple daily dosing for current PPIs despite the fact that once-daily dosing does not produce maximal acid suppression,[160] that twice-daily dosing produces greater acid suppression,[38] and that multiple daily doses or a continuous infusion may be required for upper gastrointestinal hemorrhage[39–41,161] or Zollinger-Ellison syndrome.[162] Under these circumstances, it is reasonable to consider a trial of more effective acid suppression for patients who have persistent symptoms when taking a PPI once daily.

The pharmacology of current, first-generation PPIs mitigates against day-long acid suppression or a rapid onset of action. Thus, persistent GERD symptoms and complications in patients receiving once-daily PPI therapy may respond to more prolonged acid suppression regimens, for example, with multiple daily dosing of a current PPI or single daily dosing of a new PPI that has a longer plasma residence time. Similarly, ineffective on-demand therapy may respond to IR PPIs. If increased acid suppression is ineffective, persistent symptoms may then indicate the need to address other mechanisms with, for example, prokinetics, antireflux medications, visceral sensory modulators, or mucosal protectants (**Box 3**). Based on studies to date, these agents should probably be considered as supplements to PPI therapy, tailored to the patient's symptom and disease profile and to the pharmacologic profile of the drugs.

IMPLICATIONS FOR THE FUTURE

The management of severe or persistent GERD[51–53,151,152] and its complications is likely to benefit from acid suppression agents that have a longer half-life and plasma residence time, leading to more prolonged acid suppression. The management of persistent and, possibly, extraesophageal GERD symptoms requires more sophisticated measurement tools for patient-reported outcomes to provide objective documentation of symptoms and their response to therapy in individual patients.[157,158,163,164] There will then be opportunities for additional pharmacologic therapies to address gastrointestinal sensorimotor dysfunction and also for more refined treatment strategies. Contrary to common perceptions, GERD remains an enigmatic condition, the management of which continues to challenge patients and physicians alike.

REFERENCES

1. Hanauer SB. Addicted to acid suppression. Nat Rev Gastroenterol Hepatol 2009;6:497.
2. Chiba N, De Gara CJ, Wilkinson JM, et al. Speed of healing and symptom relief in grade II to IV gastroesophageal reflux disease: a meta-analysis. Gastroenterology 1997;112(6):1798–810.
3. van Pinxteren B, Sigterman KE, Bonis P, et al. Short-term treatment with proton pump inhibitors, H2-receptor antagonists and prokinetics for gastro-oesophageal reflux disease-like symptoms and endoscopy negative reflux disease.

Cochrane Database Syst Rev 2006;3:CD002095. DOI:10.1002/14651858. CD002095.pub3:CD002095.
4. Everhart JE, Ruhl CE. Burden of digestive diseases in the United States part I: overall and upper gastrointestinal diseases. Gastroenterology 2009;136:376–86.
5. Shaheen NJ. The burden of gastrointestinal and liver diseases, 2006. Am J Gastroenterol 2006;101:2128–38.
6. Sonnenberg A. Motion-Laparoscopic Nissen fundoplication is more cost effective than oral PPI administration: arguments against the motion. Can J Gastroenterol 2002;16:627–31.
7. Swanstrom LL. Motion-Laparoscopic Nissen fundoplication is more cost effective than oral PPI administration: arguments for the motion. Can J Gastroenterol 2002;16:621–3.
8. Heikkinen TJ, Haukipuro K, Koivukangas P, et al. Comparison of costs between laparoscopic and open Nissen fundoplication: a prospective randomized study with a 3-month followup. J Am Coll Surg 1999;188:368–76.
9. Gerson LB, Robbins AS, Garber A, et al. A cost-effectiveness analysis of prescribing strategies in the management of gastroesophageal reflux disease. Am J Gastroenterol 2000;95:395–407.
10. Heidelbaugh JJ, Goldberg KL, Inadomi JM. Overutilization of proton pump inhibitors: a review of cost-effectiveness and risk. Am J Gastroenterol 2009; 104:S27–32.
11. Reimer C, Sondergaard B, Hilsted L, et al. Proton-pump inhibitor therapy induces acid-related symptoms in healthy volunteers after withdrawal of therapy. Gastroenterology 2009;137:80–7.
12. McColl KE, Gillen D. Evidence that proton-pump inhibitor therapy induces the symptoms it is used to treat. Gastroenterology 2009;137:20–2.
13. Vakil N, van Zanten SV, Kahrilas P, et al. The Montreal definition and classification of gastroesophageal reflux disease: a global evidence-based consensus. Am J Gastroenterol 2006;101:1900–20.
14. Lagergren J, Bergström R, Lindgren A, et al. Symptomatic gastroesophageal reflux as a risk factor for esophageal adenocarcinoma. N Engl J Med 1999;340: 825–31.
15. Clouse RE, Richter JE, Heading RC, et al. Functional esophageal disorders. Gut 1999;45(Suppl II):II31–6.
16. Dickman R, Bautista JM, Wong WM, et al. Comparison of esophageal acid exposure distribution along the esophagus among the different gastroesophageal reflux disease (GERD) groups. Am J Gastroenterol 2006;101:2463–9.
17. Gosselin A, Luo R, Lohoues H, et al. The impact of proton pump inhibitor compliance on health-care resource utilization and costs in patients with gastroesophageal reflux disease. Value Health 2009;12:34–9.
18. Tindall W. New approaches to adherence issues when dosing oral aminosalicylates in ulcerative colitis. Am J Health Syst Pharm 2009;66:451–7.
19. Fackler WK, Ours TM, Vaezi MF, et al. Long-term effect of H_2-RA therapy on nocturnal gastric acid breakthrough. Gastroenterology 2002;122:625–32.
20. Wilder-Smith CH, Halter F, Merki HS. Tolerance and rebound to H_2-receptor antagonists: intragastric acidity in patients with duodenal ulcer. Dig Dis Sci 1991;36:1685–90.
21. Lachman L, Howden CW. Twenty-four-hour intragastric pH: tolerance within 5 days of continuous ranitidine administration. Am J Gastroenterol 2000;95:57–61.
22. Wilder-Smith C, Halter F, Ernest T, et al. Loss of acid suppression during dosing with H_2-receptor antagonists. Aliment Pharmacol Ther 1990;4(Suppl 1):15–27.

23. Nwokolo CU, Prewett EJ, Sawyerr AF, et al. Tolerance during 5 months of dosing with ranitidine, 150 mg nightly: a placebo-controlled, double-blind study. Gastroenterology 1991;101:948–53.

24. Kahrilas PJ, Fennerty MB, Joelsson B. High- versus standard-dose ranitidine for control of heartburn in poorly responsive acid reflux disease: a prospective, controlled trial. Am J Gastroenterol 1999;94:92–7.

25. Bell NJ, Burget D, Howden CW, et al. Appropriate acid suppression for the management of gastrooesophageal reflux disease. Digestion 1992;51(Suppl 1):59–67.

26. Sachs G, Shin JM, Howden CW. Review article: the clinical pharmacology of proton pump inhibitors. Aliment Pharmacol Ther 2006;23(Suppl 2):2–8.

27. Klotz U. Pharmacokinetic considerations in the eradication of Helicobacter pylori. Clin Pharm 2000;38:243–70.

28. Shi S, Klotz U. Proton pump inhibitors: an update of their clinical use and pharmacokinetics. Eur J Clin Pharmacol 2008;64:935–51.

29. Shin JM, Sachs G. Pharmacology of proton pump inhibitors. Curr Gastroenterol Rep 2008;10:528–34.

30. Klotz U. Clinical impact of CYP2C19 polymorphism on the action of proton pump inhibitors: a review of a special problem. Int J Clin Pharmacol Ther 2006;44:297–302.

31. Saitoh T, Otsuka H, Kawasaki T, et al. Influences of CYP2C19 polymorphism on recurrence of reflux esophagitis during proton pump inhibitor maintenance therapy. Hepatogastroenterology 2009;56:703–6.

32. Armstrong D, James C, Camacho F, et al. Oral rabeprazole vs. intravenous pantoprazole: a comparison of the effect on intragastric pH in healthy subjects. Aliment Pharmacol Ther 2007;25:185–96.

33. Junghard O, Hassan-Alin M, Hasselgren G. The effect of the area under the plasma concentration vs time curve and the maximum plasma concentration of esomeprazole on intragastric pH. Eur J Clin Pharmacol 2002;58:453–8.

34. Hassan-Alin M, Andersson T, Niazi M, et al. A pharmacokinetic study comparing single and repeated oral doses of 20 mg and 40 mg omeprazole and its two optical isomers, S-omeprazole (esomeprazole) and R-omeprazole, in healthy subjects. Eur J Clin Pharmacol 2005;60:779–84.

35. Aslam N, Wright R. Dexlansoprazole MR. Expert Opin Pharmacother 2009;10:2329–36.

36. Shin JM, Homerin M, Domagala F, et al. Characterization of the inhibitory activity of tenatoprazole on the gastric H^+, K^+-ATPase in vitro and in vivo. Biochem Pharmacol 2006;71:837–49.

37. Hunt RH, Armstrong D, Yaghoobi M, et al. Predictable, prolonged suppression of gastric acidity with a novel proton pump inhibitor, AGN 201904-Z. Aliment Pharmacol Ther 2008;28:187–97.

38. Katz PO, Castell DO, Chen Y, et al. Intragastric acid suppression and pharmacokinetics of twice-daily esomeprazole: a randomized, three-way crossover study. Aliment Pharmacol Ther 2004;20:399–406.

39. Laine L, Shah A, Bemanian S. Intragastric pH with oral vs intravenous bolus plus infusion proton-pump inhibitor therapy in patients with bleeding ulcers. Gastroenterology 2008;134:1836–41.

40. Lau JY, Sung JJ, Lee KK, et al. Effect of intravenous omeprazole on recurrent bleeding after endoscopic treatment of bleeding peptic ulcers. N Engl J Med 2000;343:310–6.

41. Sung JJ, Chan FK, Lau JY, et al. The effect of endoscopic therapy in patients receiving omeprazole for bleeding ulcers with nonbleeding visible vessels or adherent clots. A randomized comparison. Ann Intern Med 2003;139:237–43.

42. Scarpignato C, Hunt RH. Proton pump inhibitors: the beginning of the end or the end of the beginning? Curr Opin Pharmacol 2008;8:677–84.
43. DeVault KR, Talley NJ. Insights into the future of gastric acid suppression. Nat Rev Gastroenterol Hepatol 2009;6:524–32.
44. Howden CW, Ballard ED, Koch FK, et al. Control of 24-hour intragastric acidity with morning dosing of immediate-release and delayed-release proton pump inhibitors in patients with GERD. J Clin Gastroenterol 2009;43:323–6.
45. Katz PO. Review article: putting immediate-release proton-pump inhibitors into clinical practice–improving nocturnal acid control and avoiding the possible complications of excessive acid exposure. Aliment Pharmacol Ther 2005;22(Suppl 3):31–8.
46. Howden CW. Review article: immediate-release proton-pump inhibitor therapy–potential advantages. Aliment Pharmacol Ther 2005;22(Suppl 3):25–30.
47. Katz PO, Koch FK, Ballard ED, et al. Comparison of the effects of immediate-release omeprazole oral suspension, delayed-release lansoprazole capsules and delayed-release esomeprazole capsules on nocturnal gastric acidity after bedtime dosing in patients with night-time GERD symptoms. Aliment Pharmacol Ther 2007;25:197–205.
48. Gralnek IM, Dulai GS, Fennerty MB, et al. Esomeprazole versus other proton pump inhibitors in erosive esophagitis: a meta-analysis of randomized clinical trials. Clin Gastroenterol Hepatol 2006;4:1452 8.
49. Kahrilas PJ, Falk GW, Johnson DA, et al. Esomeprazole improves healing and symptom resolution as compared with omeprazole in reflux oesophagitis patients: a randomized controlled trial—the esomeprazole study investigators. Aliment Pharmacol Ther 2000;14:1249–58.
50. Richter JE, Kahrilas PJ, Johanson J, et al. Efficacy and safety of esomeprazole compared with omeprazole in GERD patients with erosive esophagitis: a randomized controlled trial. Am J Gastroenterol 2001;96:656–65.
51. Castell DO, Kahrilas PJ, Richter JE, et al. Esomeprazole (40 mg) compared with lansoprazole (30 mg) in the treatment of erosive esophagitis. Am J Gastroenterol 2002;97:575–83.
52. Labenz J, Armstrong D, Lauritsen K, et al. A randomized comparative study of esomeprazole 40 mg versus pantoprazole 40 mg for healing erosive oesophagitis: the EXPO study. Aliment Pharmacol Ther 2005;21:739–46.
53. Fennerty MB, Johanson JF, Hwang C, et al. Efficacy of esomeprazole 40 mg vs. lansoprazole 30 mg for healing moderate to severe erosive oesophagitis. Aliment Pharmacol Ther 2005;21:455–63.
54. Sharma P, Shaheen NJ, Perez MC, et al. Healing of erosive oesophagitis with dexlansoprazole MR, a proton pump inhibitor with a novel dual delayed release formulation: results from two randomized controlled studies. Aliment Pharmacol Ther 2009;29:731–41.
55. Metz DC, Howden CW, Pere MC, et al. Clinical trial: dexlansoprazole MR, a proton pump inhibitor with dual delayed-release technology, effectively controls symptoms and prevents relapse in patients with healed erosive oeso-phagitis. Aliment Pharmacol Ther 2009;29:742–54.
56. Fass R, Chey WD, Zakko SF, et al. Clinical trial: the effects of the proton pump inhibitor dexlansoprazole MR on daytime and nighttime heartburn in patients with non-erosive reflux disease. Aliment Pharmacol Ther 2009;29:1261–72.
57. Howden CW, Larsen LM, Perez MC, et al. Clinical trial: efficacy and safety of dexlansoprazole MR 60 and 90 mg in healed erosive oesophagitis – maintenance of healing and symptom relief. Aliment Pharmacol Ther 2009;30:895–907.

58. Pai VG, Pai NV, Thacker HP, et al. Comparative clinical trial of S-pantoprazole versus racemic pantoprazole in the treatment of gastro-esophageal reflux disease. World J Gastroenterol 2006;12:6017–20.
59. Pai V, Pai N. A randomized, double-blind, comparative study of dexrabeprazole 10 mg versus rabeprazole 20 mg in the treatment of gastroesophageal reflux disease. World J Gastroenterol 2007;13:4100–2.
60. Zhou Q, Yan XF, Pan WS, et al. Is the required therapeutic effect always achieved by racemic switch of proton-pump inhibitors? World J Gastroenterol 2008;14:2617–9.
61. Periclou AP, Goldwater R, Lee SM, et al. A comparative pharmacodynamic study of IY-81149 versus omeprazole in patients with gastroesophageal reflux disease. Clin Pharmacol Ther 2000;68:304–11.
62. Galmiche JP, Bruley Des Varannes S, Ducrotte P, et al. Tenatoprazole, a novel proton pump inhibitor with a prolonged plasma half-life: effects on intragastric pH and comparison with esomeprazole in healthy volunteers. Aliment Pharmacol Ther 2004;19:655–62.
63. Galmiche JP, Sacher-Huvelin S, Bruley des Varannes S, et al. A comparative study of the early effects of tenatoprazole 40 mg and esomeprazole 40 mg on intragastric pH in healthy volunteers. Aliment Pharmacol Ther 2005;21:575–82.
64. Hunt RH, Armstrong D, James C, et al. Effect on intragastric pH of a PPI with a prolonged plasma half-life: comparison between tenatoprazole and esomeprazole on the duration of acid suppression in healthy male volunteers. Am J Gastroenterol 2005;100:1949–56.
65. Thomson AB, Cohen P, Ficheux H, et al. Comparison of the effects of fasting morning, fasting evening and fed bedtime administration of tenatoprazole on intragastric pH in healthy volunteers: a randomized three-way crossover study. Aliment Pharmacol Ther 2006;23:1179–87.
66. Hunt RH, Armstrong D, Yaghoobi M, et al. Pharmacodynamics and pharmacokinetics of S-tenatoprazole-Na 30 mg, 60 mg and 90 mg versus esomeprazole 40 mg in healthy male subjects. Aliment Pharmacol Ther 2010;31:648–57.
67. Yuan Y, Chen Y, Hunt RH. Dose-effect of S-tenatoprazole-Na in healthy volunteers: a meta-analysis of individual subject data from four pharmacodynamic studies [abstract: S1093]. Gastroenterology 2008;134(Suppl 1):A176.
68. Asano S, Yoshida A, Yashiro H, et al. The cavity structure for docking the K(+)-competitive inhibitors in the gastric proton pump. J Biol Chem 2004;279:13968–75.
69. Nilsson C, Albrektson E, Rydholm H, et al. Tolerability, pharmacokinetics and effects on gastric acid secretion after single oral doses of the potassium-competitive acid blocker AZD0865 in healthy male subjects [abstract]. Gastroenterology 2009;128(4 Suppl 2):A528.
70. Yu KS, Bae KS, Shon JH, et al. Pharmacokinetic and pharmacodynamic evaluation of a novel proton pump inhibitor, YH1885, in healthy volunteers. J Clin Pharmacol 2004;44:73–82.
71. Gedda K, Briving C, Svensson K, et al. Mechanism of action of AZD0865, a K+-competitive inhibitor of gastric H+, K+-ATPase. Biochem Pharmacol 2007;73:198–205.
72. Ito K, Kinoshita K, Tomizawa A, et al. Pharmacological profile of novel acid pump antagonist 7-(4-fluorobenzyloxy)-2,3-dimethyl-1-{[(1S,2S)-2-methyl cyclopropyl] methyl}-1H-pyrrolo [2,3-d]pyridazine (CS-526). J Pharmacol Exp Ther 2007;323:308–17.

73. Ito K, Kinoshita K, Tomizawa A, et al. The effect of subchronic administration of 7-(4-fluorobenzyloxy)-2,3-dimethyl-1-{[(1S,2S)-2 methylcyclopropyl] methyl}-1H-pyrrolo[2,3-d]pyridazine (CS-526), a novel acid pump antagonist, on gastric acid secretion and gastrin levels in rats. J Pharmacol Exp Ther 2008;326:163–70.

74. Simon WA, Herrmann M, Klein T, et al. Soraprazan: setting new standards in inhibition of gastric acid secretion. J Pharmacol Exp Ther 2007;321:866–74.

75. Kahrilas PJ, Dent J, Lauritsen K, et al. A randomized, comparative trial of three doses of AZD0865 and esomeprazole for healing of reflux esophagitis. Clin Gastroenterol Hepatol 2007;5:1385–91.

76. Dent J, Kahrilas PJ, Hatlebakk J, et al. A randomized, comparative trial of a potassium-competitive acid blocker (AZD0865) and esomeprazole for the treatment of patients with nonerosive reflux disease. Am J Gastroenterol 2008; 103:20–6.

77. Tran T, Lowry AM, El-Serag HB. Meta-analysis: the efficacy of over-the-counter gastroesophageal reflux disease therapies. Aliment Pharmacol Ther 2007;25: 143–53.

78. Armstrong D, Marshall JK, Chiba N, et al. Canadian Consensus Conference on the management of gastroesophageal reflux disease in adults – Update 2004. Can J Gastroenterol 2005;19:15–35.

79. Scarpignato C, Galmiche JP. The role of H2-receptor antagonists in the era of proton pump inhibitors. In: Lundell L, editor. Guidelines for management of symptomatic gastro-oesophageal reflux disease. London: Science Press; 1998. p. 55–66.

80. Rackoff A, Agrawal A, Hila A, et al. Histamine-2 receptor antagonists at night improve gastroesophageal reflux disease symptoms for patients on proton pump inhibitor therapy. Dis Esophagus 2005;18:370–3.

81. Xue S, Katz PO, Banerjee P, et al. Bedtime H_2 blockers improve nocturnal gastric acid control in GERD patients on proton pump inhibitors. Aliment Pharmacol Ther 2001;15:1351–6.

82. Ours T, Fackler W, Richter J, et al. Nocturnal acid breakthrough: clinical significance and correlation with esophageal acid exposure. Am J Gastroenterol 2003;98:545–50.

83. Fandriks L, Lonroth H, Pettersson A, et al. Can famotidine and omeprazole be combined on a once-daily basis? Scand J Gastroenterol 2007;42:689–94.

84. Ang D, Blondeau K, Sifrim D, et al. The spectrum of motor function abnormalities in gastroesophageal reflux disease and Barrett's esophagus. Digestion 2009;79: 158–68.

85. Fass R, Sifrim D. Management of heartburn not responding to proton pump inhibitors. Gut 2009;58:295–309.

86. Champion G, Richter JE, Singh S, et al. Effects of oral erythromycin on esophageal pH and pressure profiles in patients with gastroesophageal reflux disease. Dig Dis Sci 1994;39:129–37.

87. Chaussade S, Michopoulos S, Sogni P, et al. Motilin agonist erythromycin increases human lower esophageal sphincter pressure by stimulation of cholinergic nerves. Dig Dis Sci 1994;39:381–4.

88. Chrysos E, Tzovaras G, Epanomeritakis E, et al. Erythromycin enhances oesophageal motility in patients with gastro-oesophageal reflux. ANZ J Surg 2001; 71:98–102.

89. Finizia C, Lundell L, Cange L, et al. The effect of cisapride on oesophageal motility and lower sphincter function in patients with gastro-oesophageal reflux disease. Eur J Gastroenterol Hepatol 2002;14:9–14.

90. Fox M, Menne D, Stutz B, et al. The effects of tegaserod on oesophageal function and bolus transport in healthy volunteers: studies using concurrent high-resolution manometry and videofluoroscopy. Aliment Pharmacol Ther 2006;24: 1017–27.

91. Greenwood B, Dieckman D, Kirst HA, et al. Effects of LY267108, an erythromycin analogue derivative, on lower esophageal sphincter function in the cat. Gastroenterology 1994;106:624–8.

92. Inauen W, Emde C, Weber B, et al. Effects of ranitidine and cisapride on acid reflux and oesophageal motility in patients with reflux oesophagitis: a 24 hour ambulatory combined pH and manometry study. Gut 1993;34:1025–31.

93. Kahrilas PJ, Quigley EM, Castell DO, et al. The effects of tegaserod (HTF 919) on oesophageal acid exposure in gastro-oesophageal reflux disease. Aliment Pharmacol Ther 2000;14:1503–9.

94. Mertens V, Blondeau K, Pauwels A, et al. Azithromycin reduces gastroesophageal reflux and aspiration in lung transplant recipients. Dig Dis Sci 2009;54:972–9.

95. Peeters TL. Erythromycin and other macrolides as prokinetic agents. Gastroenterology 1993;105:1886–99.

96. Staiano A, Clouse RE. The effects of cisapride on the topography of oesophageal peristalsis. Aliment Pharmacol Ther 1996;10:875–82.

97. Tack J. Prokinetics and fundic relaxants in upper functional GI disorders. Curr Opin Pharmacol 2008;8:690–6.

98. Gardner JD, Rodriguez-Stanley S, Robinson M, et al. Cisapride inhibits meal-stimulated gastric acid secretion and post-prandial gastric acidity in subjects with gastro-oesophageal reflux disease. Aliment Pharmacol Ther 2002;16: 1819–29.

99. Abdulnour-Nakhoul S, Tobey NA, Nakhoul NL, et al. The effect of tegaserod on esophageal submucosal glands bicarbonate and mucin secretion. Dig Dis Sci 2008;53:2366–72.

100. Majewski M, Jaworski T, Sarosiek I, et al. Significant enhancement of esophageal pre-epithelial defense by tegaserod: implications for an esophagoprotective effect. Clin Gastroenterol Hepatol 2007;5:430–8.

101. Peeters TL. Old and new targets for prokinetic drugs: motilin and ghrelin receptors. Eur Rev Med Pharmacol Sci 2008;12(Suppl 1):136–7.

102. Sanger GJ. Motilin, ghrelin and related neuropeptides as targets for the treatment of GI diseases. Drug Discov Today 2008;13:234–9.

103. Tomita R, Tanjoh K, Munakata K. The role of motilin and cisapride in the enteric nervous system of the lower esophageal sphincter in humans. Surg Today 1997; 27:985–92.

104. Netzer P, Schmitt B, Inauen W. Effects of ABT-229, a motilin agonist, on acid reflux, oesophageal motility and gastric emptying in patients with gastro-oesophageal reflux disease. Aliment Pharmacol Ther 2002;16:1481–90.

105. van Herwaarden MA, Samsom M, Van Nispen CH, et al. The effect of motilin agonist ABT-229 on gastro-oesophageal reflux, oesophageal motility and lower oesophageal sphincter characteristics in GERD patients. Aliment Pharmacol Ther 2000;14:453–4562.

106. Pennathur A, Tran A, Cioppi M, et al. Erythromycin strengthens the defective lower esophageal sphincter in patients with gastroesophageal reflux disease. Am J Surg 1994;167:169–72.

107. Mitselos A, Peeters TL, Depoortere I. Desensitization and internalization of the human motilin receptor is independent of the C-terminal tail. Peptides 2008; 29:1167–75.

108. Dodds WJ, Dent J, Hogan WJ, et al. Mechanisms of gastroesophageal reflux in patients with reflux esophagitis. N Engl J Med 1982;307:1547–52.
109. Holloway RH, Penagini R, Ireland AC. Criteria for objective definition of transient lower esophageal sphincter relaxation. Am J Physiol 1995;268:G128–33.
110. Hirsch DP, Tytgat GN, Boeckxstaens GE. Transient lower oesophageal sphincter relaxations–a pharmacological target for gastro-oesophageal reflux disease? Aliment Pharmacol Ther 2002;16:17–26.
111. Janssens J, Sifrim D. Spontaneous transient lower esophageal sphincter relaxations: a target for treatment of gastroesophageal reflux disease. Gastroenterology 1995;109:1703–6.
112. Mittal RK, McCallum RW. Characteristics of transient lower esophageal sphincter relaxation in humans. Am J Physiol 1987;252:G636–41.
113. Sifrim D, Holloway R. Transient lower esophageal sphincter relaxations: how many or how harmful? Am J Gastroenterol 2001;96:2529–32.
114. Beaumont H, Bennink RJ, de JJ, et al. The position of the acid pocket as a major risk factor for acidic reflux in healthy subjects and patients with GORD. Gut 2010;59:441–51.
115. Cange L, Johnsson E, Rydholm H, et al. Baclofen-mediated gastro-oesophageal acid reflux control in patients with established reflux disease. Aliment Pharmacol Ther 2002;16:869–73.
116. Ciccaglione AF, Marzio L. Effect of acute and chronic administration of the GABA B agonist baclofen on 24 hour pH metry and symptoms in control subjects and in patients with gastro-oesophageal reflux disease. Gut 2003;52:464–70.
117. Koek GH, Sifrim D, Lerut T, et al. Effect of the GABA(B) agonist baclofen in patients with symptoms and duodeno-gastro-oesophageal reflux refractory to proton pump inhibitors. Gut 2003;52:1397–402.
118. Lidums I, Lehmann A, Checklin H, et al. Control of transient lower esophageal sphincter relaxations and reflux by the GABA(B) agonist baclofen in normal subjects. Gastroenterology 2000;118:7 13.
119. van Herwaarden MA, Samsom M, Rydholm H, et al. The effect of baclofen on gastro-oesophageal reflux, lower oesophageal sphincter function and reflux symptoms in patients with reflux disease. Aliment Pharmacol Ther 2002;16:1655–62.
120. Vela MF, Tutuian R, Katz PO, et al. Baclofen decreases acid and non-acid postprandial gastro-oesophageal reflux measured by combined multichannel intraluminal impedance and pH. Aliment Pharmacol Ther 2003;17:243–51.
121. Zhang Q, Lehmann A, Rigda R, et al. Control of transient lower oesophageal sphincter relaxations and reflux by the GABA(B) agonist baclofen in patients with gastro-oesophageal reflux disease. Gut 2002;50:19–24.
122. Boeckxstaens GE, Rydholm H, Lei A, et al. Effect of lesogaberan, a novel GABA-receptor agonist, on transient lower esophageal sphincter relaxations in male subjects. Aliment Pharmacol Ther 2010;31:1208–17.
123. Omari TI, Benninga MA, Sansom L, et al. Effect of baclofen on esophagogastric motility and gastroesophageal reflux in children with gastroesophageal reflux disease: a randomized controlled trial. J Pediatr 2006;149:468–74.
124. Beaumont H, Jonsson-Rylander AC, Carlsson K, et al. The role of GABA(A) receptors in the control of transient lower oesophageal sphincter relaxations in the dog. Br J Pharmacol 2008;153:1195–202.
125. Boeckxstaens GE, Hirsch DP, Fakhry N, et al. Involvement of cholecystokininA receptors in transient lower esophageal sphincter relaxations triggered by gastric distension. Am J Gastroenterol 1998;93:1823–8.

126. Penagini R, Bianchi PA. Effect of morphine on gastroesophageal reflux and transient lower esophageal sphincter relaxation. Gastroenterology 1997;113:409–14.

127. Hirsch DP, Tytgat GN, Boeckxstaens GE. Is glutamate involved in transient lower esophageal sphincter relaxations? Dig Dis Sci 2002;47:661–6.

128. Lehmann A, Blackshaw LA, Branden L, et al. Cannabinoid receptor agonism inhibits transient lower esophageal sphincter relaxations and reflux in dogs. Gastroenterology 2002;123:1129–34.

129. Beaumont H, Jensen J, Carlsson A, et al. Effect of delta9-tetrahydrocannabinol, a cannabinoid receptor agonist, on the triggering of transient lower oesophageal sphincter relaxations in dogs and humans. Br J Pharmacol 2009;156:153–62.

130. Frisby CL, Mattsson JP, Jensen JM, et al. Inhibition of transient lower esophageal sphincter relaxation and gastroesophageal reflux by metabotropic glutamate receptor ligands. Gastroenterology 2005;129:995–1004.

131. Keywood C, Wakefield M, Tack J. A proof-of-concept study evaluating the effect of ADX10059, a metabotropic glutamate receptor-5 negative allosteric modulator, on acid exposure and symptoms in gastro-oesophageal reflux disease. Gut 2009;58:1192–9.

132. Hirsch DP, Holloway RH, Tytgat GN, et al. Involvement of nitric oxide in human transient lower esophageal sphincter relaxations and esophageal primary peristalsis. Gastroenterology 1998;115:1374–80.

133. Lehmann A, Antonsson M, Bremner-Danielsen M, et al. Activation of the GABA(B) receptor inhibits transient lower esophageal sphincter relaxations in dogs. Gastroenterology 1999;117:1147–54.

134. Grossi L, Spezzaferro M, Sacco LF, et al. Effect of baclofen on oesophageal motility and transient lower oesophageal sphincter relaxations in GORD patients: a 48-h manometric study. Neurogastroenterol Motil 2008;20:760–6.

135. Beaumont H, Boeckxstaens GE. Does the presence of a hiatal hernia affect the efficacy of the reflux inhibitor baclofen during add-on therapy? Am J Gastroenterol 2009;104:1764–71.

136. Gerson LB, Huff FJ, Hila A, et al. Arbaclofen placarbil decreases postprandial reflux in patients with gastroesophageal reflux disease. Am J Gastroenterol 2010;105:1266–75.

137. Lehmann A, Brändén L, Carlsson A, et al. AZD3355, a novel GABAB receptor agonist inhibits transient lower esophageal sphincter relaxation in the dog (Abstract). Gastroenterology 2008;134:A49–50.

138. Boeckxstaens GE, Beaumont H, Hatlebakk JG, et al. Efficacy and tolerability of the novel reflux inhibitor, AZD3355, as add-on treatment in GERD patients with symptoms despite proton pump inhibitor therapy [abstract]. Gastroenterology 2009;136:A436.

139. Jensen J, Lehmann A, Uvebrant A, et al. Transient lower esophageal sphincter relaxations in dogs are inhibited by a metabotropic glutamate receptor 5 antagonist. Eur J Pharmacol 2005;519:154–7.

140. Zerbib F, Keywood C, Strabach G. Efficacy, tolerability and pharmacokinetics of a modified release formulation of ADX10059, a negative allosteric modulator of metabotropic glutamate receptor 5: an esophageal pH-impedance study in healthy subjects. Neurogastroenterol Motil 2010;22(8):859–65, e231. PMID: 20236248. DOI:10.1111/j.1365–2982.2010.01484.x.

141. Partosoedarso ER, Abrahams TP, Scullion RT, et al. Cannabinoid1 receptor in the dorsal vagal complex modulates lower oesophageal sphincter relaxation in ferrets. J Physiol 2003;550:149–58.

142. Vela MF, Camacho-Lobato L, Srinivasan R, et al. Simultaneous intraesophageal impedance and pH measurement of acid and nonacid gastroesophageal reflux: effect of omeprazole. Gastroenterology 2001;120:1599–606.
143. Clouse RE, Lustman PJ, Eckert TC, et al. Low-dose trazodone for symptomatic patients with esophageal contraction abnormalities. A double-blind, placebo-controlled trial. Gastroenterology 1987;92:1027–36.
144. Handa M, Mine K, Yamamoto H, et al. Antidepressant treatment of patients with diffuse esophageal spasm: a psychosomatic approach. J Clin Gastroenterol 1999;28:228–32.
145. Tack J, Sarnelli G. Serotonergic modulation of visceral sensation: upper gastro-intestinal tract. Gut 2002;51(Suppl 1):i77–80.
146. Sarkar S, Aziz Q, Woolf CJ, et al. Contribution of central sensitisation to the development of non-cardiac chest pain. Lancet 2000;356:1154–9.
147. Sarkar S, Hobson AR, Hughes A, et al. The prostaglandin E2 receptor-1 (EP-1) mediates acid-induced visceral pain hypersensitivity in humans. Gastroenter-ology 2003;124:18–25.
148. Willert RP, Woolf CJ, Hobson AR, et al. The development and maintenance of human visceral pain hypersensitivity is dependent on the N-methyl-D-aspartate receptor. Gastroenterology 2004;126:683 92.
149. Orlando RC, Turjman NA, Tobey NA, et al. Mucosal protection by sucralfate and its components in acid-exposed rabbit esophagus. Gastroenterology 1987;93:352–61.
150. Farré R, Cardozo L, Blondeau K, et al. Esophageal mucosal damage induced by weakly acidic solutions containing unconjugated bile acids, similar to reflux in GERD patients "on" PPI, can be prevented with anti-oxidants [abstract]. Gastroenterology 2009;136:A16.
151. Lauritsen K, Deviere J, Bigard MA, et al. Esomeprazole 20 mg and lansoprazole 15 mg in maintaining healed reflux oesophagitis: metropole study results. Aliment Pharmacol Ther 2003;17:333–41.
152. Labenz J, Armstrong D, Lauritsen K, et al. Esomeprazole 20 mg vs. pantopra-zole 20 mg for maintenance therapy of healed erosive oesophagitis: results from the EXPO study. Aliment Pharmacol Ther 2005;22:803–11.
153. Boeckxstaens GE. Reflux inhibitors: a new approach for GERD? Curr Opin Phar-macol 2008;8:1–5.
154. Johnson DA, Levy BH III. Evolving drugs in gastroesophageal reflux disease: pharmacological treatment beyond proton pump inhibitors. Expert Opin Phar-macother 2010;11:1541–8.
155. Bytzer P, Christensen PB, Damkier P, et al. Adenocarcinoma of the esophagus and Barrett's esophagus: a population-based study. Am J Gastroenterol 1999;94:86–91.
156. Jones R, Armstrong D, Malfertheiner P, et al. Does the treatment of gastroesoph-ageal reflux disease (GERD) meet patients' needs? A survey-based study. Curr Med Res Opin 2006;22:657–62.
157. Armstrong D. Symptom assessment – methods and content. J Clin Gastroenterol 2007;41(S2):S184–92.
158. Armstrong D. A critical assessment of the current state of NERD. Digestion 2008;1(Suppl 1):46–54.
159. Poh C, Gasiorowska A, Fass R, et al. Upper GI tract findings in patients with heartburn in whom proton pump inhibitor treatment failed versus those not receiving antireflux treatment. Gastrointest Endosc 2010;71:28–34.

160. Miner P, Katz O, Chen Y, et al. Gastric acid control with esomeprazole, lansoprazole, omeprazole, pantoprazole and rabeprazole: a five-way crossover study. Am J Gastroenterol 2003;98:2616–20.
161. Khuroo MS, Yattoo GN, Javid G, et al. A comparison of omeprazole and placebo for bleeding peptic ulcer. N Engl J Med 1997;336:1054–8.
162. Metz DC, Soffer E, Forsmark CE, et al. Maintenance oral pantoprazole therapy is effective for patients with Zollinger-Ellison syndrome and idiopathic hypersecretion. Am J Gastroenterol 2003;98:301–7.
163. Bardhan KD, Stanghellini V, Armstrong D, et al. Evaluation of GERD symptoms during therapy Part 1: development of the new GERD questionnaire ReQuest. Digestion 2004;69:229–37.
164. Mönnikes H, Bardhan KD, Stanghellini V, et al. Evaluation of GERD symptoms during therapy Part II: psychometric evaluation and validation of the new questionnaire ReQuest in erosive GERD. Digestion 2004;69:238–44.

The Pharmacological Therapy of Non-Variceal Upper Gastrointestinal Bleeding

Joshua Greenspoon, Alan Barkun, MD, CM, MSc (Clinical Epidemiology)*

KEYWORDS

• Gastrointestinal bleeding • Proton pump inhibitors • pH
• Histamine 2 receptor antagonists • Ulcer bleeding • Gastric pH
• Pharmacology

The modern management of patients with upper gastrointestinal bleeding includes, in selected patients, the performance of timely multimodal endoscopic hemostasis followed by profound acid suppression.[1,2] This article discusses the available data on the use of antisecretory regimens in the management of patients with bleeding peptic ulcers, which are a major cause of non-variceal upper gastrointestinal bleeding,[3] and briefly addresses other medications used in this acute setting. The most important clinically relevant data are presented, favoring fully published articles.

THE BIOLOGIC RATIONALE FOR ACID SUPPRESSION IN PATIENTS WITH UPPER GASTROINTESTINAL BLEEDING

Acid has been shown to inhibit platelet aggregation and even favors platelet disaggregation.[4] Based on in vitro and animal experiments, the pH target required to avert these deleterious effects and favor hemostasis is thought to approximate 6.0 to 6.5.[5] Acid is also known to facilitate clot lysis through the activation of pepsin, which occurs at pH levels below 2.[6,7] Acid suppression, leading to pH levels more than 4, may prevent fibrinolysis.[6] The rationale for acid suppression in upper gastrointestinal bleeding is based on the following deleterious effects of gastric acid on clot stability:

Decreased platelet aggregation, and even platelet disaggregation[4,5]
Increased clot lysis from pepsin activation by acid[7]
Increased fibrinolytic activity that is impaired by acid[8]
A pH of 6.0 to 6.5 is targeted to reverse these effects based on in vitro and animal data.[4]

Division of Gastroenterology, Montreal General Hospital site, The McGill University Health Center, 1650 Cedar Avenue, Room D16.125, Montréal, Canada H3G 1A4
* Corresponding author.
E-mail address: alan.barkun@muhc.mcgill.ca

Gastroenterol Clin N Am 39 (2010) 419–432
doi:10.1016/j.gtc.2010.08.002
0889-8553/10/$ – see front matter © 2010 Elsevier Inc. All rights reserved.

After endoscopic therapy is performed for a high-risk ulcer lesion (eg, a visible vessel or pigmented protuberance), approximately 72 hours are required for most lesions to evolve and begin to display low-risk ulcer stigmata.[18] This finding is corroborated by most clinical trials, including a recent large international study,[19] that have shown that peptic ulcer rebleeding occurs predominantly during the first 72 hours after endoscopic treatment and the initiation of high-dose intravenous proton pump inhibitor (PPI) infusion.[2]

Therefore, experts have hypothesized that acid suppression may stabilize intraluminal clots during this high-risk period, and result in a subsequent improvement of outcomes in patients with peptic ulcer bleeding. PPIs also exhibit anti-inflammatory properties of unclear clinical relevance discussed later.[20]

Box 1 lists the relevant clinical recommendations for proton pump inhibitor–related use in the acute management of patients with non-variceal upper gastrointestinal bleeding.

TRANEXAMIC ACID IS NOT RECOMMENDED IN THE ACUTE MANAGEMENT OF PATIENTS WITH PEPTIC ULCER BLEEDING

Tranexamic acid inhibits plasminogen activators, conferring its effects as an antifibrinolytic drug. Tranexamic acid is known to increase the risk of thrombosis when administered with tretinoin or coagulation factor VIIa.[21] A meta-analysis from more than 20 years ago had found that tranexamic acid decreased mortality rates by 40% relative to placebo, with no effects on rebleeding and surgery rates.[22] The meta-analysis included studies in which endoscopic hemostatic therapy was not performed, limiting the conclusions that can be drawn. Furthermore, more than 43% of the patients bled from causes other than peptic ulcers.[22] Many more randomized clinical trials would need to be conducted in accordance with current clinical procedures for a conclusion to be drawn on the efficacy of tranexamic acid in treating patients with peptic ulcer bleeding.

Box 1
Relevant clinical recommendations for proton pump inhibitor–related use in the acute management of patients with non-variceal upper gastrointestinal bleeding

Somatostatin and octreotide are not recommended for routine use in patients with acute ulcer bleeding.[2,9]

H$_2$-receptor antagonists are not recommended in the management of patients with acute upper gastrointestinal bleeding.[2,9]

An intravenous bolus followed by continuous-infusion PPI is effective in decreasing rebleeding in patients who have undergone successful endoscopic therapy.[2,9]

The use of intravenous bolus followed by continuous-infusion PPI is cost-effective after endoscopic therapy in the management of patients bleeding peptic ulcers.[10–12]

In patients awaiting endoscopy, empiric therapy with a high-dose PPI should be considered.[2,9]

Patients should be discharged with a prescription for a single daily dose of oral PPI for a duration dependent on underlying etiology.[9]

Much inappropriate use of PPIs occurs in the hospital setting.[13–17]

SOMATOSTATIN AND SOMATOSTATIN ANALOGS ARE NOT ROUTINELY RECOMMENDED IN THE ACUTE MANAGEMENT OF PATIENTS WITH PEPTIC ULCER BLEEDING

Somatostatin is initially synthesized as a pre-prohormone that is processed into two active forms: one consisting of 14 amino acids and the other consisting of 28. Somatostatin exerts many inhibitory functions throughout the body. In addition to inhibiting growth hormone and gastrointestinal secretion,[23] it decreases splanchnic blood flow, and therefore has been used in controlling upper gastrointestinal bleeding.[24] Somatostatin exerts its physiologic effects through five different G-protein–coupled receptors, and is unable to be administered orally because it is quickly inactivated by a peptidase enzyme. Octreotide is a cyclic octapeptide somatostatin analog, and is a more potent inhibitor of growth hormone, glucagon, and insulin.[23]

A study comparing the effects of a high-dose pantoprazole continuous infusion to somatostatin concluded that high-dose pantoprazole was superior.[25] This study consisted of 164 patients who received either a continuous infusion of pantoprazole, 8 mg/h, after a 40-mg bolus or a 250-μg bolus of somatostatin followed by infusion of 250 μg/h. Bleeding recurrence was significantly greater in the somatostatin group than in the pantoprazole group.[25] An earlier meta-analysis suggested that the efficacy of somatostatin was based on many trials using now-outdated diagnostic and therapeutic approaches.[26]

In a more contemporary meta-analysis, Bardou and colleagues[27] showed that neither somatostatin nor octreotide improved outcomes compared with other pharmacotherapy or endoscopic therapy. Therefore, somatostatin and octreotide are not recommended for routine use in the management of patients with acute non-variceal upper gastrointestinal bleeding,[2] but can be considered in patients with massive unresponsive bleeding, even if known to originate from a non-variceal source. These agents are, of course, the preferred approach in the management of patients with variceal bleeding in conjunction with endoscopic ligation.[28]

H₂-RECEPTOR ANTAGONISTS ARE NOT EFFICACIOUS IN THE ACUTE MANAGEMENT OF PATIENTS WITH PEPTIC ULCER BLEEDING

H$_2$-receptor antagonists bind competitively and reversibly to H$_2$ receptors on parietal cells, decreasing parietal secretions in response to histamine. H$_2$-receptor antagonists are well absorbed when given orally, but bioavailability varies.[23] A study comparing 72-hour continuous infusion of ranitidine, a H$_2$-receptor antagonist, or omeprazole, a PPI, found that the mean number of doses necessary to maintain a pH above 4 increased with ranitidine but decreased with omeprazole, suggesting decreased antisecretory effects as time progressed.[29] This conclusion was also noted by other investigators. This possibility is a serious limitation to the clinical efficacy of H$_2$-receptor antagonists because of the rapid development of pharmacologic tolerance to these medications, which can occur as early as 24 hours after the first dose and cannot be overcome by high intravenous doses greater than 500 mg per 24 hours (Fig. 1).[29–31]

An increasing serum gastrin drive to the parietal cells is one possible mechanism through which tolerance may develop.[32] One large randomized clinical trial[33] and two meta-analyses[34,35] have now confirmed that no overall benefits are attributable to the acute use of intravenous H$_2$-receptor antagonists in patients with peptic ulcer bleeding. Statistically significant but modest clinical benefits in rebleeding and decreased surgical rates have, however, been noted in a subgroup of patients with

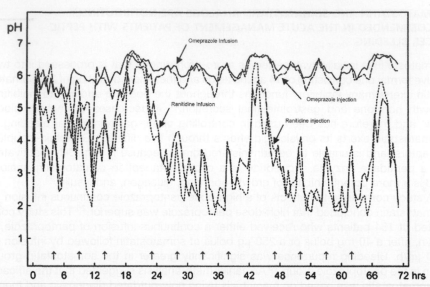

Fig. 1. Effect of omeprazole and ranitidine on intragastric pH. Doses: Omeprazole infusion, 80-mg bolus followed by continuous infusion of 8 mg/h; omeprazole injection, 80-mg bolus followed by 40 mg injection every 6 hours; ranitidine infusion, 50-mg bolus followed by continuous infusion of 25 mg/kg/h; ranitidine injection, 100-mg bolus every 6 hours. (*Adapted from* Netzer P, Gaia C, Sandoz M, et al. Effect of repeated injection and continuous infusion of omeprazole and ranitidine on intragastric pH over 72 hours. Am J Gastroenterol 1999;94:353; with permission.)

bleeding gastric ulcers.[35] The use of H_2-receptor antagonists in the routine management of patients with acute peptic ulcer bleeding is not recommended.[2]

PPIS ARE EFFICACIOUS IN MANAGING PATIENTS WITH ACUTE PEPTIC ULCER BLEEDING
Mechanism of Action

PPIs are substituted benzimidazole sulphoxides. Under the acidic conditions within the secretory canaliculus of the parietal cells, PPIs are protonated and converted to their active form, which binds covalently to cysteine residues of the H^+, K^+ ATPase enzyme of actively inserted parietal cells, leading to inactivation of the pump.[23] Pumps at rest in the cytosol of the parietal cell are not blocked. Because PPIs bind irreversibly to proton pumps, their biologic activity extends beyond their serum elimination half-life value, and the half-life of the proton pumps themselves (20–24 hours) becomes relevant[30] with synthesis of new proton pumps required for the parietal cell to secrete acid.

Optimal Intravenous Dosing

Investigators have studied a large intravenous bolus of PPIs to quickly achieve a high intragastric pH in the acute setting, followed by a high-dose intravenous route of administration to keep as many pumps as possible inhibited over time, thus achieving maximal acid suppression. Gastric pH studies have shown that bolus intravenous dosing of PPIs is suboptimal, and that a dose of 80-mg bolus followed by an 8 mg/h infusion using omeprazole is required to achieve a theoretically optimal sustained target gastric pH of around 6.[36] Similar results have been shown using comparable doses of other intravenous PPI solutions with esomeprazole,[37] lansoprazole (using shorter infusions of 90- to 120-mg bolus and 6–9 mg/h),[38,39] omeprazole,[28,36,40] pantoprazole,[41] and rabeprazole[42] in patients with acute peptic ulcer bleeding (**Fig. 2**).

Results of Randomized Trials Using Intravenous PPIs

Intravenous PPIs achieve more profound and sustained acid suppression than H_2-receptor antagonists without the development of tolerance.[36,40,41] The initial literature had shown mixed results using varying bolus doses of intravenous PPI.[30] The best designed of these studies showed no benefits attributable to the administration of omeprazole, 80 mg, intravenously immediately (before endoscopy), followed by three doses of 40 mg intravenously at 8 hourly intervals, then 40 mg orally at 12 hourly intervals for 4 days or until surgery, discharge, or death.[43]

In contrast, most well-designed and adequately powered randomized clinical trials have shown the efficacy of the high-dose infusion of an 80-mg bolus of omeprazole followed by 8 mg/h for the first 3 days of treatment, in patients having first undergone endoscopic therapy for bleeding ulcers exhibiting high-risk stigmata.[9] The landmark study by Lau and colleagues[44] showed a highly statistically and clinically significant decrease in rebleeding rate from 22.5% in the placebo group to 6.7% in the high-dose intravenous PPI group (hazard ratio, 3.9, 95% CI, 1.7–9.0). This study was stopped short of the initial enrollment for ethical reasons, given the large effect size seen in rebleeding. Nonetheless, the authors also noted trends in improvements in the proportion of patients requiring surgery or dying.

Additional trials have since confirmed the beneficial effects of this dosing, including a very recent randomized trial of high dose intravenous esomeprazole compared with placebo that involved 764 patients and confirmed the broad generalizability of these

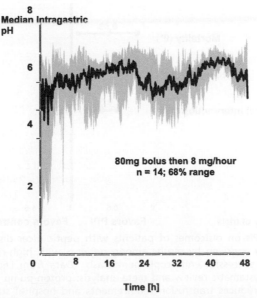

Fig. 2. Pantoprazole in patients with upper gastrointestinal bleeding after endoscopic hemostasis. (*From* van Rensburg CJ, Hartmann M, Thorpe A, et al. Intragastric pH during continuous infusion with pantoprazole in patients with bleeding peptic ulcer. Am J Gastroenterol 2003;98(12):2635–41; with permission.)

results to patients of varying races.[19] Surprisingly, the largest intravenous PPI trial conducted to date, involving 1256 patients, failed to find significant differences when comparing high-dose pantoprazole with ranitidine[45]; however, pantoprazole showed a better overall score using a composite outcome measure. Possible explanations for this unusual finding could be attributed to the very low rate of rebleeding in the ranitidine group (3.2%) in this study compared with other studies (8%–16%).[44,46] Also, the patient groups were relatively healthy in comparison with other trials, with only 4% having a history of comorbid cardiovascular disease. The authors also acknowledged potential misclassification of low-risk lesions and methodological limitations attributable to the definition of the primary outcome and the choice of statistical analysis. Significant benefits were found in patients with Forrest Ia lesions attributable to pantoprazole.

An authoritative Cochrane meta-analysis by Leontiadis and colleagues[47] including 24 randomized controlled trials and comprising 4373 patients concluded that acute PPI use (omeprazole, lansoprazole, and pantoprazole) reduced rebleeding (odds ratio[OR], 0.49; 95% CI, 0.37–0.65; number needed to treat [NNT], 13), surgical intervention (OR, 0.61; 95% CI, 0.48–0.78; NNT, 34), and repeated endoscopic treatment (OR, 0.32; 95% CI, 0.16–0.74; NNT, 34). Furthermore, assessment of the 12 trials that provided data on patients with active bleeding or a nonbleeding visible vessel showed that the PPI significantly decreased mortality (OR, 0.53; 95% CI for fixed effect, 0.31–0.91). This effect related to the results of 7 trials (including 4 high-dose intravenous and 2 high-dose oral PPIs) in which endoscopic therapy was systematically first performed, confirming that profound acid suppression should be considered an adjuvant to endoscopic hemostasis in this high-risk group (**Fig. 3**).[2,9]

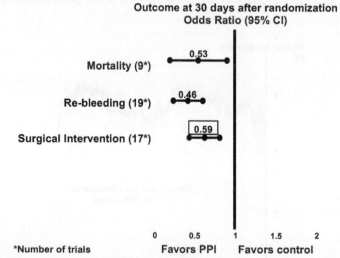

Fig. 3. Effects of PPIs on outcomes of patients with peptic ulcer disease bleeding. The benefit in mortality is driven by results among patients with high-risk stigmata having initially undergone successful endoscopic hemostasis. (*Data from* Leontiadis GI, Sharma VK, Howden CW. Systematic review and meta-analysis: proton-pump inhibitor treatment for ulcer bleeding reduces transfusion requirements and hospital stay–results from the Cochrane Collaboration. Aliment Pharmacol Ther 2006;22(3):169–74; and Barkun A, Sabbah S, Enns R, et al. The Canadian Registry on Nonvariceal Upper Gastrointestinal Bleeding and Endoscopy (RUGBE): endoscopic hemostasis and proton pump inhibition are associated with improved outcomes in a real-life setting. Am J Gastroenterol 2004;99(7):1238–46.)

The meta-analysis by Laine and McQuaid[48] found similar results, with significant benefits in rebleeding rates, surgery, and mortality with high-dose intravenous PPI therapy relative to placebo. Based on the results of two trials, recent international guidelines[9] suggest a high-dose intravenous PPI (80-mg bolus followed by 8 mg/h for 3 days) may be sufficient, even in the absence of prior endoscopic therapy, in improving the outcomes of patients with adherent clots.[48,49]

Intravenous High versus Low Dose

Surprisingly, the smallest effective dose of intravenous PPI has not been determined. High-quality evidence has shown the effectiveness of high-dose PPI regimens. Recent North American data suggest that the currently used high-dose intravenous PPI regimens may not achieve the target pH values of 6, thought to allow for clot stabilization,[39] suggesting that alternate mechanisms may also play a role in the biologic effect attributable to PPIs.[20] Additionally, results of a large trial by Andriulli and colleagues[50] comparing the high-dose intravenous regimen to single daily intravenous 40-mg bolus for 3 days suggested no dose-related difference in efficacy. Unfortunately, the validity of this conclusion was challenged because of experimental design limitations that include a systematic bias in the ascertainment of rebleeding in the high-dose intravenous PPI group, questions raised about the adequacy of blinding, confounding attributable to selective use of second-look endoscopy (with possible between-group imbalances), and a lack of statistical adjustment for each participating center to account for unmeasured variations in supportive and endoscopic therapy.[51]

A very recent meta-analysis conducted by Wang and colleagues,[52] including 1157 patients from 7 randomized studies, suggested high-dose PPIs were equivalent to non–high-dose PPIs in reducing the rates of rebleeding, surgical intervention, or mortality when used postendoscopically. However, this meta-analysis assessed studies that included patients with both high- and low-risk lesions and whose methodological quality was suboptimal. Furthermore, and perhaps most importantly, the observed effect size, total number of patients included in the meta-analysis and resulting confidence intervals are insufficient to support the claim of equivalence of low- and high-dose intravenous PPI regimens. Additional data are needed to identify the optimal intravenous dose.

Because bleeding from high-risk ulcers is associated with significant morbidity and mortality, using a less-effective therapy may place patients at risk for adverse outcomes. Although low-dose intravenous PPI regimens may be as effective as the high-dose infusion alternative, more definitive evidence showing equivalence is necessary before their use can be recommending. It currently seems reasonable to continue using a high-dose PPI infusion of a 80-mg bolus followed by an infusion of 8 mg/h for 3 days after successful endoscopic therapy, as endorsed by the recently published international consensus recommendations on non-variceal upper gastrointestinal bleeding.[9]

Results of Randomized Trials Using Oral PPI

The role of high-dose oral PPI in the acute management of patients with bleeding ulcers has remained more controversial. Results from a study conducted by Javid and colleagues[42] comparing oral omeprazole, pantoprazole, and rabeprozale did not find any significant differences with respect to raising intragastric pH above 6 for 72 hours after endoscopic hemostasis in bleeding peptic ulcers. Clinical results from trials assessing Asian populations have suggested the efficacy of high-dose oral omeprazole (a daily total of 80 mg),[53–55] whereas equivalent high-quality studies from Western Europe or North America have been few, displaying heterogeneous study methodologies and yielding discordant results,[56–58] perhaps because of racial differences in gastric acid physiology,[4] pharmacogenomics,[5,59] Helicobacter pylori infection rates, and acuity of illness.[60]

Intravenous versus Oral PPIs

Fully published head-to-head gastric pH trials comparing intravenous and oral routes of PPI administration in patients with bleeding ulcers, let alone clinical comparisons, have been very few. A pilot study comparing the effects of oral to intravenous pantoprazole consisted of only 25 patients.[61] A subsequent trial published in 2008 compared intragastric pH levels, recorded after endoscopy for 24 hours, in patients with bleeding ulcers who received either intravenous (90-mg bolus followed by an infusion of 9 mg/h) or oral lansoprazole (120-mg bolus followed by 30 mg every 3 hours).[62] A pH level greater than 6 was maintained 67.8% of the time with continuous intravenous lansoprazole, and 64.8% with the 3-hourly oral PPI. Frequent oral PPI therapy achieved similar pH values; however, use of the intravenous regimen led to a more rapid rise in pH. This study unfortunately did not evaluate pH levels after the first 24 hours, limiting interpretation of the results. A recent study by Javid and colleagues[42] randomly assigned 90 patients to six 3-day combinations that included oral omeprazole, 80 mg bolus, followed by 40 mg every 12 hours; intravenous omeprazole, 80 mg, followed by infusion of 8 mg/h; oral pantoprazole, 80 mg bolus, followed by 80 mg every 12 hours; intravenous pantoprazole, 80 mg, followed by 8 mg/h; oral rabeprazole, 80 mg, followed by 40 mg every 12 hours; or intravenous rabeprazole, 80 mg, followed by an infusion of 8 mg/h. Mean pH levels over 72 hours for oral omeprazole, pantoprazole, and rabeprazole were 6.56, 6.34, and 6.11, respectively. Mean pH levels over 72 hours for intravenous omeprazole, pantoprazole, and rabeprazole were 6.93, 6.32, and 6.18, respectively. None were statistically different, with no differences in clinical outcomes, keeping in mind the small per group patient number. Adequately powered comparative trials with clinical outcomes are needed to determine the optimal route of administration in populations of different ethnicities.

Results of PPI Use in the Real-Life Setting

In an effort to assess the generalizability of randomized controlled trial results, the benefits of using a PPI acutely in peptic ulcer bleeding were assessed in the real-life Registry of Patients with Upper Gastrointestinal Bleeding Undergoing Endoscopy (RUGBE).[3] This registry is a large national cohort that included 1869 patients with non-variceal upper gastrointestinal bleeding. Using logistic regression modeling with extensive adjustment for known confounding, independent significant improvements in clinical outcomes were attributable to both endoscopic therapy and acute PPI use.[3]

Is administration of PPIs useful in patients with upper gastrointestinal bleeding while awaiting endoscopy?

Many trials have assessed the role of acutely administering pharmacotherapy while awaiting endoscopy. A recent Cochrane systematic review reported no improvement in important clinical outcomes attributable to preendoscopic PPI treatment, yet a significant decrease in the need for endoscopic therapy (OR, 0.68; CI, 0.50–0.93) and a reduced number of patients with high-risk stigmata (OR, 0.67; CI, 0.54–0.84)[63] when these patients underwent endoscopy after varying durations of infusion (approximately 16 hours in some of the largest included trials). These summary results are based on six trials using varying doses and routes of administration, with the most widely quoted single trial reporting on a high-dose intravenous regimen.[64] This surprising finding suggests the possibility that PPI may work not only through a clot stabilizing mechanism but also by accelerating healing through other biologic effects. Several mechanisms have been proposed to account for possible anti-inflammatory actions of PPIs,[20] including antioxidant properties, scavenging of reactive oxygen species, and the induction of heme oxygenase-1. Possible effects of PPI on inflammatory cells include impaired neutrophil migration, decreased expression of adhesion molecules by neutrophils and monocytes, and impaired phagocytosis of micro-organisms by neutrophils. PPIs may also affect endothelial and epithelial cells through decreasing production of proinflammatory cytokines. Finally, PPIs may also inhibit growth of bacteria and fungi and aid in killing these microorganisms. **Box 2** summarizes non–pH-related possible mechanisms of action of PPIs.

Because the efficacy of pre-endoscopic PPI use is at best marginal, a strategy of PPI treatment while awaiting endoscopy for suspected upper gastrointestinal bleeding should not replace adequate resuscitation and the practice of early endoscopy. The most cost-effective scenarios in which pre-endoscopic PPI use may be administered include patients likely to be bleeding from a non-variceal source, especially if it is likely to be a high-risk lesion, and when a delay to endoscopy is likely to occur.[9,65]

Use of PPIs on discharge after admission for peptic ulcer bleeding
Very few data are available to guide clinicians regarding the optimal discharge acid suppression regimen after an admission for peptic ulcer bleeding. The recent international consensus conference suggested that patients should be discharged with a prescription for a single daily-dose oral PPI for a duration that should be dictated by the underlying etiology.[9]

Box 2
Possible anti-inflammatory effects of PPIs

Effect of neutrophils

Impaired neutrophil migration

Reduced phagocytosis

Suppression of oxidative burst

Decreased expression of adhesion molecules

Anti-oxidant effects

Scavenging of reactive oxygen species

Sulfhydryl molecule replenishment in the gastric mucosa

Generation of bilirubin and carbon monoxide by activation of heme-oxygenase-1

Effects on endothelial and epithelial cells

Diminished production of proinflammatory cytokines

Decreased expression of adhesion molecules

Effects on gut microflora

Selective antibacterial and antifungal effects

Data from Kedika RR, Souza RF, Spechler SJ. Potential anti-inflammatory effects of proton pump inhibitors: a review and discussion of the clinical implications. Dig Dis Sci 2009;54 (11):2312–7.

Appropriate use of PPIs

The cost-effective promise of intravenous PPI use,[9] either before or after endoscopy, can only be realized if these medications are used appropriately in the hospital setting. Unfortunately, the rates of inappropriate in-hospital antisecretory therapy prescribing are very high, ranging from 30% to 70%.[13–17] This finding is even more concerning in light of potential side effects associated with acid suppression in ill patients,[66] even if most of these associations remain controversial and exhibit very low numbers needed to harm. The risk–benefit ratio of these medications is extremely favorable, especially among patients with bleeding. Educational interventions may improve the rates of appropriate prescribing with a lesser favorable impact on overall costs.[67]

In summary, PPI use clearly decreases rates of rebleeding and the need for surgery in patients with bleeding peptic ulcers. However, the optimal route of administration and minimal dose required to produce this effect remain uncertain. The improvement in mortality attributed to PPI use has been noted in patients exhibiting high-risk stigmata and having initially undergone endoscopic therapy; for the most part, these patients have received high-dose intravenous PPI. The use of PPI before endoscopy results in much more modest benefits, if any, indicating that identification of cost-effective scenarios for its optimal use are warranted.

SUMMARY AND FUTURE AREAS OF RESEARCH

Despite a plethora of quality studies and summary data, many key questions remain regarding pharmacotherapy for the management of patients with non-variceal upper gastrointestinal bleeding, and more specifically PPIs in peptic ulcer bleeding. Additional well-designed studies are needed to determine the optimal timing, dose, and route of administration, and adequate physician education is required to fulfill the cost-effective promise of this medication class. Future comparisons will need to stratify the management of patients according to low-, intermediate-, and high-risk endoscopic lesions through assessing strategies that include sole pharmacotherapy, newer hemostatic combinations, and evolving endoscopic approaches and technologies.

REFERENCES

1. Adler DG, Leighton JA, Davila RE, et al. ASGE guideline: the role of endoscopy in acute non-variceal upper-GI hemorrhage. Gastrointest Endosc 2004;60(4): 497–504.
2. Barkun A, Bardou M, Marshall JK. Consensus recommendations for managing patients with nonvariceal upper gastrointestinal bleeding. Ann Intern Med 2003;139(10):843–57.
3. Barkun A, Sabbah S, Enns R, et al. The Canadian Registry on Nonvariceal Upper Gastrointestinal Bleeding and Endoscopy (RUGBE): endoscopic hemostasis and proton pump inhibition are associated with improved outcomes in a real-life setting. Am J Gastroenterol 2004;99(7):1238–46.
4. Green FW Jr, Kaplan MM, Curtis LE, et al. Effect of acid and pepsin on blood coagulation and platelet aggregation. A possible contributor prolonged gastroduodenal mucosal hemorrhage. Gastroenterology 1978;74(1):38–43.
5. Li Y, Sha W, Nie Y, et al. Effect of intragastric pH on control of peptic ulcer bleeding. J Gastroenterol Hepatol 2000;15(2):148–54.
6. Patchett SE, Enright H, Afdhal N, et al. Clot lysis by gastric juice: an in vitro study. Gut 1989;30(12):1704–7.

7. Berstad A. Does profound acid inhibition improve haemostasis in peptic ulcer bleeding? Scand J Gastroenterol 1997;32(4):396–8.
8. Vreeburg EM, Levi M, Rauws EA, et al. Enhanced mucosal fibrinolytic activity in gastroduodenal ulcer haemorrhage and the beneficial effect of acid suppression. Aliment Pharmacol Ther 2001;15(5):639–46.
9. Barkun AN, Bardou M, Kuipers EJ, et al. International consensus recommendations on the management of patients with nonvariceal upper gastrointestinal bleeding. Ann Intern Med 2010;152(2):101–13.
10. Barkun A, Kennedy W, Herba K, et al. The cost effectiveness of proton pump inhibitor continuous infusion (IV PPI) administered prior to endoscopy in the treatment of patients with non-variceal upper GI bleeding [abstract# 332]. Gastroenterology 2002;122:A67.
11. Erstad BL. Cost-effectiveness of proton pump inhibitor therapy for acute peptic ulcer-related bleeding. Crit Care Med 2004;32(6):1277–83.
12. Lee KK, You JH, Wong IC, et al. Cost-effectiveness analysis of high-dose omeprazole infusion as adjuvant therapy to endoscopic treatment of bleeding peptic ulcer. Gastrointest Endosc 2003;57(2):160–4.
13. Guda NM, Noonan M, Kreiner MJ, et al. Use of intravenous proton pump inhibitors in community practice: an explanation for the shortage? Am J Gastroenterol 2004;99(7):1233–7.
14. Parente F, Cucino C, Gallus S, et al. Hospital use of acid-suppressive medications and its fall-out on prescribing in general practice: a 1-month survey. Aliment Pharmacol Ther. 2003;17(12):1503–6.
15. Nardino RJ, Vender RJ, Herbert PN. Overuse of acid-suppressive therapy in hospitalized patients. Am J Gastroenterol 2000;95(11):3118–22.
16. Enns R, Andrews C, Fishman M, et al. Description of prescribing practices in patients with upper gastrointestinal bleeding receiving intravenous proton pump inhibitors: a multicentre evaluation. Can J Gastroenterol 2004;18:567–71.
17. Mat Saad A, Collins N, Lobo M, et al. Proton pump inhibitors: a survey of prescribing in an Irish general hospital. Int J Clin Pract 2005;59:31–4.
18. Lau JY, Chung SC, Leung JW, et al. The evolution of stigmata of hemorrhage in bleeding peptic ulcers: a sequential endoscopic study. Endoscopy 1998;30(6):513–8.
19. Sung JJ, Barkun A, Kuipers EJ, et al. Intravenous esomeprazole for prevention of recurrent peptic ulcer bleeding: a randomized trial. Ann Intern Med. 2009;150(7):455–64.
20. Kedika RR, Souza RF, Spechler SJ. Potential anti-inflammatory effects of proton pump inhibitors: a review and discussion of the clinical implications. Dig Dis Sci 2009;54(11):2312–7.
21. Leontiadis GI, Howden CW. Pharmacologic treatment of peptic ulcer bleeding. Curr Treat Options Gastroenterol 2007;10(2):134–42.
22. Henry DA, O'Connell DL. Effects of fibrinolytic inhibitors on mortality from upper gastrointestinal haemorrhage. BMJ 1989;298(6681):1142–6.
23. Brody TM, Larner J, Minneman KP. Brody's human pharmacology: molecular to clinical. Philadelphia: Elsevier Mosby; 2005.
24. Villanueva C, Ortiz J, Minana J, et al. Somatostatin treatment and risk stratification by continuous portal pressure monitoring during acute variceal bleeding. Gastroenterology 2001;121(1):110–7.
25. Tsibouris P, Zintzaras E, Lappas C, et al. High-dose pantoprazole continuous infusion is superior to somatostatin after endoscopic hemostasis in patients with peptic ulcer bleeding. Am J Gastroenterol 2007;102(6):1192–9.

26. Imperiale TF, Birgisson S. Somatostatin or octreotide compared with H2 antagonists and placebo in the management of acute nonvariceal upper gastrointestinal hemorrhage: a meta-analysis. Ann Intern Med 1997;127(12):1062–71.

27. Bardou M, Youseff M, Toubouti Y, et al. Newer endoscopic therapies decrease both re-bleeding and mortality in high risk patients with acute peptic ulcer bleeding: a series of meta-analyses [abstract]. Gastroenterology 2003;123:A239.

28. Garcia-Tsao G, Bosch J. Management of varices and variceal hemorrhage in cirrhosis. N Engl J Med 2010;362(9):823–32.

29. Merki HS, Wilder-Smith CH. Do continuous infusions of omeprazole and ranitidine retain their effect with prolonged dosing? Gastroenterology 1994;106(1):60–4.

30. Barkun AN, Cockeram AW, Plourde V, et al. Review article: acid suppression in non-variceal acute upper gastrointestinal bleeding. Aliment Pharmacol Ther 1999;13(12):1565–84.

31. Netzer P, Gut A, Heer R, et al. Five-year audit of ambulatory 24-hour esophageal pH-manometry in clinical practice. Scand J Gastroenterol 1999;34(7):676–82.

32. Smith JT, Gavey C, Nwokolo CU, et al. Tolerance during 8 days of high-dose H2-blockade: placebo-controlled studies of 24-hour acidity and gastrin. Aliment Pharmacol Ther 1990;4(Suppl 1):47–63.

33. Walt RP, Cottrell J, Mann SG, et al. Continuous intravenous famotidine for haemorrhage from peptic ulcer. Lancet 1992;340(8827):1058–62.

34. Collins R, Langman M. Treatment with histamine H2 antagonists in acute upper gastrointestinal hemorrhage. Implications of randomized trials. N Engl J Med 1985;313(11):660–6.

35. Levine JE, Leontiadis GI, Sharma VK, et al. Meta-analysis: the efficacy of intravenous H2-receptor antagonists in bleeding peptic ulcer. Aliment Pharmacol Ther 2002;16(6):1137–42.

36. Brunner G, Luna P, Hartmann M, et al. Optimizing the intragastric pH as a supportive therapy in upper GI bleeding. Yale J Biol Med 1996;69(3):225–31.

37. Baker DE. Peptic ulcer bleeding following therapeutic endoscopy: a new indication for intravenous esomeprazole. Rev Gastroenterol Disord 2009;9(4):E111–8.

38. Howden CW, Metz DC, Hunt B, et al. Dose-response evaluation of the antisecretory effect of continuous infusion intravenous lansoprazole regimens over 48 h. Aliment Pharmacol Ther 2006;23(7):975–84.

39. Metz DC, Amer F, Hunt B, et al. Lansoprazole regimens that sustain intragastric pH > 6.0: an evaluation of intermittent oral and continuous intravenous infusion dosages. Aliment Pharmacol Ther 2006;23(7):985–95.

40. Hasselgren G, Keelan M, Kirdeikis P, et al. Optimization of acid suppression for patients with peptic ulcer bleeding: an intragastric pH-metry study with omeprazole. Eur J Gastroenterol Hepatol 1998;10(7):601–6.

41. van Rensburg CJ, Hartmann M, Thorpe A, et al. Intragastric pH during continuous infusion with pantoprazole in patients with bleeding peptic ulcer. Am J Gastroenterol 2003;98(12):2635–41.

42. Javid G, Zargar SA, R Us, et al. Comparison of p.o. or i.v. proton pump inhibitors on 72-h intragastric pH in bleeding peptic ulcer. J Gastroenterol Hepatol 2009; 24(7):1236–43.

43. Daneshmend TK, Hawkey CJ, Langman MJ, et al. Omeprazole versus placebo for acute upper gastrointestinal bleeding: randomised double blind controlled trial. BMJ 1992;304(6820):143–7.

44. Lau JY, Sung JJ, Lee KK, et al. Effect of intravenous omeprazole on recurrent bleeding after endoscopic treatment of bleeding peptic ulcers. N Engl J Med 2000;343(5):310–6.

45. van Rensburg C, Barkun AN, Racz I, et al. Clinical trial: intravenous pantoprazole vs. ranitidine for the prevention of peptic ulcer rebleeding: a multicentre, multinational, randomized trial. Aliment Pharmacol Ther 2009;29(5):497–507.
46. Jensen DM, Pace SC, Soffer E, et al. Continuous infusion of pantoprazole versus ranitidine for prevention of ulcer rebleeding: a U.S. multicenter randomized, double-blind study. Am J Gastroenterol 2006;101(9):1991–9 [quiz: 2170].
47. Leontiadis GI, Sharma VK, Howden CW. Proton pump inhibitor therapy for peptic ulcer bleeding: Cochrane collaboration meta-analysis of randomized controlled trials. Mayo Clin Proc 2007;82(3):286–96.
48. Laine L, McQuaid KR. Endoscopic therapy for bleeding ulcers: an evidence-based approach based on meta-analyses of randomized controlled trials. Clin Gastroenterol Hepatol 2009;7(1):33–47 [quiz: 31–32].
49. Kahi CJ, Jensen DM, Sung JJ, et al. Endoscopic therapy versus medical therapy for bleeding peptic ulcer with adherent clot: a meta-analysis. Gastroenterology 2005;129(3):855–62.
50. Andriulli A, Loperfido S, Focareta R, et al. High- versus low-dose proton pump inhibitors after endoscopic hemostasis in patients with peptic ulcer bleeding: a multicentre, randomized study. Am J Gastroenterol 2008;103(12):3011–8.
51. Barkun AN, Kuipers EJ, Sung JJ. It is premature to recommend low-dose intravenous proton pump inhibition after endoscopic hemostasis in patients with bleeding ulcers. Am J Gastroenterol 2009;104(8):2120–1.
52. Wang CH, Ma MH, Chou HC, et al. High-dose vs non-high-dose proton pump inhibitors after endoscopic treatment in patients with bleeding peptic ulcer: a systematic review and meta-analysis of randomized controlled trials. Arch Intern Med 2010;170(9):751–8.
53. Khuroo MS, Yattoo GN, Javid G, et al. A comparison of omeprazole and placebo for bleeding peptic ulcer. N Engl J Med 1997;336(15):1054–8.
54. Javid G, Masoodi I, Zargar SA, et al. Omeprazole as adjuvant therapy to endoscopic combination injection sclerotherapy for treating bleeding peptic ulcer. Am J Med 2001;111(4):280–4.
55. Kaviani MJ, Hashemi MR, Kazemifar AR, et al. Effect of oral omeprazole in reducing re-bleeding in bleeding peptic ulcers: a prospective, double-blind, randomized, clinical trial. Aliment Pharmacol Ther 2003;17(2):211–6.
56. Coraggio F, Rotondano G, Marmo R, et al. Somatostatin in the prevention of recurrent bleeding after endoscopic haemostasis of peptic ulcer haemorrhage: a preliminary report. Eur J Gastroenterol Hepatol 1998;10(8):673–6.
57. Fasseas P, Leybishkis B, Rocca G. Omeprazole versus ranitidine in the medical treatment of acute upper gastrointestinal bleeding: assessment by early repeat endoscopy. Int J Clin Pract 2001;55(10):661–4.
58. Michel P, Duhamel C, Bazin B, et al. Lansoprazole versus ranitidine in the prevention of early recurrences of digestive hemorrhages from gastroduodenal ulcers. Randomized double-blind multicenter study. Gastroenterol Clin Biol 1994;18(12):1102–5 [in French].
59. Goldstein JA. Clinical relevance of genetic polymorphisms in the human CYP2C subfamily. Br J Clin Pharmacol 2001;52(4):349–55.
60. Leontiadis GI, Sharma VK, Howden CW. Proton pump inhibitor treatment for acute peptic ulcer bleeding. Cochrane Database Syst Rev 2006;1:CD002094.
61. Bajaj JS, Dua KS, Hanson K, et al. Prospective, randomized trial comparing effect of oral versus intravenous pantoprazole on rebleeding after nonvariceal upper gastrointestinal bleeding: a pilot study. Dig Dis Sci 2007;52(9):2190–4.

62. Laine L, Shah A, Bemanian S. Intragastric pH with oral vs intravenous bolus plus infusion proton-pump inhibitor therapy in patients with bleeding ulcers. Gastroenterology 2008;134(7):1836–41.

63. Sreedharan A, Martin J, Leontiadis GI, et al. Proton pump inhibitor treatment initiated prior to endoscopic diagnosis in upper gastrointestinal bleeding. Cochrane Database of Systematic Reviews 2006;4:CD005415. DOI: 10.1002/14651858.CD005415.pub2.

64. Lau JY, Leung WK, Wu JC, et al. Omeprazole before endoscopy in patients with gastrointestinal bleeding. N Engl J Med 2007;356(16):1631–40.

65. Barkun AN. Should every patient with suspected upper GI bleeding receive a proton pump inhibitor while awaiting endoscopy? Gastrointest Endosc 2008; 67(7):1064–6.

66. Dial S, Alrasadi K, Manoukian C, et al. Risk of Clostridium difficile diarrhea among hospital inpatients prescribed proton pump inhibitors: cohort and case–control studies. Can Med Assoc J 2004;171:33–8.

67. Kaplan GG, Bates D, McDonald D, et al. Inappropriate use of intravenous pantoprazole: extent of the problem and successful solutions. Clin Gastroenterol Hepatol 2005;3(12):1207–14.

Nonsteroidal Antiinflammatory Drug-Related Injury to the Gastrointestinal Tract: Clinical Picture, Pathogenesis, and Prevention

Carmelo Scarpignato, MD, DSc (Hons), PharmD (h.c.), FRCP (Lond), FCP, FACG[a,b,*],
Richard H. Hunt, FRCP, FRCPEd, FRCPC, FACG, AGAF[c]

KEYWORDS

- Nonsteroidal antiinflammatory drug • Gastrointestinal tract
- Pathogenesis • Injury • Prevention

Increasing life expectancy in developed countries has led to a growing prevalence of arthritic disorders, which has been accompanied by increasing prescriptions for nonsteroidal antiinflammatory drugs (NSAIDs).[1] These are the most widely used agents for musculoskeletal and arthritic conditions, representing more than 7.7% of all prescriptions in Europe.[1] However, these figures are probably underestimated, because over-the-counter (OTC) use is not included. In absolute terms, in 2004, there were 111 million NSAID prescriptions in the United States.[2] The reason for such widespread use is the clinical effectiveness of NSAIDs, which have been consistently shown to be more effective than acetaminophen (paracetamol) for the management of osteoarthritis (OA),[3,4] and the fact that NSAIDs are endorsed in current OA management guidelines.[5,6]

Conflict of interest statement. The authors have received consulting and/or lecture fees from several pharmaceutical companies and other organizations. The authors have also received research support from charities and government sources at various times. No author has any direct stock holding in any pharmaceutical company.
[a] Division of Gastroenterology, Department of Clinical Sciences, University of Parma, Italy
[b] Laboratory of Clinical Pharmacology, School of Medicine & Dentistry, University of Parma, Via Volturno, 39, 43100 Parma, Italy
[c] Division of Gastroenterology, Department of Medicine, McMaster University and Farncombe Family Digestive Health Research Institute, Hamilton, Ontario, Canada
* Corresponding author.
E-mail address: scarpi@tin.it

Gastroenterol Clin N Am 39 (2010) 433–464
doi:10.1016/j.gtc.2010.08.010
0889-8553/10/$ – see front matter © 2010 Elsevier Inc. All rights reserved.

gastro.theclinics.com

Although NSAIDs are effective, their use is associated with a broad spectrum of adverse reactions in the liver, kidney, cardiovascular (CV) system, skin, and gut.[7] Gastrointestinal (GI) side effects are the most common and range from dyspepsia, heartburn, and abdominal discomfort to more serious events such as peptic ulcer with the life-threatening complications of bleeding and perforation.[8,9] The dilemma for the physician prescribing NSAIDs is, therefore, to maintain the antiinflammatory and analgesic benefits, while reducing or preventing GI side effects.

NSAIDs are usually given orally, although intravenous, intramuscular, rectal, or topical administrations are used if specifically designed formulations are available. With the exception of renal colic, in which NSAIDs act faster when given intravenously,[10] in all other pain conditions there is no evidence that injected NSAIDs are superior to oral.

Despite the oral route being the most widely used, and allowing self-medication, it is the most challenging in terms of absorption and drug- and food-drug interactions.[11] Moreover, oral intake allows direct contact between the drug and the entire GI tract mucosa, thus exposing it to topical damage until absorption. However, injury may continue after drug absorption if the mucosa is further exposed as a result of enterohepatic circulation of the NSAID.

The GI tract, like the skin and the respiratory system, is in continuous and direct interaction with the environment. The functions of the GI tract as a protective barrier are as important as digestion and absorption.[12] The large surface area and prolonged exposure increase the risk of drug-mediated damage, and increased permeability (often found in some inflammatory conditions) may augment this. The remarkable tolerance of the GI mucosa to damaging agents including NSAIDs relies on rapid epithelial repair, which depends on restitution and cell replication. When repair fails, erosions and ulcers develop, disrupting the basement membrane, forming persistent ulcers, which then increase the risk of clinically relevant events.[13]

EPIDEMIOLOGY OF NSAID-ASSOCIATED MUCOSAL INJURY

In the United States, a national prescription audit showed an annual NSAID consumption of 111,400,000 at a cost of $4.8 billion, with further sales of OTC oral analgesics of $3 billion. A survey of NSAID use among people older than 65 years showed that 70% were taking an NSAID at least once a week and half of these were taking an NSAID daily.[14] A study in Europe reported an NSAID consumption of 42.82 to 74.17 defined daily dose/1000 inhabitants in 2007, increasing by 25.1% between 2002 and 2007. Diclofenac and ibuprofen were the most prescribed agents, with a notable increase in nimesulide and meloxicam use. Trends for consumption of selective cyclooxygenase-2 (COX-2) inhibitors differed within countries.[15]

Recent data from US veterans older than 65 years shows an overall mortality of 5.5 per 1000 person years after an upper GI event, rising to 17.7 per 1000 person years following a myocardial infarction and 21.8 per 1000 person years following a cardiovascular accident. Predictors of mortality were advancing age, comorbidities, increased COX-2 inhibitor use, and failure to provide gastroprotection.[16]

In the United Kingdom, a previous study[17] reported an overall mortality in patients with GI bleeding of 12%. A more recent systematic review of studies published since 1997 shows that upper GI bleeding or perforation still carries a finite risk of death. Differences in study design, population characteristics, risk factors, definition of mortality, and reporting of outcomes imposes limitations on interpreting effect size. Data published since 1997 suggest that mortality in patients suffering from an upper

GI bleed or perforation has fallen to 1 in 13 overall, but remains higher, at about 1 in 5, in those exposed to NSAIDs or aspirin.[18]

There have also been serious consequences to the post-Vioxx anxieties about the use of COX-2 selective drugs. There has been a move back to the use of nonselective NSAIDs (ns-NSAIDs) by rheumatologists in North America. A recent study has shown that COX-2 inhibitor withdrawals also resulted in a rapid decline in NSAID gastroprotection prescribed by US rheumatologists despite the availability of different gastroprotective options. Channeling toward nonselective NSAID use was widespread, also among patients at increased CV risk. Longer-term follow-up is required to determine the clinical significance of these changes in NSAID prescribing, particularly for NSAID-related GI and CV-related toxicities.[19]

There has also been a changing pattern to the location of GI bleeding in patients taking NSAIDs, with increasing reports of bleeding lesions located in the small intestine. However, it is not yet clear whether this reflects increased awareness and ascertainment bias or a real increase in small bowel lesions. A study of hospitalized patients in Spain[20] shows that, in the past decade, there has been a progressive change in the overall picture of GI events leading to hospitalization, with a decreasing trend in upper GI events and a significant increase in lower GI events, causing the rates of these GI complications to converge. Overall mortality has also decreased, but the in-hospital case fatality rate from upper or lower GI complications has remained constant. It will be a challenge to improve care unless new strategies can be developed to reduce the number of events originating in the lower GI tract, as well as reducing associated mortality.[20]

The high risk in elderly patients taking NSAIDs has been repeatedly confirmed, and a study from Argentina in 324 adults with a mean age of 74 years and a similar number of controls found that NSAID exposure increased the risk of hospitalization for peptic ulcer disease (PUD, odds ratio [OR] 5.20; 95% confidence interval [CI] 3.31–8.15). A history of upper GI complications was independently associated with hospitalization for PUD (OR 14.62; 95% CI 6.70–31.91). Thus, ns-NSAIDs are a significant risk factor for PUD-related hospitalizations among older adults.[21]

The use of all medications increases with age and the elderly are at increased risk of adverse drug reactions. The risk of these complications depends on the presence of risk factors, the most frequent and relevant of which is age. Thus, patients at risk should be on prevention strategies including the lowest effective dose of NSAID, cotherapy with a gastroprotective drug, or the use of a COX-2 selective agent. Although the best strategy to prevent lower GI complications has yet to be defined, treatment of associated *Helicobacter pylori* infection is also important when starting treatment with ns-NSAIDs or aspirin, especially in the presence of an ulcer history.[22,23]

A recent study exploring gastroprotective strategies among 1.5 million patients in the AGIS database indicated that both the prevalence of NSAID prescriptions and the risk of gastric complications is increasing steadily. Although the number of patients receiving gastroprotective medication increased from 39.6% in 2001 to 69.9% in 2007, more than 30% of patients at risk for GI complications were left unprotected in 2007. To enhance protection rates in patients using NSAIDs and to decrease NSAID-related hospital admissions in the future, the implementation of gastroprotection guidelines needs to be improved.[24]

NSAID-ASSOCIATED MUCOSAL DAMAGE TO THE GI TRACT
NSAID-associated Esophageal Injury

NSAIDs may cause damage throughout the GI tract. Although the stomach and duodenum are well-recognized sites of damage, esophageal injury is common.

Despite esophageal mucosa possessing several intrinsic mechanisms of epithelial defense[25] and an efficient clearing system, nearly 100 medications have been implicated as causes of esophageal mucosal damage.[26] Of 92 patients with pill-induced esophageal injury, NSAIDs were causative in 41% (38 of 92) of them.[27] The prevalence of esophagitis in patients with arthritis taking NSAIDs was 21%,[28] and a case-control study[29] indicated that, together with hiatal hernia, NSAID intake represents a significant ($P = .021$) risk factor (OR 1.87; 95% CI 1.10–3.19) for esophageal ulcer.

Retrosternal or substernal chest pain is the most common complaint in patients with pill esophagitis, and is present in more than 60% of cases, occurring immediately or several hours after ingestion of medication. Other common complaints are odynophagia and dysphagia, which are present in 50% and 40% of patients, respectively. Symptoms usually develop within the first few days of starting a new medication, but frequently occur with the first dose.[30] If left unrecognized and NSAID intake persists, the acute injury can be complicated by esophageal bleeding, stricture, and even fatal perforation. Drug-induced esophageal injury tends to occur at the anatomic site of narrowing, with the middle third behind the left atrium predominating (75.6%). At endoscopy, erosions, kissing ulcers, and multiple areas of ulceration with bleeding may be seen.[27] The presence of exudates with thickening of the esophageal wall suggests a chemical esophagitis. Moreover, 50% of patients with acute necrotizing esophagitis, a previously considered rare cause of upper gastrointestinal bleeding (UGIB), had taken NSAIDs.[31]

NSAID-associated Gastroduodenal Symptoms and Lesions

The 2 most common causes of PUD are infection with H pylori and use of NSAIDs.[32] The term NSAID gastropathy was first introduced in 1986 to differentiate between classic PUD and the unique range of gastric mucosal lesions associated with long-term NSAID therapy.[33] However, because NSAIDs also damage duodenal mucosa, NSAID-induced gastroduodenal damage is a more appropriate term to describe NSAID-associated lesions. This definition encompasses the true ulcers, which are mucosal lesions that penetrate the muscularis mucosa, and the erosions that are limited to the mucosa. Injury from NSAIDs usually occurs within the first few weeks of treatment but also seems to be associated with long-term use.[8] Upper GI symptoms associated with NSAID use include dyspepsia, heartburn, bloating or cramping, nausea, and vomiting in up to 40% to 50% of patients taking NSAIDs.[34] These symptoms prompt a change in therapy in 10% of patients. However, symptoms associated with NSAIDs have little relationship to erosions or ulcerations seen endoscopically, which are often asymptomatic, and patients with symptoms often have no identifiable lesions. The first sign of NSAID-induced GI damage in asymptomatic individuals may be a life-threatening complication.[8]

Endoscopic examination of NSAID users can reveal subepithelial hemorrhages, erosions, and ulceration, or a combination. Mucosal damage is seen in 30% to 50% of patients taking NSAIDs,[34] but most lesions are of little clinical significance and disappear or reduce in number with continued use, probably because of mucosal adaptation.[35] Only 15% to 30% of NSAIDs users have endoscopically confirmed ulcers, with the gastric antrum being the most frequently affected.

GI complications occur in 1% to 1.5% of patients in the first year of treatment with ns-NSAIDs and, when symptomatic ulcers are included, this figure increases to 4% to 5%.[34] The average relative risk of developing a serious GI complication is three- to fivefold greater among NSAIDs users than among non users. Aspirin is also associated with both gastric and duodenal ulcers, and upper GI complications occur even with the lowest dose of 75 mg/d.[36] Although some studies suggest that the first 2 months of treatment is the period of greatest risk for complications, with a relative risk of 4.5% (95% CI 2.9–7.0), evidence from both randomized clinical trials (RCTs) and observational studies indicate that the risk of GI complications is present with both short-term and long-term use of ns-NSAIDs from the first dose.[37] Thus, even a short course of NSAID therapy (eg, for postoperative pain or acute musculoskeletal injury) carries a risk equivalent to that of long-term treatment. Thus, strategies to prevent GI complications should be implemented regardless of the duration of therapy, especially in patients at high GI risk.

The worst GI outcome with NSAIDs is UGIB, which may result in death. However, mortality data associated with NSAIDs are scarce. Current mortality incidence was estimated at 15.3 deaths per 100,000 among NSAID/aspirin users in a large Spanish study. This mortality is lower than previously quoted, likely because of a decline in the rate of complications in the last 5 to 10 years associated with increasing use of prevention strategies for NSAID-induced GI damage and a decline in the prevalence of *H pylori* infection.[20,34]

COX-2 selective NSAIDs (often incorrectly referred to as coxibs[38]) have an improved upper GI safety profile compared with traditional (nonselective) NSAIDs, as extensively shown in endoscopy and clinical outcomes studies.[9,24,37] The evidence is strong, with consistent reductions in events of about 50% in large RCTs, meta-analyses of RCTs, and large observational studies in clinical practice.[39]

The prevalence of dyspepsia in users of ns-NSAIDs and COX-2 selective inhibitors was examined in a meta-analysis of 26 RCTs,[40] which revealed a 12% relative risk reduction in dyspeptic symptoms for COX-2 selective *versus* ns-NSAIDs. Compared with ns-NSAIDs, the number needed to treat with a COX-2 inhibitor to prevent 1 patient from developing dyspepsia was 27. Dyspepsia reduction with COX-2 inhibitor therapy may not be substantial, and patients on COX-2 selective NSAIDs may need cotherapy with proton pump inhibitors (PPIs) to obtain the same symptom improvement as those taking ns-NSAIDs.[41] However, experience indicates that, in the individual patient, the lower dyspepsia rate with coxibs compared with ns-NSAIDs, although not large, could be clinically relevant.[37]

Large outcome studies, as well as endoscopic and epidemiologic studies, confirm that low-dose aspirin (LD-ASA) increases the risk of UGIB in NSAID and COX-2 inhibitor users and attenuates the GI benefits of COX-2 selective NSAIDs. A COX-2 inhibitor plus aspirin was associated with a nonsignificantly lower ulcer and lower ulcer complication rate when compared with ns-NSAIDs alone.[37,39] Moreover, a COX-2 inhibitor plus LD-ASA was associated with lower GI risk than an ns-NSAID plus LD-ASA. Thus, combination of aspirin plus a COX-2 inhibitor should be the preferred option, compared with aspirin plus an ns-NSAID, for patients at high GI risk who require CV prophylaxis. Future RCTs, specifically designed to compare the GI and CV safety of a COX-2 inhibitor plus aspirin and an ns-NSAID plus aspirin, are needed to confirm these conclusions.[37]

NSAID-associated Bowel Injury

The small bowel is more common than the stomach as a site for adverse effects of NSAIDs, producing NSAID enteropathy.[42] The pathogenesis and clinical implications of adverse effects at the two sites have many similarities but differ in some important aspects. NSAID enteropathy, rather than being life threatening, often leads to complications that call for extensive investigation, and needs to be differentiated from other newly discovered enteropathies.[43] In particular, a common problem is to distinguish between ileitis in association with spondyloarthropathy, NSAID enteropathy, and Crohn disease. Moreover, the frequency of life-threatening complications in the lower

GI tract represent one-third of all GI complications associated with NSAIDs. In the last 10 years, there has been a decreasing trend in hospitalizations because of upper GI complications, in contrast with an increasing trend of lower GI complications, and the clinical effect and severity of lower GI events were greater than for upper GI events.[20]

Most patients with NSAID enteropathy are asymptomatic and can be diagnosed by demonstrating increased intestinal permeability,[44] increased fecal calprotectin,[45] or by wireless capsule enteroscopy.[46] However, the capsule findings (mucosal breaks, reddened folds, petechiae or red spots, denuded mucosa, and blood in the lumen without a visualized source) are not pathognomonic for NSAID injury, and similar changes are seen in a variety of small bowel diseases. In particular, it is sometimes impossible to differentiate NSAID enteropathy from that of Crohn disease. The most common indication leading to a diagnosis of NSAID enteropathy is iron deficiency anemia. Endoscopy and colonoscopy may fail to provide an adequate explanation for the anemia, and capsule enteroscopy is likely to provide a diagnosis when luminal blood may be evident.[47]

The spectrum of abnormalities that are detected range from subclinical damage, including increased mucosal permeability, mucosal inflammation, fecal occult blood loss, ileal dysfunction, and malabsorption, to clinical features including anemia, mucosal diaphragms and strictures, small bowel, colonic, and rectal ulceration, colitis, as well as bleeding and perforation.[42,43,48] Increased mucosal permeability is silent and observed within 24 hours of ingestion with almost all NSAIDs, except the coxibs and ns-NSAIDs not undergoing enterohepatic recirculation.[44]

The lack of intestinal damage with selective COX-2 inhibitors seen in animal experiments has been confirmed in clinical studies. Most patients taking either meloxicam[49] or nimesulide,[50] two preferential COX-2 inhibitors, had normal intestinal permeability and no increase in intestinal inflammation compared with control patients. In studies in healthy volunteers, rofecoxib[51] and etoricoxib,[52] compared with the ns-NSAID, ibuprofen, did not increase fecal blood loss. Furthermore, the incidence of anemia with celecoxib was significantly less than that seen with ns-NSAIDs.[53,54] Although some case reports of acute colitis or lower intestinal complications have been associated with COX-2 inhibitors, post hoc analysis of the Vioxx GI Outcomes Research (VIGOR) study showed that the benefits of rofecoxib 50 mg/d compared with naproxen (500 mg twice a day) were present in both the upper and the lower GI tract, with a risk reduction for serious lower GI events of 50% and 60%, respectively.[55,56] In the recent CONDOR study, comparing celecoxib with slow-release diclofenac plus omeprazole, celecoxib was superior to the NSAID plus PPI in reducing the risk of clinical outcomes throughout the GI tract.[57] The study used as primary end point a novel composite score (clinically significant upper and/or lower gastrointestinal events [CSULGIEs]), which is discussed later. Etoricoxib, which is an acidic (pK_a 4.5) COX-2 selective compound, did not achieve a significant decrease in lower GI clinical events compared with diclofenac in the RCTs belonging to the Multinational Etoricoxib and Diclofenac Arthritis Long-term (MEDAL) program.[58]

Colonoscopy studies confirm that NSAIDs are associated with isolated and diffuse colonic ulceration that may be associated with occult or major intestinal bleeding and/or perforation. Diffuse colitis has been observed after mefenamic acid, ibuprofen, piroxicam, naproxen, and aspirin.[48] NSAID colopathy (ulceration or stricture formation) usually involves the right colon, but the rectum may also be involved.[59] Patients may present with diarrhea, bleeding, anemia, weight loss, or obstruction.[60] Ileoscopy may show an ulcerative ileitis, whose features overlap with Crohn ileitis, but differentiation is critical for appropriate management.[61] Although some patients with inflammatory bowel disease (IBD) can tolerate NSAIDs,[62] they may reactivate quiescent disease[63], exacerbate preexisting lesions, including colonic diverticula,[64] and trigger intestinal bleeding from angiodysplasia lesions.[65]

Coxibs also seem to be better tolerated in the colon than ns-NSAIDs. A retrospective study[66] reported the long-term (median 9 months) safety of these agents in patients with IBD, whereas 2 prospective, placebo-controlled studies with celecoxib[67] or etoricoxib[68] did not show any significant increase in relapse rate, at least in the short-term.

NSAID USERS: WHO IS AT RISK OF GI COMPLICATIONS?

Because symptoms are not a reliable indicator of mucosal damage, it is important to identify factors that increase the risk of GI events in NSAID users. Risk factors for UGIB associated with NSAID use are well defined by several studies[69] and are summarized in **Fig. 1**. The most important are age and prior history of complicated ulcer. Older age is common in NSAID users, and those older than 70 years carry a risk similar to those with a history of peptic ulcer. Advancing age increases risk by about 4% per year, probably because of the presence of other associated risk factors.[70] The role of *H pylori* infection in patients taking NSAIDs, and the potential benefit of eradication on upper GI risk in infected NSAIDs users, has been controversial. A meta-analysis of case-control studies showed synergism for the development of complicated and uncomplicated ulcer between *H pylori* infection and NSAIDs.[71] *H pylori* is also a risk factor in LD-ASA users,[72] and a *post hoc* analysis of the VIGOR trial suggested that the GI benefits of coxibs are lower in patients with the infection than in those without.[70] Concomitant aspirin use increases the risk of GI events in patients taking ns-NSAIDs[73] or selective COX-2 inhibitors.[74] The presence of multiple risk factors greatly increases the risk of GI complications. When combinations of these risk factors are considered, the logistic regression model predicts that, in 6 months, patients with none of the 4 factors considered (age>75 years, history of PUD, history of GI bleed, CV disease) have a risk for having one of the defined GI complications of only 0.4%, patients with any single factor, a risk of 0.9%, and patients with all 4 factors, a risk of 9% (**Fig. 2**).[75]

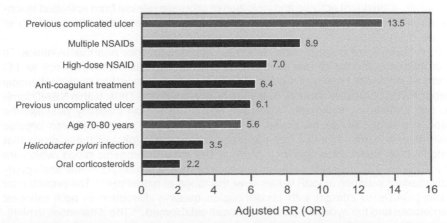

Fig. 1. Established risk factors for upper GI bleeding associated with NSAID use. (*From* Lanas A. A review of the gastrointestinal safety data - a gastroenterologist's perspective. Rheumatology (Oxford) 2010;49(Suppl 2):ii15; with permission.)

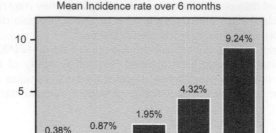

Fig. 2. NSAID-associated GI complications: incidence by number of risk factors. (*Data from* Silverstein FE, Graham DY, Senior JR, et al. Misoprostol reduces serious gastrointestinal complications in patients with rheumatoid arthritis receiving nonsteroidal anti-inflammatory drugs. A randomized, double-blind, placebo-controlled trial. Ann Intern Med 1995;123:241–9.)

MECHANISMS OF MUCOSAL INJURY
General Pharmacology and Physicochemical Properties of NSAIDs

For more than 100 years, analgesic agents have been integral to the management of musculoskeletal disorders. The clinical benefits and adverse effects of aspirin, indomethacin, phenylbutazone, and the newer propionic acid drugs were well established by the end of the 1960s, but it was only after 1971 that the late Professor Sir John Vane established the key mechanism of action of NSAIDs as inhibitors of prostaglandin (PG) synthesis.[76] Neither all the benefits nor untoward reactions are solely caused by inhibition of PG synthesis because weak inhibitors, such as nonacetylated salicylates, are equipotent to aspirin in inflammatory joint disease. Some NSAIDs display a broad spectrum of other pharmacologic activities (eg, inhibition of histamine release from basophils, antioxidant activity, and inhibition of protease release from activated leucocytes), which contribute to both the desirable and undesirable effects of these drugs.[77]

Most NSAIDs are organic acids, which is important for their pharmacokinetics, GI ulcerogenicity, and for certain biochemical actions, especially their potency as PG synthesis inhibitors. However, there are important differences in their physicochemical properties that probably underlie variations in ulcerogenicity. Thus, within NSAID families (eg, salicylates, fenamates, arylacetic acids) there is an interplay between the respective lipophilic (as measured by the partitioning of drugs between organic solvents and water to yield a logP) and acidic properties (pK_a) of these drugs that underlie their gastric ulcerogenicity. Many of the more ulcerogenic drugs (which are also COX-1/COX-2 inhibitors) are carboxylic acids with a low pK_a (2.8–4.4) and apparently marked variation in logP values over the range of acidic pH.[77] The potential for acidic NSAIDs to interact with phospholipids causing disruption in both mucosal membranes and the hydrophobic barrier is well established.[78] The differences in physicochemical properties determine the topical irritancy in the GI mucosa and also their systemic bioavailability, especially in relation to protein binding. Thus, the systemic bioavailability in the GI mucosa is expected to contribute to ulcerogenic activity.

The physicochemical properties also underlie the potential for interactions with the active sites of COX-1 and COX-2, respectively.[79] Selective COX-2 inhibitors are different from most ns-NSAIDs, being nonacidic, with much higher pK_a values.[8] This major difference may account for the low mucosal irritancy observed with these drugs separately from their lack of or low inhibitory activity on COX-1 in the stomach. Acidic selective COX-2 inhibitors (eg, etoricoxib) increase gastric potential difference (an index of mucosal integrity), whereas nonacidic selective COX-2 inhibitors (eg, celecoxib) do not (Scarpignato and colleagues, unpublished results).

Topical and Systemic Toxicity

Gastroduodenal mucosa possesses many defensive mechanisms and NSAIDs have a deleterious effect on most of them.[8,80] This results in a mucosa less able to cope with even a reduced acid load. The presence of acid seems to be a *conditio sine qua non* for NSAID injury, which is pH dependent.[81] Acid injures the mucosa by H^+ ion back diffusion from the lumen causing tissue acidosis and also increases drug absorption, which is inversely proportional to drug ionization. NSAIDs cause gastroduodenal damage by 2 main mechanisms: a physiochemical disruption of the gastric mucosal barrier and systemic inhibition of gastric mucosal protection, through inhibition of cyclooxygenase (PG endoperoxide G/H synthase, COX) activity of the GI mucosa. A reduced synthesis of mucus and bicarbonate, an impairment of mucosal blood flow, and an increase in acid secretion are the main consequences of NSAID-induced PG deficiency.[8,80] There is mounting evidence to suggest that gastric damage induced by ns-NSAIDs does not occur because of COX-1 inhibition; dual suppression of COX-1 and COX-2 is necessary for damage. However, against a background of COX inhibition by antiinflammatory doses of NSAIDs, their physicochemical properties, in particular their acidity, underlie the topical effect, leading to short-term damage.[82] Gastric injury (quantitated by Lanza score) correlated significantly with the pK_a of the single compound (**Fig. 3**): the lower the acidity of the drug, the less the mucosal damage.

Additional mechanisms may contribute to damage, including uncoupling of oxidative phosphorylation leading to ATP depletion, reduced mucosal cell proliferation and DNA synthesis, as well as neutrophil activation.[8,80]

NSAID inhibition of the so-called cytoprotective PGs has been regarded as a major factor for mucosal damage. However, diversion of arachidonate through the lipoxygenase (LOX) pathway enhances leukotriene (LT) synthesis. These mediators cause vasoconstriction and release oxygen free radicals, which add to damage caused by the impairment of mucosal defense.[80] Enhanced gastric mucosal leukotriene B_4 (LTB_4) synthesis is seen in patients taking NSAIDs,[83] corroborating the animal data. A summary of the mechanisms involved in NSAID-associated upper GI mucosal damage is presented in **Fig. 4**.

Nitric oxide (NO) and hydrogen sulfide (H_2S) are endogenously generated gaseous mediators, important in maintaining gastric mucosal integrity, which share many biologic effects with PGs.[84,85] Evidence suggests that NSAIDs may also induce GI damage by interference with the mucosal synthesis and availability of these mediators.

Being COX-1 sparing, selective COX-2 inhibitors, such as rofecoxib, do not impair gastric mucosal PG synthesis or serum thromboxane A_2 in humans,[86] nor do they affect platelet aggregation and bleeding time.[87] Thus, endoscopy studies show that ulcer incidence with these drugs overlaps that seen with placebo.[34,38,67] However, biochemical selectivity is only one of several important determinants of the risk of experiencing a serious GI complication during long-term NSAID therapy. Selective COX-2 inhibitors, besides sparing PG synthesis in the GI mucosa, do not uncouple oxidative

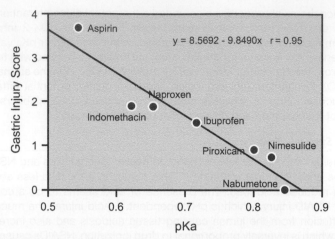

Fig. 3. Short-term gastric injury (expressed as Lanza score) versus acidity (expressed as pK$_a$) for some widely used ns-NSAIDs. (*Data from* Scarpignato C, Bjarnason I, Bretagne J-F, et al. Working team report: towards a GI safer antiinflammatory therapy. Gastroenterology International 1999;12:186–215.; and Bjarnason I, Scarpignato C, Takeuchi K, et al. Determinants of the short-term gastric damage caused by NSAIDs in man. Aliment Pharmacol Ther 2007;26:95–106.)

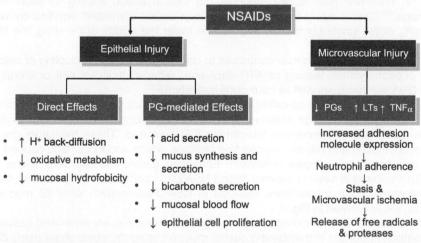

Fig. 4. Mechanisms of NSAID-induced gastric damage. NSAIDs cause both epithelial and microvascular injury, which occur early in the series of pathophysiologic events leading to gross lesion formation. This injury is mainly caused by increased LT mucosal concentration, with consequent increased expression of adhesion molecules, leading to microvascular ischemia and free radical release. Epithelial damage is caused by both topical (direct) and systemic (PG-mediated) effects of NSAIDs. Reduction in PG mucosal concentration is followed by an impairment of the gastric mucosal barrier and an increase in acid secretion, which tips the balance between aggressive and defensive factors toward the former. (*Modified from* Scarpignato C, Bjarnason I, Bretagne J-F, et al. Working team report: towards a GI safer antiinflammatory therapy. Gastroenterology International 1999;12:194.)

phosphorylation, because they are nonacidic, nor do they increase gastric permeability.[49,88] Therefore, they do not significantly affect these 2 basic biochemical mechanisms of NSAID-induced damage, which accounts for their remarkable GI safety.[8]

The reduction in the gastroduodenal safety of coxibs when given to patients taking aspirin[35] might be caused by the suppression of a class of lipid mediators produced by the interaction of aspirin with the COX-2 isoenzyme, the aspirin-triggered lipoxins (ATLs). ATLs are generated in the gastric mucosa in response to aspirin, and are involved in gastric adaptation to aspirin. Inhibition of COX-2 activity by ns-NSAIDs and selective COX-2 inhibitors interferes with the adaptation of the gastric mucosa to aspirin, and exacerbates mucosal injury. Experiments in healthy volunteers suggest that this mechanism operates in the human stomach.[89]

The pathogenesis of small intestinal damage with NSAIDs is less well understood. Although inhibition of mucosal PG synthesis during NSAID use occurs along the entire digestive tract, there are significant differences between the distal and proximal GI tract in the concurrence of other pathogenic factors that may add to mucosal damage. The most evident of these differences are the absence of acid (which plays a pivotal role in upper GI damage) and the presence of bacteria and bile in the intestine, which may trigger specific NSAID-related pathogenic mechanisms in the distal GI tract.[90]

Increasing experimental evidence suggests that inhibition of both COX-1 and COX-2 is necessary to cause significant GI damage.[42,43,82,91] However, NSAID-induced damage to the intestinal epithelium is started by direct effects of the drug after oral administration, a persistent local action caused by enterohepatic recirculation and systemic effects after absorption. Initial cellular damage is caused by the entrance of the usually acidic NSAID into the cell via damage to the brush border cell membrane, and disruption of mitochondrial processes of oxidative phosphorylation, with consequent ATP deficiency.[42,43,82,91] This deficiency leads to increased mucosal permeability,[44] which facilitates entry and actions of luminal factors such as dietary macromolecules, bile acids, components of pancreatic juice, and bacteria, activating the inflammatory cascade.[42,43,82,91]

Among luminal aggressors, intestinal bacteria are the main neutrophil chemoattractants. Several studies[48] show that antimicrobials (tetracycline, kanamycin, metronidazole or neomycin, plus bacitracin) attenuate NSAID enteropathy, further supporting the pathogenic role of enteric bacteria. In addition, indirect support for the role of gut bacteria in the pathogenesis of NSAID enteropathy comes from the similarity between indomethacin-induced intestinal damage and Crohn disease. Not only are the lesions both macro- and microscopically similar, they are also sensitive to the same drugs (eg, sulfasalazine, corticosteroids, immunosuppressives, and antibiotics).[92] The multiple mechanisms involved in the generation of NSAID-associated small bowel injury are shown in **Fig. 5**.

NSAID-associated intestinal damage is a pH-independent phenomenon. As a consequence, coadministration of antisecretory drugs is not expected to be able to either prevent or treat mucosal lesions. Video capsule studies show that combination of a PPI with an ns-NSAID does not prevent intestinal damage associated with short-term administration of naproxen or ibuprofen.[93,94] Celecoxib was better tolerated than ns-NSAIDs by the intestinal mucosa, and was associated with significantly fewer small bowel mucosal breaks than ns-NSAIDs plus PPI.

The lack of acidity (ie, lack of free carboxylic groups) in the celecoxib molecule seems to be an important determinant of GI safety not only in the upper, but also the lower, GI tract. Celecoxib does not increase intestinal permeability[95] or inflammation[94] and does not initiate the sequence of pathophysiologic events leading to mucosal damage with consequent loss of blood and protein.

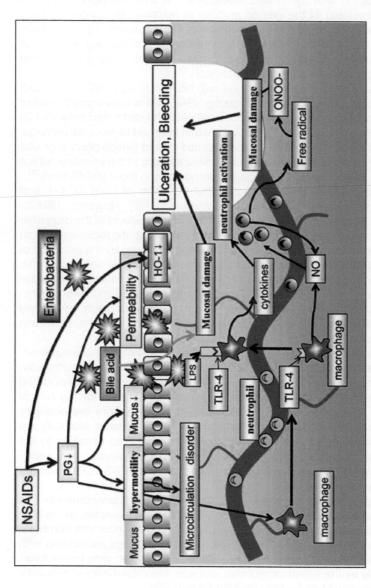

Fig. 5. Mechanisms of NSAID-induced small bowel injury. NSAIDs decrease mucosal endogenous PG, resulting in the reduction of intestinal mucus, microcirculatory disturbances accompanying abnormally increased intestinal motility, the disruption of intercellular junctions, and increased mucosal permeability. Mucosal injury can be caused by penetration of bile acids, proteolytic enzymes, intestinal bacteria, or toxins. At the same time, the expression inflammatory cytokines (via activation of TLR4 by bacterial-derived LPS) is induced and neutrophil infiltration occurs. HO-1, heme oxygenase-1; LPS, lipopolysaccharide, TLR4, toll-like receptor 4. (*From* Higuchi K, Umegaki E, Watanabe T, et al. Present status and strategy of NSAIDs-induced small bowel injury. J Gastroenterol 2009;44:882; with permission.)

The Role of Mucosal Inflammation

There is increasing interest in the role of the immune system in regulating the host response to noxious agents. We have recently shown in a mouse model that Th2-predominant Balb/c mice are more susceptible to NSAIDs gastropathy than Th1-predominant C57BL/6 mice and that this is associated with strain-specific PG differences.[96] Moreover, acid secretion in C57BL/6 mice is not inhibited by PGs because they have a fivefold lower expression of EP_3 receptors on the parietal cell compared with Balb/c mice, so that, in the Black/6, acid secretion is unchanged despite inhibition of prostaglandin E_2 by NSAIDs and there is less mucosal damage compared with Balb/c mice. This finding suggests the importance of the host immune response to NSAIDs and potentially offers an alternative explanation for the increased incidence of myocardial infarction seen with both ns-NSAIDs and selective inhibitors of COX-2.[97]

Enterobacteria and the mucosal inflammatory response, involving cellular response and cytokine production, both play their roles in the pathophysiology of NSAID-induced enteropathy. Toll-like receptor (TLR) 4 recognizes lipopolysaccharide (LPS) expressed by bacteria, which results in activation of an inflammatory cascade, acting through accessory protein MyD88. In a recent study,[98] rats treated with indomethacin were also given the antibiotics ampicillin, aztreonam, or vancomycin orally or intraperitoneal LPS, which is a TLR4 ligand, or neutralizing antibodies against neutrophils, tumor necrosis factor (TNF)-α, or monocyte chemotactic protein 1 (MCP-1). Intestinal ulcerogenicity of indomethacin was also examined in TLR4-mutant mice. Indomethacin-induced small intestinal damage was associated with the expression of TNF-α and MCP-1. Antibodies against neutrophils, TNF-α, and MCP-1 prevented the damage by 83%, 67%, and 63%, respectively. Ampicillin and aztreonam also inhibited this damage, and decreased the number of gram-negative bacteria in the rat small intestine, but vancomycin showed no activity against bacteria, nor any protective effect.[98] This understanding of how indomethacin may injure the small intestine through a TLR4/MyD88-dependent pathway offers potential new targets for protection (**Fig. 6**).[90]

EVALUATION OF MUCOSAL INJURY
Noninvasive Assessment

Upper GI endoscopy is the gold standard for assessing NSAID-induced GI damage, because it is generally believed that NSAID damage is usually confined to the gastroduodenal mucosa. Endoscopy is widely available, precise, sensitive, and easy to perform. However, the technique is invasive, not completely devoid of complications, and unsuitable as a routine screening test because it is time consuming and expensive. Furthermore, an ideal test should be able to detect NSAID-induced lesions before development of clinically significant sequelae and the need for hospitalization. Substantial efforts have been made to develop noninvasive methods to detect GI abnormalities, with permeability tests being the most widely used methodology.[44,99]

There are many ways to assess gastric and/or small intestinal permeability in humans. Although the methods to quantify bowel permeability have been available and developed for some time, those evaluating gastric permeability are recent. Sucrose represents an ideal probe molecule to detect increased gastroduodenal permeability in a site-specific manner. Because this disaccharide is rapidly degraded within the small intestine, it does not detect small intestinal damage, making it specific for the upper GI tract,[100] and making the test more sensitive than endoscopy in that it is able to detect subclinical mucosal damage.[101] Sucrose permeability is also sensitive enough to differentiate the effect of nonacidic selective COX-2 inhibitors (namely

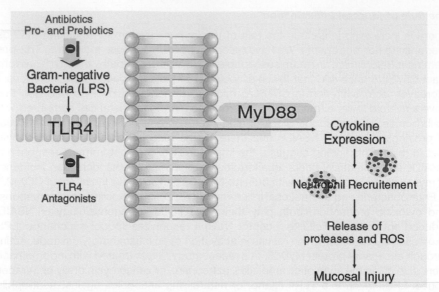

Fig. 6. Potential new targets for prevention of NSAID-associated bowel injury. Once the mucosal barrier has been disrupted by NSAIDs, luminal gram-negative bacteria can enter the cell and are then recognized by the transmembrane TLR4 because of their LPS component. MyD88-dependent activation of TLR4 induces cytokine mucosal expression, which triggers neutrophil recruitment, with subsequent release of proteases and reactive oxygen species, leading ultimately to mucosal injury. The bacteria-induced inflammatory cascade might be blunted either via manipulation of microbial ecology (via antibiotics, pre- or probiotics) or through blockade of TLR4. (*From* Scarpignato C. NSAID-induced intestinal damage: are luminal bacteria the therapeutic target? Gut 2007;57:146; with permission.)

celecoxib), which do not affect gastric permeability, from ns-NSAIDs, which significantly increase it.[48,88]

The best way of assessing intestinal permeability is to use ^{51}Cr-ethylenediaminetetraacetic acid (^{51}Cr-EDTA) as a permeability probe (maximum sensitivity) or the differential urinary excretion of ingested di- and monosaccharides (such as lactulose/L-rhamnose) for maximum specificity. Using these methods, all ns-NSAIDs increase intestinal permeability within 24 hours of ingestion.[44] The only exceptions are the prodrugs sulindac and nabumetone, as well as the nonacidic COX-2 selective inhibitors.[44]

NSAID enteropathy can be detected by measurement of fecal calprotectin.[45] Inflammatory diseases, including IBD, show a higher loss of leukocytes in feces.[102] Excretion of autologous ^{111}In-labeled granulocytes in feces has been used as an index to quantitate disease activity in IBD. Constant leucocyte shedding in feces of patients with inflammatory conditions led to the idea that an increased translocation of granulocytes into the intestinal mucosa might translate into increased levels of proteins originating from such cells in fecal samples. Calprotectin is a 36-kDa calcium-binding protein, derived predominantly from neutrophils and, to a lesser extent, from monocytes and reactive macrophages. Calprotectin is found in neutrophil cytoplasm, adding up to 60% of the cytosolic proteins from granulocytes.[102] Thus, the presence of calprotectin in feces is directly proportional to neutrophil migration to the intestinal tract. There is a close correlation between fecal calprotectin concentration and excretion of ^{111}In-labeled leukocytes.[45,103]

By using this simple test, Tibble and colleagues[45] found a prevalence of enteropathy in 44% of patients with arthritis taking short-term NSAIDs. In all those taking a slow-release formulation of diclofenac, fecal calprotectin concentrations increased, with 75% of patients having levels greater than the upper limits of the normal.[46] However, fecal calprotectin concentrations did not correlate with capsule endoscopy (CE) results, likely because mucosal breaks cannot be measured with certainty. Administration of celecoxib[94] or lumiracoxib,[104] did not cause any significant change in fecal calprotectin levels compared with placebo. In both studies, ns-NSAIDs (ibuprofen and naproxen, respectively) plus a PPI significantly increased fecal calprotectin.

Evaluation of Anemia and Blood Loss

Patients taking NSAIDs are often found to be anemic and this has commonly been attributed mistakenly to the anemia of chronic disease. Patients usually show a typical microcytic, iron-deficient picture with a reduced hematocrit. Blood loss is seldom enough to produce frank rectal bleeding or melena, and fecal occult blood testing with Hemoccult is unreliable to determine intestinal blood loss above the ileocecal valve because this test was designed to detect colonic bleeding in screening programs for colorectal neoplasia. Fecal blood loss can be accurately determined by ^{51}Cr-labeled red cells but this is seldom practical in the clinical setting. Nevertheless, the technique has been useful to understanding intestinal blood loss in patients taking an ns-NSAIDs or COX-2 selective inhibitors.[51,52,105] In comparative randomized control studies in healthy volunteers, both rofecoxib and etoricoxib did not increase fecal blood loss and were not different from controls in 1 month of treatment. In contrast, ibuprofen 800 mg three times a day was associated with a significant blood loss in 87% of subjects, and this occurred in an intermittent manner. Bleeding began within 3 to 5 days of starting treatment and, in some instances, exceeded 65 mL/d, which was the upper limit of accurate measurement.[105]

Upper GI endoscopy is often used to determine the presence of an ulcer or erosions as a cause of iron deficiency anemia. The standard of care for postmenopausal women and men older than 50 years is to exclude a GI source of bleeding and to rule out any GI neoplasm. However, this group often includes surreptitious NSAID or aspirin takers as well as those being prescribed antiinflammatory drugs. Green and Rockey[106] identified 111 premenopausal women, with a mean age of 42.5 years, undergoing endoscopy for the sole indication of iron deficiency anemia. Lesions, which were the potential cause of iron deficiency anemia, were found in 22 patients (20%), with upper GI lesions present in 14 patients (13%), only 1 of which was an erosive lesion. Lower GI lesions were detected in 8 patients (7.2%) and included colon cancer (2.7%), IBD (3.6%), and a colonic ulcer larger than 1 cm (0.9%). Patients with upper GI lesions were more likely to be taking aspirin and/or NSAIDs (11/14, 79%) than those with no lesions (26/89, 23%; $P = .043$). Occult blood was more common in patients with lower GI lesions 8/8 (100%) and patients with upper GI lesions (9/14, 64%) than in patients without lesions (28/89, 31%; $P = .037$ and 0.039).[106] As a consequence, patients with anemia or GI symptoms, fecal occult blood, and/or weight loss should always undergo endoscopy.

Persistent iron deficiency anemia or a positive occult blood test in the face of negative upper GI endoscopy and colonoscopy is termed obscure GI bleeding. Lesions responsible may be situated in the small bowel and, when suspected, CE[107] or double-balloon enteroscopy (DBE)[108] is indicated. CE and DBE have comparable diagnostic yields in obscure GI bleeding of 50% to 60%.[109] DBE has 2 advantages.

The first is that interventional procedures such as biopsy or hemostasis may be performed. The second is relevant to patients on NSAIDs, who may have strictures or diaphragm-like lesions in their small intestine, and the capsule endoscope may impact and cause intestinal obstruction requiring surgical removal.

Composite Scores as End Points in RCTs with NSAIDs

Although upper GI endoscopy is sensitive to assess NSAID-associated gastroduodenal mucosal damage, it does not quantify injury. To this end, scores have been developed, the most widely used being the Lanza score.[110] Typically, the number of erosions and petechial hemorrhages are counted as end points, and a score is then derived. A binary end point is usually presented (typically the proportion of subjects with Lanza grade ≥2; ie, at least 1 erosion). With the advent of modern technologies, endoscopic findings are recorded and two or more different endoscopists review the video images to reach a consensus.

In a series of painstaking endoscopic studies in which Lanza himself conducted virtually all the endoscopies, he showed that aspirin and nonaspirin NSAIDs caused acute mucosal erosions, although some NSAIDs, such as nabumetone and etodolac, did not.[111] Some confusion has arisen in the literature because several different but related scores have emanated from Lanza's group. Provided the number of volunteers is large enough, a quantal response (ie, the number of subjects with or without a given mucosal lesion) could be adopted.

Biopsy specimens can be taken from three points: greater curvature of the gastric antrum, lesser curvature of the lower part of the gastric corpus, and greater curvature of the upper part of the gastric corpus. Gastric biopsy specimens are stained with hematoxylin-eosin, and severity of gastritis and inflammation is assessed according to the updated Sydney[112] or the new Operative Link on Gastritis Assessment (OLGA) system.[113] Histologically, a chemical gastritis is described, but some investigators fail to distinguish between inflammations induced by H pylori and by NSAIDs.[114]

The evaluation of NSAID injury has focused primarily on the upper GI tract and has often neglected the lower GI tract. With the advent of selective COX-2 inhibitors and the related large outcome trials, evaluation has moved from simple assessment of visible upper GI complications to more thorough evaluation of bleeding. A team of experts[115] has recently developed a novel composite end point (ie, CSULGIEs) to evaluate the GI effects of NSAIDs throughout the GI tract. CSULGIEs extends the traditional perforation, obstruction, and bleeding assessment of upper GI complications by including events in the lower GI tract (small/large bowel) such as perforation, bleeding, and clinically significant anemia.[2] CSULGIEs have been used as the primary end point in the CONDOR trial[57] and are being used in the ongoing GI Randomized Event and Safety Open-label NSAID (GI-REASONS) study.[116] By providing clinicians with a new, descriptive language for adverse events throughout the GI tract, the CSULGIEs end point has the potential to become a standard tool for evaluating the GI effects of novel antiinflammatory drugs or new preventive strategies.

PREVENTION OF NSAID-ASSOCIATED MUCOSAL INJURY
Drug Formulations and Chemical Modification of NSAID Molecules

Attempts have been made to reduce NSAID-induced gastroduodenal damage.[117,118] These include enteric-coated preparations or soluble formulations of NSAIDs to reduce the gastric residence time (and thus contact with gastric mucosa), buffered preparations, and nonacidic prodrugs (like, for instance, droxicam and nabumetone).

Rectal or parenteral administration of NSAIDs has also been advocated. Some evidence suggests that enteric coating reduces acute aspirin-induced gastric injury, whereas significant damage to the gastric mucosa is seen with both regular and buffered aspirin, and there is no significant difference between them. However, a multi-center case-control study found that low doses of enteric-coated or buffered aspirin carries a threefold increase in the risk of major UGIB.[73] Therefore, the assumption that these formulations are less harmful than plain aspirin may be mistaken. Although enteric coating or increase of intragastric pH may reduce topical irritancy, once the drug is absorbed, injury may develop from the systemic effects of COX inhibition. Moreover, sustained-release NSAID formulations may shift the damage from the upper to the lower GI tract and increase morbidity.[118]

Because gastric acidity is pivotal in triggering topical irritancy, the development of nonacidic NSAIDs was attempted in the hope of reducing NSAID-associated mucosal injury. Nonacidic compounds cannot dissociate in the stomach after oral administration and do not concentrate in the gastric mucosa by the so-called ion trapping phenomenon.[8] This is the case for nabumetone or etodolac, which do not cause acute mucosal lesions.[111] Recent selective COX-2 inhibitors (namely celecoxib, rofecoxib, and valdecoxib) are also nonacidic, which provides an additional reason for their improved GI safety.

Rainsford[77] showed that esterification of acidic NSAIDs suppresses their gastrotoxicity without adversely affecting antiinflammatory activity. More recently, this avenue has been followed with the synthesis of new GI-sparing compounds, in which the ns-NSAIDs are combined with NO- or H_2S-releasing moieties (see later discussion).

Another way to develop NSAIDs with better GI tolerability is to complex these molecules with cyclodextrins, which have a lipophilic interior and a hydrophilic exterior. They form inclusion complexes with hydrophobic guest molecules by trapping them within their interior. The molecules are trapped by noncovalent intermolecular forces, such as Van der Waals, hydrogen bonding, and hydrophobic solvent forces. These inclusion complexes can have physical, chemical, and biologic properties that are different from either those of the drug or the cyclodextrin. Complexation of NSAIDs with β-cyclodextrin potentially leads to a more rapid onset of action after oral administration and improved GI tolerability because of minimization of the drug's gastric effects.[119] One such drug, piroxicam-β-cyclodextrin, has been used in Europe for more than 20 years.[120] Recently, such an approach has been applied to selective COX-2 inhibitors.[121]

Acid Suppression versus Mucosal Protection

There are four strategies to reduce the risk of gastroduodenal mucosal injury that occurs with antiinflammatory drug treatment. These are cotherapy with an ns-NSAID and an acid-suppressing drug or misoprostol, the use of a selective COX-2 inhibitor, cotherapy with a selective COX-2 inhibitor and acid-suppressing drug or misoprostol, and eradication of *H pylori* infection.

PPIs are significantly superior to H_2-receptor antagonists (H_2-RAs) for both prevention and treatment of acid-related disease in relation to NSAIDs.[122,123] Moreover, there is insufficient evidence to support the use of H_2-RAs for the prevention of upper GI bleeding because they have not been shown to be consistently effective at standard doses. Double-dose H_2-RA reduced both gastric and duodenal ulcers[122] as well as erosive esophagitis in patients taking LD-ASA.[124] However, a recent paper[125] showed that, in patients with aspirin-related peptic ulcers/erosions, high-dose famotidine (40 mg twice a day) therapy is inferior to pantoprazole (20 mg once a day) in preventing recurrent dyspeptic symptoms or bleeding ulcers/erosions.

The careful meta-analyses undertaken for the Cochrane Review[122] and for the Canadian Consensus guidelines[123] provide excellent direction for the standard of care in patients who require antiinflammatory drug therapy. PPIs reduce the risk of ns-NSAID–related endoscopic duodenal ulcer by 81% and gastric ulcer by 61%, but there is less evidence for a reduction in bleeding events.

After ulcer healing, maintenance therapy with a PPI was more effective at reducing recurrent bleeding than eradication of *H pylori* infection alone, emphasizing the importance of continuing antisecretory therapy in patients at risk of rebleeding. In patients with a history of prior GI bleeding, treatment with a selective COX-2 inhibitor or ns-NSAID combined with a PPI is still associated with a clinically significant risk of recurrent ulcer bleeding (**Fig. 7**).[126–128] The combination of celecoxib and a PPI in one small trial over one year reduced the risk of upper GI bleeding at 0% while with a selective COX-2 inhibitor alone the rate of bleeding was still 8.9%,[129] and this strategy is supported by pooled analysis of the Verification of Esomeprazole for NSAID Ulcers and Symptoms (VENUS) and Prevention of Latent Ulceration Treatment Options (PLUTO) studies in patients at high risk.[130] Thus, patients at high risk need to be closely monitored for the risk of rebleeding, and withholding the antiinflammatory drug may need to be considered in selected clinical cases.

Based on the pharmacokinetics and pharmacodynamics of PPIs, a twice-daily regimen may be worthwhile. All currently available PPIs have a short plasma half-life of 1 to 1.5 hours, and the antisecretory effect is about 4 to 5 hours, during which any active H^+,K^+-ATPase inserted into the secretory canalicular membrane is blocked. However, after that time, any pump that is at rest in the cytosol of the parietal cell or is newly synthesized, has the capacity to secrete acid. Thus, a PPI given once daily, in the morning before breakfast, has no meaningful effect on acid secretion during the subsequent evening or night. Healthy volunteers taking esomeprazole 40 mg every morning experience a pH of less than 2 for 40% of the time between midnight and 07:00 AM.[131] Most preventive strategies with PPIs as cotherapy to date have given the PPI once daily, despite the NSAIDs being given twice daily or

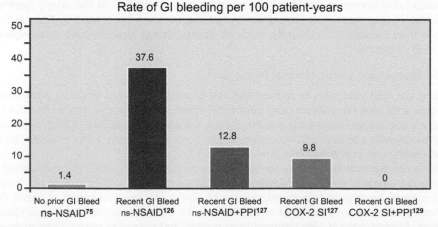

Rate of GI bleeding per 100 patient-years

Fig. 7. NSAID-associated upper GI bleeding rate in patients without prior GI bleed, taking ns-NSAIDs, or with a previous bleeding episode and taking different antiinflammatory drug regimens, such as nonselective or COX-2 selective NSAIDs, with or without a PPI. Figures have been calculated on ITT populations, assuming a constant rate of complications (*Data from* Refs.[75,126,127,129]).

even at bedtime. Naproxen, one of the most frequently prescribed ns-NSAIDs in the United States, has a plasma half-life of 12 to 15 hours, is given twice daily, and also displays a marked enterohepatic circulation. It would therefore be more logical to give the PPI twice a day, before breakfast and dinner. Indeed, a new combination of immediate-release esomeprazole (20 mg) and enteric-coated naproxen (500 mg), referred to as PN400 or Vimovo, given twice a day has recently been approved by the US Food and Drug Administration. Two pivotal studies showed that in patients at risk, compared with enteric-coated naproxen alone, PN400 significantly reduced the incidence of gastric ulcers (3.0% vs 28.4%, $P<.001$) regardless of low-dose aspirin use and duodenal ulcer.[132]

High-dose misoprostol also reduces the risk of upper GI complications from ns-NSAIDs,[75,133,134] and a Cochrane meta-analysis of placebo RCTs confirms a reduction of endoscopic gastric and duodenal ulcers by 74% and 53% respectively.[122] Despite the efficacy of misoprostol in clinical trials for the reduction of endoscopic ulcer in patients taking ns-NSAIDs, misoprostol at doses of 200 µg four times a day is more effective than lower doses. However, adverse events, including nausea, abdominal pain, and diarrhea, are common and occur significantly more than with PPI therapy.[122,134]

With antisecretory treatment, NSAID-associated ulcers heal at the same rate as non–NSAID-induced ulcers, provided that the NSAID is discontinued. However, healing is faster with PPIs compared with H_2-RAs. PPIs are therefore the treatment of choice for ulcers not only after NSAID discontinuation but also in those requiring ongoing NSAID therapy. A PPI is also associated with prevention of recurrence in patients requiring long-term NSAID therapy.[135]

ns-NSAID–associated intestinal damage is not pH dependent, and coadministration of antisecretory drugs neither prevents nor treats lower GI mucosal lesions beyond the proximal duodenum. Although recent experimental evidence[37] suggests a protective activity of PPIs on indomethacin-induced intestinal damage acting through antioxidant and antiinflammatory properties, video capsule studies[93,94] show that this is not the case in humans. Because COX-2 selective inhibitors may induce less or no damage to the distal GI tract compared with ns-NSAIDs, their use should be considered as a strategy of prophylaxis.[37]

BALANCING GI AND CV RISKS OF NONSELECTIVE AND COX-2 SELECTIVE NSAIDs

Several publications have raised concerns about the CV complications associated with selective COX-2 inhibitors, particularly rofecoxib, and the drug was withdrawn in 2004 because of an increase in the rate of acute myocardial infarction (AMI). The putative mechanisms involved an imbalance between antithrombotic (prostacyclin I_2) and prothrombotic (thromboxane A_2) prostanoids resulting in AMI.[136,137] Subsequently, these concerns were extended to all selective COX-2 inhibitors and a review and meta-analyses provided evidence for and against the increased risk with selective COX-2 inhibition.[138,139] Evidence then began to suggest that this increase in AMI was not restricted to selective COX-2 inhibitors when the National Institutes of Health stopped the Alzheimer Disease Anti-inflammatory Prevention Trial (ADAPT) study prematurely because of an increased rate of AMI in patients taking naproxen.[140] This was followed by further observational studies,[141–145] systematic reviews of observational studies,[146,147] and a meta-analysis of RCTs,[148] all of which concluded that both selective COX-2 inhibitors and ns-NSAIDs share similar CV risks with an increase in AMI, congestive heart failure, and sudden death.

These findings now obligate those prescribing antiinflammatory drugs to tailor therapy to the individual patient, balancing the analgesic and antiinflammatory benefits and improved quality of life with not only the GI but also the CV risks. The choices to optimize this approach are summarized in **Table 1**.[35]

Many patients taking NSAIDs also require LD-ASA for CV prophylaxis. Aspirin, even at low dose, increases the risk for GI bleeding by about 2.5-fold[149] and increases the risk of upper GI complications when combined with an ns-NSAID or COX-2 inhibitor.[150] Although debate continues on the extent to which LD-ASA compromises the benefit of a selective COX-2 inhibitor, large outcome studies indicate that LD-ASA plus a selective COX-2 inhibitor is associated with a numerically, but not significantly, lower complication rate than LD-ASA plus an ns-NSAID.[151] Moreover, hospital admissions for upper GI bleeding are significantly lower for LD-ASA users who are also taking a selective COX-2 inhibitor, compared with those taking ns-NSAIDs.[152] Thus, a selective COX-2 inhibitor plus LD-ASA is the preferred option for patients at high GI risk who require aspirin for CV prophylaxis.

The last important point centers on a clinically relevant interaction between low-dose aspirin and ns-NSAIDs. Ibuprofen, when given concomitantly with LD-ASA, attenuates the benefit of aspirin, because the binding of ibuprofen to COX-1 blocks

Table 1
Recommendations and levels of evidence for individual patients with different levels of risk who need NSAIDs

GI Risk Factors	CV Risk Factors (Aspirin Use)	Recommendation	Grade of Evidence	Level of Recommendation
No	No	ns-NSAID	1a	A
No	Yes	NSAID+PPI/MSP Coxib+PPI[a]	2b	B
Yes	No	Coxib NSAID+PPI/MSP	1a 1c/1b	A
Yes	Yes	NSAID+IBP/MSP Coxib+PPI[a]	3b	B
Ulcer bleeding Hx	No	Coxib+PPI HP test/treat	2b 2a	B B
Ulcer bleeding Hx	Yes	Avoid NSAID/ coxib use Coxib+PPI	5	D
Lower GI bleeding Hx	No	Coxib	2b	B
Lower GI bleeding Hx	Yes	Coxib	5	D

Both NSAIDs and coxibs should be used at the lowest effective dose and for the shortest period of time. Grade of evidence and level of recommendation follow the guidelines given by the Cochrane Collaboration.[122]

Abbreviations: HP, *Helicobacter pylori*; Hx, history; MSP, misoprostol; PPI, proton pump inhibitor.

[a] *Post hoc* analysis of randomized outcome trials suggest that the incidence of upper GI complication events is not statistically different in patients taking LD-ASA and ns-NSAIDs or LD-ASA and coxibs. Endoscopy ulcer studies show a lower incidence of endoscopic ulcer in patients taking coxibs and LD-ASA than in those taking LD-ASA and ns-NSAIDs. One epidemiologic study suggests a lower risk of serious upper GI events in patients taking celecoxib+LD-ASA, than ns-NSAIDs+ LD-ASA.

Data from Lanas A, Hunt R. Prevention of anti-inflammatory drug-induced gastrointestinal damage: benefits and risks of therapeutic strategies. Ann Med 2006;38:423.

access of aspirin to the serine binding site at the apex of the COX-1 hydrophobic channel[136] and has important clinical relevance by significantly reducing CV protection and increasing all-cause and CV mortality.[153] Celecoxib treatment did not adversely influence aspirin-related protection.[154]

NOVEL ANTIINFLAMMATORY COMPOUNDS: A LOOK TO THE FUTURE

Although cotherapy with misoprostol or PPIs is effective in preventing NSAID-induced GI damage, a more appealing approach would be to develop drugs that are devoid of, or have reduced, GI toxicity. Several attempts have been disappointing, and selective COX-2 inhibitors represent a step forward; new, potentially GI safe, antiinflammatory agents are imminent.

The protective properties of NO and H_2S in the GI tract make them attractive candidates for coupling with NSAIDs. The release of small amounts of one of these gaseous mediators over prolonged periods of time might compensate, in terms of mucosal defense, for inhibition of gastric PG synthesis.[84,85] By counteracting the detrimental effects of the NSAID part of the molecule, this may be effective for reducing GI toxicity. In this respect, two new generations of antiinflammatory drugs have been developed: ns-NSAIDs combined with NO- or H_2S-releasing moieties.[155] Being ns-COX inhibitors, NO-releasing NSAIDs have been named cycloxygenase inhibiting NO donors (CINODs).

Although several compounds are under preclinical investigation, naxproxicinod (ie, NO-releasing naproxen) has completed phase III clinical trials in OA. The combination of a slightly enhanced GI safety, a reduced risk of GI ulcers in the safety, tolerability and efficacy of AR - P900758XX study,[156] and enhanced CV safety with little or no effect on blood pressure makes naproxcinod an effective alternative to ns-NSAIDs and coxibs in a subset of patients who require NSAIDs, although there is an enhanced risk for CV events. CINODs are likely to be the first-choice therapy for those patients. However, because CINODs still cause GI injury at a rate that is greater than that of selective COX-2 inhibitors, comedication with a PPI will likely be required.

Because acidic ns-NSAIDs interact with phospholipids causing disruption to mucosal membranes and the hydrophobic barrier,[157] preassociating ns-NSAIDs with zwitterionic phospholipids (eg, phosphatidylcholine [PC]) before administration reduces their ulcerogenicity. PC-ibuprofen proved to be safer than regular ibuprofen in a proof-of-concept study.[158]

Because LTs are important in the genesis of mucosal damage and LOX inhibitors reduce the severity of NSAID-induced injury,[8,80] drugs that inhibit both COX-1 and COX-2 as well as 5-LOX, often referred to as dual-acting NSAIDs, could have reduced GI toxicity.[159] One such drug (licofelone) showed a gastroduodenal tolerability similar to that of placebo.[160]

Other molecular targets downstream of COX-2 are also being considered for novel NSAIDs. These NSAIDs include terminal PG synthase (in particular mPGES-1) inhibitors and selective E prostanoid receptor (EP_4) antagonists. Compared with COX-2 inhibitors, these agents might display effective antiinflammatory action with fewer likely atherothrombotic complications.[161]

TOWARDS A SAFER ANTIINFLAMMATORY THERAPY

NSAIDs are an essential part of our therapeutic armamentarium despite their well-characterized GI and CV risk profiles. Increasing appreciation of these relationships and new knowledge, as discussed in this article, should allow a safer and more effective use of these drugs.

Physicians should not prescribe NSAIDs before taking a careful history and performing a physical examination so they have the information they need to balance the risks and benefits for individual patients. When GI and/or CV risk factors are present, appropriate preventive strategies (ie, PPI use or LD-ASA) should be implemented from the beginning, and compliance with treatment assessed regularly,[162,163] especially in the elderly.[164] The appropriateness of NSAID prescription should be emphasized, namely to control inflammation and pain, rather than to control pain alone.[165] Only then can the expanding NSAID epidemic of adverse events be limited.

SUMMARY

NSAIDs are widely prescribed and, although they represent an effective class of drugs, their use is associated with a broad spectrum of untoward reactions in the liver, kidney, CV system, skin, and gut. GI problems constitute a wide range of clinical features, from symptoms of dyspepsia, heartburn, and abdominal discomfort to more serious events, including peptic ulcer and its life-threatening complications, bleeding and perforation. In the past decade, there has been a progressive change in the overall picture of GI events leading to hospitalization, with a decreasing trend in upper GI events and a significant increase in lower GI events, causing the rates of these 2 GI complications to converge. Overall mortality has also decreased, but the in-hospital case fatality rate from upper or lower GI complications has remained constant.

Gastroduodenal mucosa possesses many defensive mechanisms and NSAIDs have a deleterious effect on most of them, resulting in a mucosa that is less able to cope with even a reduced acid load. The presence of acid is a *conditio sine qua non* for NSAID injury, which is pH dependent. Acid not only injures the mucosa by H^+ ion back diffusion from the lumen causing tissue acidosis but also increases drug absorption, which is inversely proportional to drug ionization. NSAIDs cause gastroduodenal damage by a physiochemical disruption of the gastric mucosal barrier and systemic inhibition of gastric mucosal protection, through inhibition of COX activity of the GI mucosa. The pathogenesis of small intestinal damage by NSAIDs is less well understood. Although inhibition of mucosal PG synthesis with NSAID use occurs along the entire digestive tract, there are significant differences between the distal and the proximal GI tract in the concurrence of pathogenic factors that add to mucosal damage. Among them, the absence of acid and the presence of bacteria and bile in the intestine, which may trigger specific NSAID-related pathogenic mechanisms in the distal GI tract, are the most evident.

There are 4 strategies to reduce the risk of gastroduodenal mucosal injury with anti-inflammatory drugs. These are cotherapy with an ns-NSAID and an acid-suppressing drug or misoprostol, the use of a selective COX-2 inhibitor, cotherapy with a selective COX-2 inhibitor and acid-suppressing drug or misoprostol, and eradication of H pylori infection. PPIs are significantly superior to H_2-RAs for both prevention and treatment of acid-related disease in relation to NSAIDs. Since NSAID-associated intestinal damage is not pH-dependent, antisecretory cotherapy is unable to prevent or treat lower GI mucosal lesions. COX-2 selective inhibitors induce less or no damage to the distal GI tract compared with ns- NSAIDs.

The challenge for those attempting to develop safer NSAIDs is to shift from a focus on GI toxicity to the increasingly more appreciated CV toxicity. Currently, physicians should not prescribe NSAIDs before taking a careful history and performing a full physical examination to have the essential information to balance the risks and benefits for individual patients. When GI and/or CV risk factors are present, appropriate preventive strategies (ie, PPI use or LD-ASA) should be implemented from the beginning and compliance with treatment assessed regularly. Only then can the expanding NSAID epidemic of adverse events be managed.

Note added in proof: While this paper was being typeset the American College of Gastroenterology published the updated Guidelines for Prevention of NSAID-related ulcer complications.[166] Owing to the volume of new data on the topic, it was elected by the Committee of Experts to confine these guidelines to upper GI injury and to leave post-duodenal injury as the subject of a separate guideline. These guidelines contain, however, important evidence-based recommendations for clinical practice.

Conversely from upper GI tract, where co-therapy with PPIs is highly effective, the NSAID-related small bowel injury is difficult to prevent. However, a recent single-blind, controlled study[167] showed that co-therapy with misoprostol is able to reduce the incidence of small-intestinal lesions (as seen at capsule endoscopy) induced by a 2-week administration of diclofenac. These findings are in line with the drug ability to attenuate the increase of intestinal permeability[168] as well as anemia[169] induced by ns-NSAIDs. Although preliminary, these data are encouraging and call for a large trial with lower GI events as an outcome.

In accordance with animal data, manipulation of intestinal microecology via a probiotic mixture (VSL#3) does reduce fecal calprotectin shedding in healthy volunteers.[170] While giving further, albeit indirect, support for the role of gut bacteria in the pathogenesis of NSAID-enteropathy these results suggest that further studies in this area would be worthwhile.

ACKNOWLEDGMENTS

We are indebted to Simone Bertolini, MSc, PhD (Department of Clinical Sciences, University of Parma) for his help in drawing the figures and managing the references.

REFERENCES

1. Jones R. Nonsteroidal anti-inflammatory drug prescribing: past, present, and future. Am J Med 2001;110(Suppl 1A):4S–7S.
2. Shaheen NJ, Hansen RA, Morgan DR, et al. The burden of gastrointestinal and liver diseases, 2006. Am J Gastroenterol 2006;101:2128–38.
3. Pincus T, Koch G, Lei H, et al. Patient preference for placebo, acetaminophen (paracetamol) or celecoxib efficacy studies (PACES): two randomised, double blind, placebo controlled, crossover clinical trials in patients with knee or hip osteoarthritis. Ann Rheum Dis 2004;63:931–9.
4. Geba GP, Weaver AL, Polis AB, et al. Efficacy of rofecoxib, celecoxib, and acetaminophen in osteoarthritis of the knee. JAMA 2002;287:64–71.
5. Jordan KM, Arden NK, Doherty M, et al. EULAR recommendations 2003: an evidence based approach to the management of knee osteoarthritis: report of a task force of the standing committee for international clinical studies including therapeutic trials (ESCISIT). Ann Rheum Dis 2003;62:1145–55.
6. American College of Rheumatology Subcommittee on Osteoarthritis Guidelines. Recommendations for the medical management of osteoarthritis of the hip and knee: 2000 update. Arthritis Rheum 2000;43:1905–15.
7. Aronson JK. Meyler's side effects of analgesics and anti-inflammatory drugs. Amsterdam: Elsevier; 2010. p. 1–702.
8. Scarpignato C, Bjarnason I, Bretagne J-F, et al. Working team report: towards a GI safer antiinflammatory therapy. Gastroenterology International 1999;12:186–215.

9. Lanas A, Hunt R. Prevention of anti-inflammatory drug-induced gastrointestinal damage: benefits and risks of therapeutic strategies. Ann Med 2006;38: 415–28.

10. Tramèr MR, Williams JE, Carroll D, et al. Comparing analgesic efficacy of non-steroidal anti-inflammatory drugs given by different routes in acute and chronic pain: a qualitative systematic review. Acta Anaesthesiol Scand 1998;42:71–9.

11. Baxter K. Stockley's drug interactions. 9th edition. London: Pharmaceutical Press; 2010. p. 1–1792.

12. Marchiando AM, Graham WV, Turner JR. Epithelial barriers in homeostasis and disease. Annu Rev Pathol 2010;5:119–4413.

13. Laine L, Takeuchi K, Tarnawski A. Gastric mucosal defense and cytoprotection: bench to bedside. Gastroenterology 2008;135:41–60.

14. Laine L. Approach to non steroidal anti-inflammatory drug use in the high risk patient. Gastroenterology 2001;120:594–606.

15. Inotai A, Hanko B, Meszaros A. Trends in the non-steroidal anti-inflammatory drug market in six central-eastern European countries based on retail information. Pharmacoepidemiol Drug Saf 2010;19:183–90.

16. Abraham NS, Castillo DL, Hartman C. National mortality following upper gastrointestinal or cardiovascular events in older veterans with recent nonsteroidal anti-inflammatory drug use. Aliment Pharmacol Ther 2008;28:97–106.

17. Tramèr MR, Moore RA, Reynolds DJ, et al. Quantitative estimation of rare adverse events which follow a biological progression: a new model applied to chronic NSAIDs use. Pain 2000;85:169–82.

18. Straube S, Tramèr MR, Moore RA, et al. Mortality with upper gastrointestinal bleeding and perforation: effects of time and NSAID use. BMC Gastroenterol 2009;9:41.

19. Greenberg JD, Fisher MC, Kremer J, et al. The COX-2 inhibitor market withdrawals and prescribing patterns by rheumatologists in patients with gastrointestinal and cardiovascular risk. Clin Exp Rheumatol 2009;27:395–401.

20. Lanas A, Garcia-Rodriguez LA, Polo-Tomas M, et al. Time trends and impact of upper and lower gastrointestinal bleeding and perforation in clinical practice. Am J Gastroenterol 2009;104:1633–41.

21. Insua J, Mavros P, Hunsche E, et al. Exposure to nonsteroidal anti-inflammatory drugs among older adult patients hospitalized for peptic ulcer disease in Argentina: a case-control study. Am J Geriatr Pharmacother 2006;4:251–9.

22. Hunt RH, Bazzoli F. Review article: should NSAID/low-dose aspirin takers be tested routinely for *H. pylori* infection and treated if positive? Implications for primary risk of ulcer and ulcer relapse after initial healing. Aliment Pharmacol Ther 2004;19(Suppl 1):9–16.

23. Kiltz U, Zochling J, Schmidt WE, et al. Use of NSAIDs and infection with *Helicobacter pylori* - what does the rheumatologist need to know? Rheumatology (Oxford) 2008;47:1342–7.

24. Helsper CW, Smeets HM, Numans ME, et al. Trends and determinants of adequate gastroprotection in patients chronically using NSAIDs. Pharmacoepidemiol Drug Saf 2009;18:800–6.

25. Orlando RC. The pathogenesis of gastroesophageal reflux disease: the relationship between epithelial defense, dysmotility, and acid exposure. Am J Gastroenterol 1997;92(Suppl 4):3S–5S.

26. Tutuian R. Adverse effects of drugs on the esophagus. Best Pract Res Clin Gastroenterol 2010;24:91–7.

27. Abid S, Mumtaz K, Jafri W, et al. Pill-induced esophageal injury: endoscopic features and clinical outcomes. Endoscopy 2005;37:740–4.
28. Avidan B, Sonnenberg A, Schnell TG, et al. Risk factors of oesophagitis in arthritic patients. Eur J Gastroenterol Hepatol 2001;13:1095–9.
29. Avidan B, Sonnenberg A, Schnell TG, et al. Risk factors for erosive reflux esophagitis: a case-control study. Am J Gastroenterol 2001;96:41–6.
30. Winstead NS, Bulat R. Pill esophagitis. Curr Treat Options Gastroenterol 2004;7: 71–6.
31. Yasuda H, Yamada M, Endo Y, et al. Acute necrotizing esophagitis: role of nonsteroidal anti-inflammatory drugs. J Gastroenterol 2006;41:193–7.
32. Yuan Y, Padol IT, Hunt RH. Peptic ulcer disease today. Nat Clin Pract Gastroenterol Hepatol 2006;3:80–9.
33. Roth SH. NSAID gastropathy. A new understanding. Arch Intern Med 1996;156: 1623–8.
34. Sostres C, Gargallo CJ, Arroyo MT, et al. Adverse effects of non-steroidal anti-inflammatory drugs (NSAIDs, aspirin and coxibs) on upper gastrointestinal tract. Best Pract Res Clin Gastroenterol 2010;24:121–32.
35. Lanas A, García-Rodríguez LA, Arroyo MT, et al. Risk of upper gastrointestinal ulcer bleeding associated with selective cyclo-oxygenase-2 inhibitors, traditional non-aspirin non-steroidal anti-inflammatory drugs, aspirin and combinations. Gut 2006;55:1731–8.
36. Yeomans ND, Hawkey CJ, Brailsford W, et al. Gastroduodenal toxicity of low-dose acetylsalicylic acid: a comparison with non-steroidal anti-inflammatory drugs. Curr Med Res Opin 2009;25:2785–93.
37. Hunt RH, Lanas A, Stichtenoth DO, et al. Myths and facts in the use of anti-inflammatory drugs. Ann Med 2009;8:1–16.
38. Wallace JL. Selective cyclooxygenase-2 inhibitors: after the smoke has cleared. Dig Liver Dis 2002;34:89–94.
39. Moore RA, Derry S, Phillips CJ, et al. Nonsteroidal anti-inflammatory drugs (NSAIDs), cyclooxygenase-2 selective inhibitors (coxibs) and gastrointestinal harm: review of clinical trials and clinical practice. BMC Musculoskelet Disord 2006;7:79.
40. Spiegel BM, Farid M, Dulai GS, et al. Comparing rates of dyspepsia with Coxibs vs NSAID+PPI: a meta-analysis. Am J Med 2006;119:448, e27–36.
41. Hawkey C, Talley NJ, Yeomans ND, et al. Improvements with esomeprazole in patients with upper gastrointestinal symptoms taking non-steroidal antiinflammatory drugs, including selective COX-2 inhibitors. Am J Gastroenterol 2005; 100:1028–36.
42. Adebayo D, Bjarnason I. Is non-steroidal anti-inflammaory drug (NSAID) enteropathy clinically more important than NSAID gastropathy? Postgrad Med J 2006;82:186–91.
43. Smale S, Tibble J, Sigthorsson G, et al. Epidemiology and differential diagnosis of NSAID-induced injury to the mucosa of the small intestine. Best Pract Res Clin Gastroenterol 2001;15:723–38.
44. Bjarnason I, Takeuchi K. Intestinal permeability in the pathogenesis of NSAID-induced enteropathy. J Gastroenterol 2009;44(Suppl 19):23–9.
45. Tibble JA, Sigthorsson G, Foster R, et al. High prevalence of NSAID enteropathy as shown by a simple faecal test. Gut 1999;45:362–6.
46. Maiden L, Thjodleifsson B, Theodors A, et al. A quantitative analysis of NSAID-induced small bowel pathology by capsule enteroscopy. Gastroenterology 2005;128:1172–8.

47. Bermejo F, García-López S. A guide to diagnosis of iron deficiency and iron deficiency anemia in digestive diseases. World J Gastroenterol 2009;15:4638–43.
48. Lanas A, Scarpignato C. Microbial flora in NSAID-induced intestinal damage: a role for antibiotics? Digestion 2006;73(Suppl 1):136–50.
49. Smecuol E, Bai JC, Sugai E, et al. Acute gastrointestinal permeability responses to different non-steroidal anti-inflammatory drugs. Gut 2001;49:650–5.
50. Shah AA, Thjodleifsson B, Murray FE, et al. Selective inhibition of COX-2 in humans is associated with less gastrointestinal injury: a comparison of nimesulide and naproxen. Gut 2001;48:339–46.
51. Hunt RH, Bowen B, Mortensen ER, et al. A randomized trial measuring fecal blood loss after treatment with rofecoxib, ibuprofen, or placebo in healthy subjects. Am J Med 2000;109:201–6.
52. Hunt RH, Harper S, Callegari P, et al. Complementary studies of the gastrointestinal safety of the cyclo-oxygenase-2-selective inhibitor etoricoxib. Aliment Pharmacol Ther 2003;17:201–10.
53. Silverstein FE, Faich G, Goldstein JL, et al. Gastrointestinal toxicity with celecoxib vs nonsteroidal anti-inflammatory drugs for osteoarthritis and rheumatoid arthritis: the CLASS study: a randomized controlled trial. celecoxib long-term arthritis safety study. JAMA 2000;284:1247–55.
54. Burke TA, Zabinski RA, Pettitt D, et al. A framework for evaluating the clinical consequences of initial therapy with NSAIDs, NSAIDs plus gastroprotective agents, or celecoxib in the treatment of arthritis. Pharmacoeconomics 2001; 19(Suppl 1):33–47.
55. Bombardier C, Laine L, Reicin A, et al. Comparison of upper gastrointestinal toxicity of rofecoxib and naproxen in patients with rheumatoid arthritis. N Engl J Med 2000;343:1520–8.
56. Laine L, Connors LG, Reicin A, et al. Serious lower gastrointestinal clinical events with nonselective NSAID or coxib use. Gastroenterology 2003;124:288–92.
57. Chan FK, Lanas A, Scheiman J, et al. Celecoxib versus omeprazole and diclofenac in patients with osteoarthritis and rheumatoidarthritis (CONDOR): a randomised trial. Lancet 2010;376:173–9.
58. Laine L, Curtis SP, Langman M, et al. Lower gastrointestinal events in a double-blind trial of the cyclo-oxygenase-2 selective inhibitor etoricoxib and the traditional non steroidal anti-inflammatory drug diclofenac. Gastroenterology 2008; 135:1517–25.
59. Kurahara K, Matsumoto T, Iida M, et al. Clinical and endoscopic features of nonsteroidal anti-inflammatory drug-induced colonic ulcerations. Am J Gastroenterol 2001;96:473–80.
60. El Hajj I, Hawchar M, Sharara A. NSAID-induced colopathy: case report and review of the literature. J Med Liban 2009;57:274–6.
61. Lengeling RW, Mitros FA, Brennan JA, et al. Ulcerative ileitis encountered at ileocolonoscopy: likely role of nonsteroidal agents. Clin Gastroenterol Hepatol 2003; 1:160–9.
62. Bonner GF, Walczak M, Kitchen L, et al. Tolerance of nonsteroidal antiinflammatory drugs in patients with inflammatory bowel disease. Am J Gastroenterol 2000;95:1946–8.
63. Kefalakes H, Stylianides TJ, Amanakis G, et al. Exacerbation of inflammatory bowel diseases associated with the use of nonsteroidal anti-inflammatory drugs: myth or reality? Eur J Clin Pharmacol 2009;65:963–70.
64. Morris CR, Harvey IM, Stebbings WS, et al. Epidemiology of perforated colonic diverticular disease. Postgrad Med J 2002;78:654–8.

65. Faucheron JL, Parc R. Non-steroidal anti-inflammatory drug-induced colitis. Int J Colorectal Dis 1996;11:99–101.

66. Mahadevan U, Loftus EV Jr, Tremaine WJ, et al. Safety of selective cyclooxygenase-2 inhibitors in inflammatory bowel disease. Am J Gastroenterol 2002;97: 910–4.

67. Sandborn WJ, Stenson WF, Brynskov J, et al. Safety of celecoxib in patients with ulcerative colitis in remission: a randomized, placebo-controlled, pilot study. Clin Gastroenterol Hepatol 2006;4:203–11.

68. El Miedany Y, Youssef S, Ahmed I, et al. The gastrointestinal safety and effect on disease activity of etoricoxib, a selective cox-2 inhibitor in inflammatory bowel diseases. Am J Gastroenterol 2006;101:311–7.

69. Lanas A. A review of the gastrointestinal safety data - a gastroenterologist's perspective. Rheumatology (Oxford) 2010;49(Suppl 2):3–10, ii.

70. Laine L, Bombardier C, Hawkey CJ, et al. Stratifying the risk of NSAID-related upper gastrointestinal clinical events: results of a double-blind outcomes study in patients with rheumatoid arthritis. Gastroenterology 2002;123:1006–12.

71. Huang JQ, Sridhar S, Hunt RH. Role of *Helicobacter pylori* infection and non-steroidal anti-inflammatory drugs in peptic-ulcer disease: a meta-analysis. Lancet 2002;359:14–22.

72. Lanas A, Fuentes J, Benito R, et al. *Helicobacter pylori* increases the risk of upper gastrointestinal bleeding in patients taking low-dose aspirin. Aliment Pharmacol Ther 2002;16:779–86.

73. Laine L. Review article: gastrointestinal bleeding with low-dose aspirin - what's the risk? Aliment Pharmacol Ther 2006;24:897–908.

74. Dubois RW, Melmed GY, Henning JM, et al. Risk of upper gastrointestinal injury and events in patients treated with cyclooxygenase (COX)-1/COX-2 nonsteroidal antiinflammatory drugs (NSAIDs), COX-2 selective NSAIDs, and gastroprotective cotherapy: an appraisal of the literature. J Clin Rheumatol 2004;10: 178–89.

75. Silverstein FE, Graham DY, Senior JR, et al. Misoprostol reduces serious gastrointestinal complications in patients with rheumatoid arthritis receiving nonsteroidal anti-inflammatory drugs. A randomized, double-blind, placebo-controlled trial. Ann Intern Med 1995;123:241–9.

76. Vane JR. Inhibition of prostaglandin synthesis as a mechanism of action for aspirin-like drugs. Nature 1971;231:232–5.

77. Rainsford KD. Profile and mechanisms of gastrointestinal and other side effects of nonsteroidal anti-inflammatory drugs (NSAIDs). Am J Med 1999;107:27S–35S.

78. Lichtenberger LM, Zhou Y, Dial EJ, et al. NSAID injury to the gastrointestinal tract: evidence that NSAIDs interact with phospholipids to weaken the hydrophobic surface barrier and induce the formation of unstable pores in membranes. J Pharm Pharmacol 2006;58:1421–8.

79. Michaux C, Charlier C. Structural approach for COX-2 inhibition. Mini Rev Med Chem 2004;4:603–15.

80. Wallace JL. Pathogenesis of NSAID-induced gastroduodenal mucosal injury. Best Pract Res Clin Gastroenterol 2001;15:691–703.

81. Scarpignato C, Pelosini I. Prevention and treatment of non-steroidal anti-inflammatory drug-induced gastro-duodenal damage: rationale for the use of antisecretory compounds. Ital J Gastroenterol Hepatol 1999;31(Suppl 1):S63–72.

82. Bjarnason I, Scarpignato C, Takeuchi K, et al. Determinants of the short-term gastric damage caused by NSAIDs in man. Aliment Pharmacol Ther 2007;26: 95–106.

83. Hudson N, Balsitis M, Everitt S, et al. Enhanced gastric mucosal leukotriene B4 synthesis in patients taking non-steroidal anti-inflammatory drugs. Gut 1993;34: 742–7.
84. Wallace JL, Miller MJ. Nitric oxide in mucosal defense: a little goes a long way. Gastroenterology 2000;119:512–20.
85. Wallace JL. Physiological and pathophysiological roles of hydrogen sulfide in the gastrointestinal tract. Antioxid Redox Signal 2010;12:1125–33.
86. Wight NJ, Gottesdiener K, Garlick NM, et al. Rofecoxib, a COX-2 inhibitor, does not inhibit human gastric mucosal prostaglandin production. Gastroenterology 2001;120:867–73.
87. Patrono C, Patrignani P, García Rodríguez LA. Cyclooxygenase-selective inhibition of prostanoid formation: transducing biochemical selectivity into clinical read-outs. J Clin Invest 2001;108:7–13.
88. Ekenel M, Avşar E, Imeryüz N, et al. Effects of selective COX-2 inhibitors on the gastric permeability of sucrose: a controlled study with placebo and ibuprofen. Eur J Gastroenterol Hepatol 2003;15:403–6.
89. Wallace JL, de Lima OM Jr, Fiorucci S. Lipoxins in gastric mucosal health and disease. Prostaglandins Leukot Essent Fatty Acids 2005;73:251–5.
90. Scarpignato C. NSAID-induced intestinal damage: are luminal bacteria the therapeutic target? Gut 2007;57:145–8.
91. Higuchi K, Umegaki E, Watanabe T, et al. Present status and strategy of NSAIDs-induced small bowel injury. J Gastroenterol 2009;44:879–88.
92. Scarpignato C, Pelosini I. Rifaximin, a poorly absorbed antibiotic: pharmacology and clinical potential. Chemotherapy 2005;51(Suppl 1):36–66.
93. Goldstein JL, Eisen GM, Lewis B, et al. Video capsule endoscopy to prospectively assess small bowel injury with celecoxib, naproxen plus omeprazole, and placebo. Clin Gastroenterol Hepatol 2005;3:133–41.
94. Goldstein JL, Eisen GM, Lewis B, et al. Small bowel mucosal injury is reduced in healthy subjects treated with celecoxib compared with ibuprofen plus omeprazole, as assessed by video capsule endoscopy. Aliment Pharmacol Ther 2007; 25:1211–22.
95. Tibble JA, Sigthorsson G, Foster R, et al. Comparison of the intestinal toxicity of celecoxib, a selective COX-2 inhibitor, and indomethacin in the experimental rat. Scand J Gastroenterol 2000;35:802–7.
96. Padol IT, Hunt RH. Host specific differences in the physiology of acid secretion related to prostaglandins may play a role in gastric inflammation and injury. Am J Physiol Gastrointest Liver Physiol 2005;288:G1110–7.
97. Padol IT, Hunt RH. Association of myocardial infarctions with COX-2 inhibition may be related to the immunomodulation towards Th1 response resulting in atheromatous plaque instability: an evidence based interpretation. Rheumatology 2010;49:837–43.
98. Watanabe T, Higuchi K, Kobata A, et al. Non-steroidal anti-inflammatory drug-induced small intestinal damage is toll-like receptor 4 dependent. Gut 2008; 57:181–7.
99. Davies NM. Review article: non-steroidal anti-inflammatory drug-induced gastrointestinal permeability. Aliment Pharmacol Ther 1998;12:303–20.
100. Meddings JB, Sutherland LR, Byles NI, et al. Sucrose: a novel permeability marker for gastroduodenal disease. Gastroenterology 1993;104: 1619–26.
101. Erlacher L, Wyatt J, Pflugbeil S, et al. Sucrose permeability as a marker for NSAID-induced gastroduodenal injury. Clin Exp Rheumatol 1998;16:69–71.

102. Tibble JA, Bjarnason I. Non-invasive investigation of inflammatory bowel disease. World J Gastroenterol 2001;7:460–5.
103. Roseth AG, Schmidt PN, Fagerhol MK. Correlation between faecal excretion of indium-111-labelled granulocytes and calprotectin, a granulocyte marker protein, in patients with inflammatory bowel disease. Scand J Gastroenterol 1999;34:50–4.
104. Hawkey CJ, Ell C, Simon B, et al. Less small-bowel injury with lumiracoxib compared with naproxen plus omeprazole. Clin Gastroenterol Hepatol 2008;6: 536–44.
105. Bowen B, Yuan Y, James C, et al. Time course and pattern of blood loss with ibuprofen treatment in healthy subjects. Clin Gastroenterol Hepatol 2005;3: 1075–82.
106. Green BT, Rockey DC. Gastrointestinal endoscopic evaluation of pre-menopausal women with iron deficiency anemia. J Clin Gastroenterol 2004;38:104–9.
107. Maiden L. Capsule endoscopic diagnosis of nonsteroidal antiinflammatory drug-induced enteropathy. J Gastroenterol 2009;44(Suppl 19):64–71.
108. Ohmiya N, Yano T, Yamamoto H, et al. Diagnosis and treatment of obscure GI bleeding at double balloon endoscopy. Gastrointest Endosc 2007; 66(Suppl 3):S72–7.
109. Westerhof J, Weersma RK, Koornstra JJ. Investigating obscure gastrointestinal bleeding: capsule endoscopy or double balloon enteroscopy? Neth J Med 2009;67:260–5.
110. Lanza FL, Graham DY, Davis RE, et al. Endoscopic comparison of cimetidine and sucralfate for prevention of naproxen-induced acute gastroduodenal injury. Effect of scoring method. Dig Dis Sci 1990;35:1494–9.
111. Lanza FL. Gastrointestinal toxicity of newer NSAIDs. Am J Gastroenterol 1993; 88:1318–23.
112. Stolte M, Meining A. The updated Sydney system: classification and grading of gastritis as the basis of diagnosis and treatment. Can J Gastroenterol 2001;15: 591–8.
113. Rugge M, Meggio A, Pennelli G, et al. Gastritis staging in clinical practice: the OLGA staging system. Gut 2007;56:631–6.
114. Aabakken L. Clinical symptoms, endoscopic findings and histologic features of gastroduodenal non-steroidal anti-inflammatory drugs lesions. Ital J Gastroenterol Hepatol 1999;31(Suppl 1):S19–22.
115. Chan FK, Cryer B, Goldstein JL, et al. A novel composite endpoint to evaluate the gastrointestinal (GI) effects of non steroidal antiinflammatory drugs through the entire GI tract. J Rheumatol 2010;37:167–74.
116. Available at: ClinicalTrials.gov. GI-Reasons. A trial of GI safety of celecoxib compared with non-selective nonsteroidal antiinflammatory drugs (NSAIDs). Available at: http://www.clinicaltrials.gov/ct2/show/NCT00373685?term=GI-reasons& rank=1. Accessed September 10, 2010.
117. Lancaster C. Effective nonsteroidal anti-inflammatory drugs devoid of gastrointestinal side effects: do they really exist? Dig Dis 1995;13(Suppl 1):40–7.
118. Davies NM. Sustained release and enteric coated NSAIDs: are they really GI safe? J Pharm Pharm Sci 1999;2:5–14.
119. Rainsford KD. NSAID gastropathy: novel physicochemical approaches for reducing gastric mucosal injury by drug complexation with cyclodextrins. Drug Investig 1990;2(Suppl 4):3–10.
120. Lee CR, Balfour JA. Piroxicam-beta-cyclodextrin. A review of its pharmacodynamic and pharmacokinetic properties, and therapeutic potential in rheumatic diseases and pain states. Drugs 1994;48:907–29.

121. Ventura CA, Giannone I, Paolino D, et al. Preparation of celecoxib-dimethyl-beta-cyclodextrin inclusion complex: characterization and in vitro permeation study. Eur J Med Chem 2005;4:624–31.
122. Rostom A, Dube C, Wells G, et al. Prevention of NSAID-induced gastroduodenal ulcers. Cochrane Database Syst Rev 2002;4:CD002296.
123. Rostom A, Moayyedi P, Hunt R. Canadian consensus guidelines on long-term nonsteroidal anti-inflammatory drug therapy and the need for gastroprotection: benefits versus risks. Aliment Pharmacol Ther 2009;29:481–96.
124. Taha AS, McCloskey C, Prasad R, et al. Famotidine for the prevention of peptic ulcers and oesophagitis in patients taking low-dose aspirin (FAMOUS): a phase III, randomised, double-blind, placebo-controlled trial. Lancet 2009;374:119–25.
125. Ng FH, Wong SY, Lam KF, et al. Famotidine is inferior to pantoprazole in preventing recurrence of aspirin-related peptic ulcers or erosions. Gastroenterology 2010;138:82–8.
126. Chan FK, Chung SC, Suen BY, et al. Preventing recurrent upper gastrointestinal bleeding in patients with helicobacter pylori infection who are taking low-dose aspirin or naproxen. N Engl J Med 2001;344:967–73.
127. Chan FK, Hung LC, Suen BY, et al. Celecoxib versus diclofenac and omeprazole in reducing the risk of recurrent ulcer bleeding in patients with arthritis. N Engl J Med 2002;347:2104–10.
128. Lai KC, Chu KM, Hui WM, et al. Celecoxib compared with lansoprazole and naproxen to prevent gastrointestinal ulcer complications. Am J Med 2005;118:1271–8.
129. Chan FK, Wong VW, Suen BY, et al. Combination of a cyclo-oxygenase-2 inhibitor and a proton-pump inhibitor for prevention of recurrent ulcer bleeding in patients at very high risk: a double-blind, randomised trial. Lancet 2007;369:1621–6.
130. Scheiman JM, Yeomans ND, Talley NJ, et al. Prevention of ulcers by esomeprazole in at-risk patients using non-selective NSAIDs and COX-2 inhibitors. Am J Gastroenterol 2006;101:701–10.
131. Wang C, Yuan Y, Hunt RH. . Night-time pH holding time: What is hidden by the % time pH ≤4? Am J Gastroenterol 2008;103(Suppl 1):S50.
132. Goldstein JL, Hochberg MC, Fort JG, et al. Clinical trial: the incidence of NSAID-associated endoscopic gastric ulcers in patients treated with PN 400 (naproxen plus esomeprazole magnesium) vs enteric-coated naproxen alone. Aliment Pharmacol Ther 2010;32:401–13.
133. Hawkey CJ, Karrasch JA, Szczepañski L, et al. Omeprazole compared with misoprostol for ulcers associated with nonsteroidal antiinflammatory drugs. Omeprazole versus Misoprostol for NSAID-induced Ulcer Management (OMNIUM) Study Group. N Engl J Med 1998;338:727–34.
134. Wilson DE. Antisecretory and mucosal protective actions of misoprostol. Potential role in the treatment of peptic ulcer disease. Am J Med 1987;83:2–8.
135. Arora G, Singh G, Triadafilopoulos G. Proton pump inhibitors for gastroduodenal damage related to nonsteroidal anti-inflammatory drugs or aspirin: twelve important questions for clinical practice. Clin Gastroenterol Hepatol 2009;7:725–35.
136. Catella-Lawson F, Crofford LJ. Cyclooxygenase inhibition and thrombogenicity. Am J Med 2001;110(Suppl 3A):28S–32S.
137. Mitchell JA, Warner TD. COX isoforms in the cardiovascular system: understanding the activities of non-steroidal anti-inflammatory drugs. Nat Rev Drug Discov 2006;5:75–86.

138. Scott PA, Kingsley GH, Smith CM, et al. Non-steroidal anti-inflammatory drugs and myocardial infarctions: comparative systematic review of evidence from observational studies and randomised controlled trials. Ann Rheum Dis 2007; 66:1296–304.
139. Joshi GP, Gertler R, Fricker R. Cardiovascular thromboembolic adverse effects associated with cyclooxygenase-2 selective inhibitors and nonselective antiinflammatory drugs. Anesth Analg 2007;105:1793–804.
140. ADAPT Research Group. Cardiovascular and cerebrovascular events in the randomized, controlled Alzheimer's Disease Anti-inflammatory Prevention Trial (ADAPT). PLoS Clin Trials 2006;1:e33.
141. Hudson M, Richard H, Pilote L. Differences in outcomes of patients with congestive heart failure prescribed celecoxib, rofecoxib, or non-steroidal anti-inflammatory drugs: population based study. Br Med J 2005;1370:330.
142. Hippisley-Cox J, Coupland C. Risk of myocardial infarction in patients taking cyclo-oxygenase-2 inhibitors or conventional non-steroidal anti-inflammatory drugs: population based nested case-control analysis. BMJ 2005;330:1366.
143. Johnsen SP, Larsson H, Tarone RE, et al. Risk of hospitalization formyocardial infarction among users of rofecoxib, celecoxib, and other NSAIDs: a population-based case-control study. Arch Intern Med 2005;165:978–84.
144. Chan AT, Manson JE, Albert CM, et al. Non steroidal anti-inflammatory drugs, acetaminophen, and the risk of cardiovascular events. Circulation 2006;113:1578–87.
145. Abraham NS, El-Serag HB, Hartman C, et al. Cyclooxygenase-2 selectivity of non-steroidal anti-inflammatory drugs and the risk of myocardial infarction and cerebrovascular accident. Aliment Pharmacol Ther 2007;25:913–24.
146. McGettigan P, Henry D. Cardiovascular risk and inhibition of cyclooxygenase: a systematic review of the observational studies of selective and nonselective inhibitors of cyclooxygenase-2. JAMA 2006;296:1633–44.
147. Singh G, Wu O, Langhorne P, et al. Risk of acute myocardial infarction with nonselective non-steroidal anti-inflammatory drugs: a meta-analysis. Arthritis Res Ther 2006;8:R153.
148. Solomon SD, Wittes J, Finn PV, et al. Cardiovascular risk of celecoxib in 6 randomized placebo-controlled trials: the cross trial safety analysis. Circulation 2008;117:2104–13.
149. Derry S, Loke YK. Risk of gastrointestinal haemorrhage with long term use of aspirin: meta-analysis. BMJ 2000;321:1183–7.
150. Goldstein JL, Aisenberg J, Zakko SF, et al. Endoscopic ulcer rates in healthy subjects associated with use of aspirin (81 mg q.d.) alone or coadministered with celecoxib or naproxen: a randomized, 1-week trial. Dig Dis Sci 2008;53:647–56.
151. Moore RA, Derry S, Makinson GT, et al. Tolerability and adverse events in clinical trials of celecoxib in osteoarthritis and rheumatoid arthritis: systematic review and meta-analysis of information from company clinical trial reports. Arthritis Res Ther 2005;7:R644–65.
152. Rahme E, Bardou M, Dasgupta K, et al. Gastrointestinal effects of rofecoxib and celecoxib versus NSAIDs among patients on low dose aspirin. Gastroenterology 2004;126(Suppl 2):A1–2.
153. MacDonald TM, Wei L. Effect of ibuprofen on cardioprotective effect of aspirin. Lancet 2003;361:573–4.
154. Renda G, Tacconelli S, Capone ML, et al. Celecoxib, ibuprofen, and the antiplatelet effect of aspirin in patients with osteoarthritis and ischemic heart disease. Clin Pharmacol Ther 2006;80:264–74.

155. Fiorucci S. Prevention of nonsteroidal anti inflammatory drug-induced ulcer: looking to the future. Gastroenterol Clin North Am 2009;38:315–32.
156. Lohmander LS, McKeith D, Svensson O, et al. A randomised, placebo controlled, comparative trial of the gastrointestinal safety and efficacy of AZD3582 versus naproxen in osteoarthritis. Ann Rheum Dis 2005;64:449–56.
157. Lichtenberger LM, Barron M, Marathi U. Association of phosphatidylcholine and NSAIDs as a novel strategy to reduce gastrointestinal toxicity. Drugs Today (Barc) 2009;45:877–90.
158. Lanza FL, Marathi UK, Anand BS, et al. Clinical trial: comparison of ibuprofen phosphatidylcholine and ibuprofen on the gastrointestinal safety and analgesic efficacy in osteoarthritic patients. Aliment Pharmacol Ther 2008;28: 431–42.
159. Leone S, Ottani A, Bertolini A. Dual acting anti-inflammatory drugs. Curr Top Med Chem 2007;7:265–75.
160. Bias P, Buchner A, Klesser B, et al. The gastrointestinal tolerability of the LOX/ COX inhibitor, licofelone, is similar to placebo and superior to naproxen therapy in healthy volunteers: results from a randomized, controlled trial. Am J Gastroenterol 2004;99:611–88.
161. Patrono C, Rocca B. Nonsteroidal antiinflammatory drugs: past, present and future. Pharmacol Res 2009;59:285–9.
162. Van der Linden MW, Gaugris S, Kuipers EJ, et al. Gastroprotection among new chronic users of non-steroidal anti-inflammatory drugs: a study of utilization and adherence in the Netherlands. Curr Med Res Opin 2009;25:195–204.
163. Herlitz J, Tóth PP, Naesdal J. Low-dose aspirin therapy for cardiovascular prevention: quantification and consequences of poor compliance or discontinuation. Am J Cardiovasc Drugs 2010;10:125–41.
164. Lanas A, Ferrandez A. Inappropriate prevention of NSAID-induced gastrointestinal events among long-term users in the elderly. Drugs Aging 2007;24:121–31.
165. Hunt RH, Choquette D, Craig BN, et al. Approach to managing musculoskeletal pain: acetaminophen, cyclooxygenase-2 inhibitors, or traditional NSAIDs? Can Fam Physician 2007;53:1177–84.
166. Lanza FL, Chan FK, Quigley EM. Practice Parameters Committee of the American College of Gastroenterology. Guidelines for prevention of NSAID-related ulcer complications. Am J Gastroenterol 2009;104:728–38.
167. Fujimori S, Seo T, Gudis K, et al. Prevention of nonsteroidal anti-inflammatory drug-induced small-intestinal injury by prostaglandin: a pilot randomized controlled trial evaluated by capsule endoscopy. Gastrointest Endosc 2009; 69:1339–46.
168. Bjarnason I, Smethurst P, Fenn CG, et al. Misoprostol reduces indomethacin-induced changes in human small intestinal permeability. Dig Dis Sci 1989;34: 407–11.
169. Morris AJ, Murray L, Sturrock RD, et al. Short report: the effect of misoprostol on the anaemia of NSAID enteropathy. Aliment Pharmacol Ther 1994;8:343–6.
170. Montalto M, Gallo A, Curigliano V, et al. Clinical trial: the effects of a probiotic mixture on non-steroidal anti-inflammatory drug enteropathy - a randomized, double-blind, cross-over, placebo-controlled study. Aliment Pharmacol Ther 2010;32:209–14.

Pharmacologic Aspects of Eradication Therapy for *Helicobacter pylori* Infection

Takahisa Furuta, MD, PhD[a],*, David Y. Graham, MD, PhD[b]

KEYWORDS

- CYP2C19 • *Helicobacter pylori* • Pharmacogenomics
- Proton pump inhibitor • Rapid metabolizer
- Intermediate metabolizer • Poor metabolizer

A close relationship has been found between *Helicobacter pylori* infection and upper gastrointestinal disorders such as peptic ulcer diseases, gastric cancer, and gastric mucosa–associated lymphoid tissue lymphoma.[1] Eradication of *H pylori* is a part of the effective treatment and/or prevention of these disorders and also reduces the occurrence of new gastric cancers after endoscopic resection.[2–8] At present, the most common methods for the eradication of *H pylori* infection consist of the administration of a proton pump inhibitor (PPI) and antimicrobial agents, such as amoxicillin, clarithromycin, metronidazole, fluoroquinolone, or tetracycline. Each of these agents has its own characteristics in respect to pharmacokinetics, pharmacodynamics, and pharmacogenomics, which theoretically affect treatment success attained with the different therapeutic regimens. This article describes the pharmacologic characteristics of the common agents used for eradication of *H pylori* infection. This knowledge should be helpful for clinicians trying to achieve optimal eradication of *H pylori* infection and investigators designing new treatment protocols.

Disclosure: See last page of article.
[a] Center for Clinical Research, Hamamatsu University School of Medicine, 1-20-1 Handayama, Higsahi-Ku, Hamamatsu 431-3192, Japan
[b] Molecular Virology and Microbiology, Michael E. DeBakey Veterans Affairs Medical Center, Baylor College of Medicine, 2002 Holcombe Boulevard Room 3A-320 (111D), Houston, TX 7730, USA
* Corresponding author.
E-mail address: furuta@hama-med.ac.jp

Gastroenterol Clin N Am 39 (2010) 465–480
doi:10.1016/j.gtc.2010.08.007
0889-8553/10/$ – see front matter © 2010 Elsevier Inc. All rights reserved.

PHARMACOLOGIC CHARACTERISTICS OF REPRESENTATIVE THERAPEUTIC AGENTS INVOLVED IN REGIMENS FOR ERADICATION OF *H PYLORI* INFECTION
Proton Pump Inhibitor

PPIs potentially play a major role in an *H pylori* eradication therapy by (1) increasing the intragastric pH, which improves antibiotic stability and bioavailability[9]; (2) increasing the intragastric pH to 6 or more, which prompts *H pylori* to replicate and thus become more sensitive to antibiotics that are effective only against replicating bacteria, such as amoxicillin[10,11]; (3) suppressing acid secretion, which increases the concentration of antibiotics in the stomach[12]; and (4) having an anti-*H pylori* effect.[13]

PPIs are primarily metabolized by cytochrome P450 (CYP) 2C19 (CYP2C19) (**Fig. 1**). The genetic polymorphisms of CYP2C19 are classified into 3 groups: rapid metabolizer (RM: *1/*1), intermediate metabolizer (IM: *1/*X), and poor metabolizer (PM: *X/*X), (*1 = wild type allele and *X = mutated allele). Recently, the *CYP2C19*17* allele has been found in the ultrarapid extensive metabolizer genotype of CYP2C19.[14] However, the clinical effect of *CYP2C19*17* remains to be elucidated.[15]

Although various genetic mutations involved in the CYP2C19 polymorphisms have been discovered from different ethnic populations, the differences in the activity of CYP2C19 can be explained in most cases by the combination of 2 point mutations, *CYP2C19*2* of exon 5 and *CYP2C19*3* of exon 4.[16–18] There are interethnic differences in the frequencies of PM genotypes of this enzyme.[19–21] Representative frequencies of phenotypes and alleles in different ethnic groups are summarized in **Table 1**.

When omeprazole, 20 mg, is given as a single dose, plasma omeprazole concentrations differ among the 3 different CYP2C19 genotypic groups (RM, IM, and PM) (**Fig. 2**).[22] Plasma omeprazole levels in the PM group are sustained for a longer time after dosing. The pharmacokinetic data in relation to CYP2C19 genotypes are summarized in **Table 2**. When a PPI (ie, omeprazole, 20 mg) is administered, the intragastric

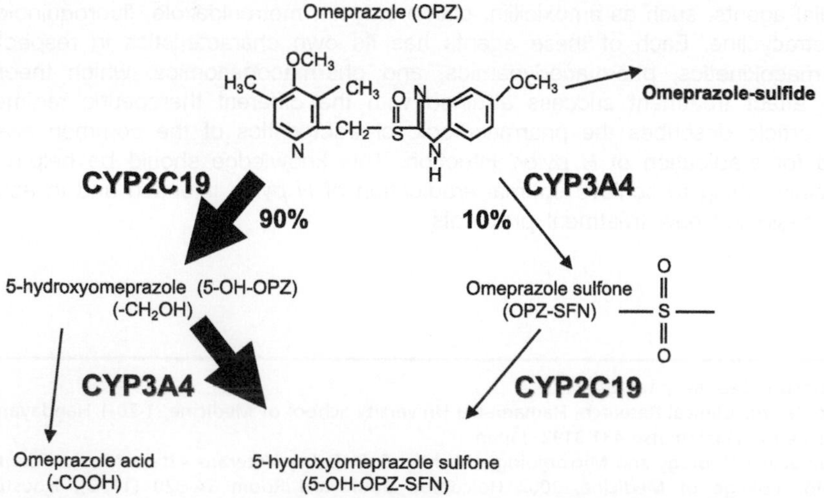

Fig. 1. Metabolism of omeprazole (OPZ) in relation to cytochrome (CYP) P450 isoenzymes. Thickness of arrows indicates the relative contribution of different enzyme pathways. OPZ is mainly metabolized by CYP2C19 to 5-hydroxyomeprazole (5-OH-OPZ), which is then metabolized to 5-hydroxyomeprazole sulfone (5-OH-OPZ-SFN). OPZ is also metabolized by CYP3A4 to omeprazole sulfone (OPZ-SFN), which is then metabolized by CYP2C19 to 5-OH-OPZ-SFN.

Table 1
Frequencies of CYP2C19 phenotypes and alleles in different populations

Ethnicity	Phenotype Frequency			Allele Frequency			References
	RM	IM	PM	*1	*2	*3	
Africans	0.68	0.28	0.04	0.823	0.173	0.004	19
Asians	0.35	0.46	0.19	0.58	0.29	0.13	20
Caucasians	0.69	0.28	0.03	0.83	0.17	0	21

IM of CYP2C19 (*1/*2 or *1/*3), PM of CYP2C19 (*2/*2, *2/*3, or *3/*3), and RM of CYP2C19 (*1/*1).

pH profile also differs among the 3 different genotypic groups (**Fig. 3**). The mean 24-hour intragastric pH of the RM group is the lowest, the IM group comes next, and the PM group is the highest.[22] Several reports on intragastric pH profiles after PPI dosing are summarized in **Table 3**. The differences in acid inhibition by a PPI among the different CYP2C19 genotypic groups are considered to result from the different plasma concentrations of the PPI among the different genotypic groups.[23,24]

When lansoprazole, 30 mg, is given 4 times daily to sustain the plasma lansoprazole levels all day long (**Fig. 4**A), near-complete acid inhibition can be achieved, even among the RM genotypes (see **Fig. 4**B). The peak plasma concentration (Cmax) of lansoprazole is not increased in the RM group with lansoprazole, 30 mg, given 4 times daily when compared with that of once daily administration of lansoprazole, 30 mg, (see **Fig. 4**A) and is not as high as that observed in the PM group. Therefore, the dosing regimen of a PPI is a key element when attempting to attain sustained levels of high intragastric pH. Clinically, one would wish to be able to estimate the effectiveness of a PPI dosing regimen irrespective of the CYP2C19 genotype (see later discussion).

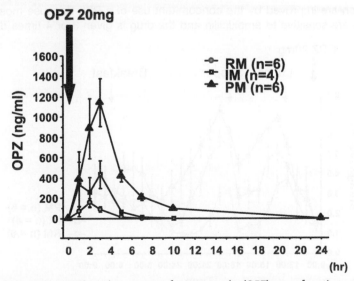

Fig. 2. Plasma concentration time curve of omeprazole (OPZ) as a function of CYP2C19 genotype. Plasma concentration of OPZ was highest in the PM group, intermediate in the IM group, and lowest in the RM group. (*Data from* Furuta T, Ohashi K, Kosuge K, et al. CYP2C19 genotype status and effect of omeprazole on intragastric pH in humans. Clin Pharmacol Ther 1999;65(5):552–61.)

Table 2
CYP2C19 genotypic groups and area under the curve$_{0-24 h}$ (ng·h/mL) of PPIs

Regimen	RM	IM	PM	RM/IM/PM ratio	References
OPZ, 20 mg, day 1	421	1403	5109	1:3.3:12.2	[22]
OPZ, 20 mg, day 1	524	1096	5607	1:2.1:10.7	[23]
OPZ, 20 mg, day 8	1057	2418	7153	1:2.3:6.8	[23]
RPZ, 20 g, day 1	696	1609	2329	1:2.3:3.3	[23]
RPZ, 20 mg, day 8	464	1398	2437	1:3.0:5.3	[23]
LPZ, 30 mg, day 8	1980	4775	10,663	1:2.4:5.4	[63]

IM of CYP2C19 (*1/*2 or *1/*3), PM of CYP2C19 (*2/*2, *2/*3, or *3/*3), and RM of CYP2C19 (*1/*1).
Abbreviations: LPZ, lansoprazole; OPZ, omeprazole; RPZ, rabeprazole.

Amoxicillin

Amoxicillin is a penicillin derivative that inhibits the synthesis of the bacterial cell wall. Therefore, amoxicillin's bactericidal effect requires the bacteria to be replicating.

Amoxicillin is excreted by the kidneys, the plasma half-life is approximately 1 hour, and the bactericidal effect is time dependent. Moreover, amoxicillin has little postantibiotic effect (PAE) on gram-negative bacteria, such as *H pylori*. Therefore, theoretically, amoxicillin should be given 3 or 4 times daily to maximize the time above minimal inhibitory concentration (MIC) (**Fig. 5**). However, in most *H pylori* eradication therapies, amoxicillin is given twice daily, where the estimated time above MIC attained by twice daily dosing is insufficient for amoxicillin. Therefore, if a patient infected with clarithromycin-resistant strain of *H pylori* is treated with triple therapy with PPI/amoxicillin/clarithromycin twice daily, the chance of eradication of *H pylori* infection is low.

Amoxicillin is also somewhat acid labile, and both its stability and bioavailability in the stomach are improved by the concomitant use of a PPI. Because most strains of *H pylori* are sensitive to amoxicillin and the drug is given 3 or 4 times daily with

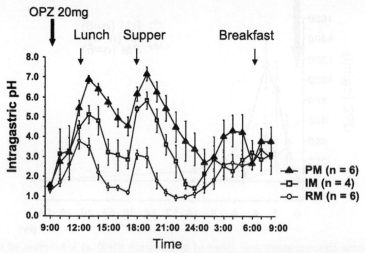

Fig. 3. Profiles of intragastric pH values as a function of CYP2C19 genotypic status for omeprazole (OPZ), 20 mg, dosing. (*Data from* Furuta T, Ohashi K, Kosuge K, et al. CYP2C19 genotype status and effect of omeprazole on intragastric pH in humans. Clin Pharmacol Ther 1999;65(5):552–61.)

Table 3
Intragastric pH attained by a PPI as a function of CYP2C19 genotypic status

Regimen	RM	IM	PM	References
OPZ, 20 mg, day 1	2.1	3.3	4.5	22
OPZ, 20 mg, day 1	2.3	3.3	4.1	23
OPZ, 20 mg, day 8	4.1	4.7	5.9	23
LPZ, 30 mg, day 8	4.4	4.9	5.4	24
RPZ, 20 mg, day 1	3.3	4.2	5.3	23
RPZ, 20 mg, day 8	4.8	5.0	6.0	23

IM of CYP2C19 (*1/*2 or *1/*3), PM of CYP2C19 (*2/*2, *2/*3, *3/*3), and RM of CYP2C19 (*1/*1).
Abbreviations: LPZ, lansoprazole; OPZ, omeprazole; RPZ, rabeprazole.

appropriate dosing of a PPI to attain sufficient acid inhibition, high eradication rates can been achieved with dual PPI/amoxicillin therapy as discussed later.

Clarithromycin

Clarithromycin is a macrolide and often included in the standard regimens for the eradication of *H pylori* infection. The plasma half-life of clarithromycin is relatively long (around 5 hours),[25] such that a twice daily dosing is an appropriate dosing schedule. The prevalence of clarithromycin-resistant *H pylori* strains is increasing all over the world,[26] and this increase has resulted in a decrease in the eradication rates with clarithromycin-containing regimens, such as the combination of PPI/amoxicillin/clarithromycin. Bacterial resistance to clarithromycin can be estimated by the measurement of point mutations of the 23S ribosomal RNA (rRNA) gene at positions 2142 and 2143.[27,28]

Clarithromycin is a strong inhibitor of CYP3A4. Therefore, clinicians must pay attention to the risk of drug-drug interactions in patients who are treated with other drugs that are metabolized by the CYP3A4 pathway. Plasma levels of a PPI are also increased by clarithromycin,[29] which also inhibits P-glycoprotein (MDR1),[30] resulting in the increased risk of adverse events with drugs that are also substrates of MDR1, such as digoxin.

Metronidazole

Metronidazole has been used widely for the eradication of *H pylori* infection together with amoxicillin or clarithromycin and a PPI. The bactericidal mechanism of metronidazole is unique. Metronidazole is a prodrug, and the nitro moiety of metronidazole is reduced by bacteria, which induces DNA double-strand breaks resulting in cell death.[31] The plasma half-life of metronidazole is around 8 hours. Therefore, a twice or thrice daily dosing is appropriate.

There are marked geographic differences in the distribution of metronidazole-resistant strains of *H pylori*.[32] Resistance to metronidazole is associated with decreased eradication rates when metronidazole-based regimens are used. However, metronidazole is unique among the commonly used antibiotics because resistance to this drug can be partially overcome by increasing the dose and duration of therapy.

Metronidazole also inhibits CYP3A4 and CYP2C9. Therefore, clinicians should pay attention to drug-drug interactions with substrates of CYP3A4 and CYP2C9, such as warfarin, when metronidazole is given.[33] Metronidazole also inhibits aldehyde dehydrogenase in the metabolic process of alcohol breakdown, resulting in an increase in blood acetaldehyde levels and thus can cause a disulfiram (Antabuse)-like

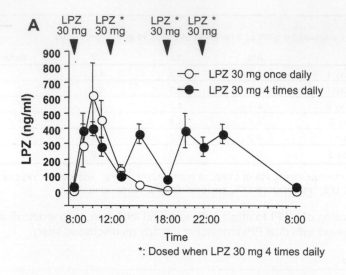

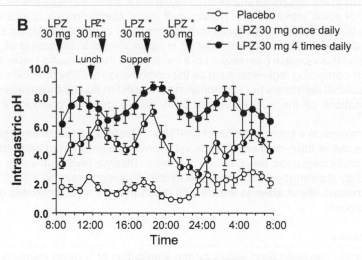

Fig. 4. Mean (± SE) plasma concentration versus time (*A*) and mean (± SE) intragastric pH values versus time course curves (*B*) for lansoprazole (LPZ) after the final dosing of LPZ, 30 mg once daily, and LPZ, 30 mg 4 times daily, for 8 days in the 5 subjects with RM genotype. With LPZ, 30 mg 4 times daily, plasma levels of LPZ are sustained during each of the dosing intervals in the 5 subjects with RM genotype and complete acid inhibition (ie, intragastric pH around 7.0) can be achieved. (*Data from* Furuta T, Shirai N, Xiao F, et al. Effect of high-dose lansoprazole on intragastric pH in subjects who are homozygous extensive metabolizers of cytochrome P4502C19. Clin Pharmacol Ther 2001;70(5):484–92.)

reaction.[34] Patients are advised not to drink alcohol while taking metronidazole or the similar nitroimidazole, tinidazole.

Fluoroquinolones

Fluoroquinolones, such as levofloxacin, are now used for eradication of *H pylori* infection. Fluoroquinolones disturb the function of gyrase in bacteria, which is an essential

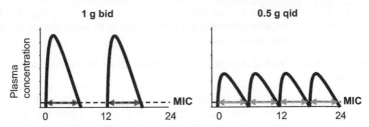

Fig. 5. The relationship between time above MIC and dosing scheme of amoxicillin. The time above MIC in the 0.5-g 4-times-daily dosing is longer than that in the 1-g twice-daily dosing.

enzyme for DNA replication, resulting in the induction of DNA breaks and cell death. Fluoroquinolone-containing regimens are often used in rescue regimens after failure of standard regimens.[35] However, the worldwide overuse of fluoroquinolones has led to a rapid increase in resistance such that it is unlikely that this group of drug will be a useful anti-*H pylori* agent without prior susceptibility testing.

The bactericidal effect of fluoroquinolones depends on the Cmax and the area under the curve and not on the time above MIC. Fluoroquinolones have PAE, the duration of which depends on Cmax. Therefore, a higher dose of the fluoroquinolone given once daily is the best dosing scheme (**Fig. 6**). Di Caro and colleagues[36] reported that levofloxacin, 500 mg once daily, was as effective as levofloxacin, 500 mg twice daily, when used with amoxicillin and esomeprazole. Therefore, the authors suggest that fluoroquinolones should be dosed once daily at a higher dose.

Tetracycline/Minocycline

Tetracycline antibiotics (eg, tetracycline and minocycline) bind to the bacterial 70S rRNA and disturb the aminoacyl transfer RNA from combining with the messenger RNA and ribosome composite, resulting in the inhibition of protein synthesis. Tetracycline was involved in the classical triple therapy with bismuth subcitrate and tinidazole. The incidence of tetracycline-resistant strains of *H pylori* is very low in most countries. The plasma half-life of tetracycline is around 6 hours, and therefore, twice daily dosing is theoretically an appropriate dosing scheme for tetracycline. However, the most studied tetracycline-containing regimen (tetracycline hydrochloride, metronidazole,

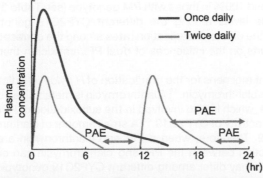

Fig. 6. The relationship between Cmax and dosing scheme of a quinolone. The bactericidal effect of quinolone and the duration of PAE depend on Cmax. Therefore, once-daily dosing with the higher dose is the best dosing scheme for quinolone.

bismuth, and a PPI) used tetracycline, 500 mg, 4 times a day. This regimen has not been adequately tested in a head-to-head comparison with twice-a-day tetracycline regimens. Such studies are clearly needed.

Combinations of Antimicrobial Agents for Regimens Used in Eradication of H pylori Infection

In the most effective eradication regimens, 2 or 3 antimicrobial agents are used. However, clinicians must pay attention to the combination of antimicrobial agents. When amoxicillin is taken together with tetracycline, the latter may theoretically decrease the ability of amoxicillin to kill bacteria.

Both clarithromycin and levofloxacin have effects on cardiac electric signaling. When clarithromycin and levofloxacin are used together, the effect of either drug on the heart may be increased or prolonged, resulting in the alteration of cardiac rhythm, which may be dangerous or potentially life threatening.

On the positive side, metronidazole has an additional or a synergistic bactericidal effect on the eradication of H pylori infection with any of the antimicrobial agents mentioned earlier.

Therefore, commonly used regimens for the eradication of H pylori infection include (1) amoxicillin and clarithromycin, (2) amoxicillin and metronidazole, (3) amoxicillin and a fluoroquinolone, (4) clarithromycin and metronidazole, (5) a fluoroquinolone and metronidazole, and (6) tetracycline and metronidazole. These combinations of antimicrobial agents are administered with a PPI. The combination of clarithromycin and tetracycline was also reported to achieve a high eradication rate.[37] There have been few studies on the combinations of tetracycline and fluoroquinolones.

Sequential therapy (PPI/amoxicillin followed by PPI/metronidazole/clarithromycin) has been found to achieve sufficient eradication rates.[38,39] However, concomitant therapy with a PPI, amoxicillin, metronidazole, and clarithromycin has also been found to achieve the high eradication rates attained by sequential therapy.[40]

PHARMACOGENETICS IN H PYLORI ERADICATION THERAPY
CYP2C19 Genotypic Status as the Therapeutic Determinant of PPI-Containing Eradication Therapy for H pylori Infection

The first report on the influence of CYP2C19 polymorphisms on H pylori eradication rates was with the dual PPI/amoxicillin therapy. The eradication rates for H pylori infection by dual therapy with omeprazole, 20 mg once daily, and amoxicillin, 500 mg 4 times daily, for 2 weeks are around 30% in those with the RM genotype, 60% in those with IM genotype, and 100% in those with PM genotype (see **Table 3**).[41] Differences in plasma omeprazole levels among the different CYP2C19 genotypic groups are assumed to reflect the different eradication rates among the correspondent genotypic groups. Other reports on the influences of dual PPI/amoxicillin therapy are summarized in **Table 4**.

One of the current regimens for the eradication of H pylori infection is triple therapy with PPI/amoxicillin/clarithromycin.[42] Clarithromycin is metabolized by and is a potent inhibitor of CYP3A4, which is also involved in the sulfoxidation of PPIs.[43] Clarithromycin also affects the activity of CYP2C19.[44] A small amount of clarithromycin is metabolized by CYP2C19. Therefore, when a PPI and clarithromycin are taken together, a drug-drug interaction between the PPI and clarithromycin can occur and plasma clarithromycin levels may differ among different CYP2C19 genotypic groups.[29]

Differences in plasma clarithromycin and PPI levels among the different CYP2C19 genotypic groups can result in different eradication rates for H pylori infection. In the study by Furuta and colleagues,[45] eradication rates for H pylori infection by a triple

Table 4
Eradication rates of *H pylori* infection by PPI-based regimens as a function of CYP2C19 genotypic status

Regimen	RM (%)	IM (%)	PM (%)	References
OPZ, 20 mg qd, + AMPC, 500 mg qid, for 2 wk	29	60	100	41
OPZ, 20 mg bid, + AMPC, 500 mg tid, for 1 wk	40	42	100	64
RPZ, 10 mg bid, + AMPC, 500 mg tid, for 2 wk	61	92	94	58
OPZ, 20 mg bid; or LPZ, 30 mg bid, + AMPC, 500 mg tid, + CAM, 200 mg tid, for 1 wk	73	92	98	45
OPZ, 20 mg bid, + AMPC, 1000 mg bid, + CAM, 500 mg bid, for 1 wk	60	84	100	65

Abbreviations: AMPC, amoxicillin; CAM, clarithromycin; LPZ, lansoprazole; OPZ, omeprazole; RPZ, rabeprazole.

therapy with daily doses of omeprazole, 40 mg, or lansoprazole, 60 mg; amoxicillin, 1500 mg; and clarithromycin, 600 mg, for 1 week were 73% in the RM group, 92% in the IM group, and 98% in the PM group (**Fig. 7**). The prevalence of the RM genotype was higher in the group without eradication or with therapeutic failure, whereas the prevalence of the PM genotype in patients without eradication was very low. Other reports on the influence of CYP2C19 polymorphisms on the eradication rates by a triple therapy are summarized in **Table 4**. Some reports have not shown a statistical significance in the eradication rates among different CYP2C19 genotypic groups,[46,47] but the CYP2C19 genotype-dependent trends in eradication rates is reported in most of such articles. A recent meta-analysis by Zhao and colleagues[48] demonstrated that CYP2C19 is the significant factor associated with therapeutic outcomes with triple therapy with PPI/amoxicillin/clarithromycin. Taken together, one of the reasons for eradication failures of *H pylori* infection by triple therapy with PPI/amoxicillin/clarithromycin is an insufficient dose of the PPI (omeprazole or lansoprazole) in the RM group.

Another important factor associated with the success or failure of eradication of *H pylori* infection by a triple therapy with PPI/amoxicillin/clarithromycin is bacterial resistance to clarithromycin. Bacterial resistance to clarithromycin is caused by mutation in the 23S rRNA, which can be detected directly by genetic testing, even using stool samples.[49–52] The eradication rate in patients with RM genotype infected with clarithromycin-resistant strains of *H pylori* was reportedly dramatically low (7.1%).[45] Therefore, it could be concluded that the major factors associated with the success or failure of eradication of *H pylori* infection by a triple regimen with PPI/amoxicillin/clarithromycin are not only CYP2C19 genotypic status of patients but also bacterial resistance of *H pylori* strains to clarithromycin.

Pharmacogenomics-Based Rescue Regimens After Eradication Failure with Standard PPI/Amoxicillin/Clarithromycin Therapy at the Usual Dose

Most recommendations for rescue regimens after failure of initial therapy consist of different antimicrobial agents that were not used in the initial therapy. Another strategy for rescue regimens is to carefully consider the pharmacology underlying the eradication therapy.

Most patients who fail eradication of *H pylori* infection by PPI/amoxicillin/clarithromycin therapy at the usual standard doses have the RM genotype of CYP2C19 and/or are infected with a clarithromycin-resistant strain of *H pylori*. Amoxicillin-resistant strains of *H pylori* are rare,[53] and therefore, well-designed amoxicillin-based

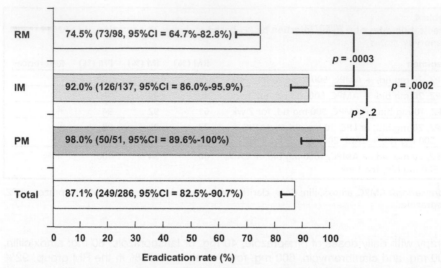

Fig. 7. Eradication rates of *H pylori* with a daily dose of 30 mg of lansoprazole, 600 mg of clarithromycin, and 1500 mg of amoxicillin for 1 week in the different CYP2C19 genotypic groups. Bars indicate 95% confidence intervals (CIs). There was a significant difference in the eradication rates among the 3 different CYP2C19 genotypic groups, RM, IM, and PM. (*Data from* Furuta T, Shirai N, Xiao F, et al. Effect of high-dose lansoprazole on intragastric pH in subjects who are homozygous extensive metabolizers of cytochrome P4502C19. Clin Pharmacol Ther 2001;70(5):484–92.)

regimens may succeed in the eradication of *H pylori* infection in patients who have experienced therapeutic failure. Bayerdorffer and colleagues[54] reported an eradication rate of approximately 90% with dual therapy with omeprazole, 40 mg thrice daily, and amoxicillin, 750 mg thrice daily, for 2 weeks. As noted earlier, amoxicillin alone is both theoretically[55,56] and practically an effective anti-*H pylori* single agent if a near neutral intragastric pH can be maintained. For example, dual therapy with lansoprazole, 30 mg, or rabeprazole, 10 mg, and amoxicillin, 500 mg, administered 4 times daily for 2 weeks attained eradication rates greater than 90%.[45,57,58] The reported eradication rates for *H pylori* infection with 3 or 4 times daily dosing of PPI and amoxicillin are summarized in **Table 5**.

Table 5
Cure rates of *H pylori* infection by treatment with high doses of a PPI plus amoxicillin (PP analysis)

Regimen	Eradication Rates (%) (PP Analysis)	References
OPZ, 40 mg tid, + AMPC, 750 mg tid, for 2 wk	91.0	54
LPZ, 30 mg qid, + AMPC, 500 mg qid, for 2 wk	96.7	45
RPZ, 10 mg qid, + AMPC, 500 mg qid, for 2 wk	100.0	57,58
RPZ, 10 mg qid, + AMPC, 500 mg qid, for 2 wk	93.8	66
OPZ, 40 mg qid, + AMPC, 750 mg qid, for 2 wk	83.8	67
ESO, 40 mg tid, + AMPC, 750 mg tid, for 2 wk	74.2	68

Abbreviations: AMPC, amoxicillin; ESO, esomeprazole; LPZ, lansoprazole; OPZ, omeprazole; PP, per protocol; RPZ, rabeprazole.

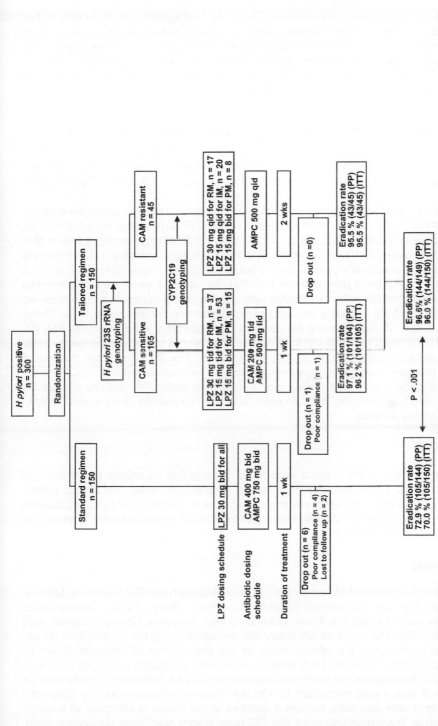

Fig. 8. Flowchart for patients who test positive for *H pylori* and enrolled in standard and tailored regimen groups. AMPC, amoxicillin; CAM, clarithromycin; ITT, intention to treat; LPZ, lansoprazole; PP, per protocol. (*Data from* Furuta T, Shirai N, Kodaira M, et al. Pharmacogenomics-based tailored versus standard therapeutic regimen for eradication of *H. pylori*. Clin Pharmacol Ther 2007;81(4):521–8.)

There are alternate ways to achieve a sustained intragastric pH more than 6. For example, it is more efficient and practical to increase pH levels with antacids than to attempt to inhibit all parietal cells for an extended time; alternative approaches would be to directly increase the intragastric pH with antacids such as sodium bicarbonate,[59] to use a new long acting PPI, or a combination of both.[60] A third option to overcome the persistent state other than by increasing the pH level would be to increase the duration of the standard dose dual therapy (eg, to 6 weeks).[55,61]

The Pharmacogenomics-Tailored Strategy for Eradication of H pylori Infection

The principles underlying the strategy for H pylori eradication can be summarized as follows: first, to select the antibacterial agent to which H pylori is sensitive and second, to optimize the environmental condition in the stomach for the selected antibacterial agent.

A strategy was tailored for the eradication of H pylori infection, in which the susceptibility of H pylori strains to clarithromycin and the CYP2C19 status were determined by genotyping.[62] Japanese patients infected with clarithromycin-sensitive strains of H pylori were treated with clarithromycin, 200 mg thrice daily, amoxicillin, 500 mg thrice daily, and personalized doses of lansoprazole (ie, 30 mg thrice daily, 15 mg thrice daily, and 15 mg twice daily in those with RM, IM, and PM genotypes, respectively) for 1 week, whereas patients infected with clarithromycin-resistant strains received amoxicillin, 500 mg 4 times a day, and personalized dose of lansoprazole (ie, 30 mg 4 times a day, 15 mg 4 times a day, and 15 mg twice daily in patients with RM, IM, and PM genotypes, respectively) for 2 weeks. This tailored strategy achieved the sufficient eradication rates in H pylori infection (ie, 96%) (**Fig. 8**). If a regimen that would reliably produce a sustained high intragastric pH irrespective of the CYP2C19 genotype and allow convenient dosing (eg, a truly long acting PPI with or without an antacid) can be developed, it would seem likely that amoxicillin alone would be sufficient for most patients.

SUMMARY

Each agent used in the H pylori eradication therapy has its unique pharmacologic characteristics. Eradication regimens should be designed based on a good understanding of the pharmacologic aspects of each agent used in the H pylori eradication therapy, and such eradication regimens can lead to the optimal tailored treatment to eradicate H pylori infection.

DISCLOSURE

Dr Graham is supported in part by the Office of Research and Development, Medical Research Service, Department of Veterans Affairs; Public Health Service grant DK56338, which funds the Texas Medical Center Digestive Diseases Center; and R21DK067366. The contents are solely the responsibility of the authors and do not necessarily represent the official views of the Department of Veterans Affairs or National Institutes of Health. Dr Graham is an unpaid consultant for Novartis in relation to vaccine development for treatment or prevention of Helicobacter pylori infection. Dr Graham is also a paid consultant for Otsuka Pharmaceuticals regarding diagnostic testing, and until July 2007, he was a member of the Board of Directors of Meretek Diagnostics, the manufacturer of the ^{13}C-urea breath test. Until November 2009, Dr Graham received royalties on the Baylor College of Medicine patent covering materials related to ^{13}C-urea breath test. Dr Furuta declares no conflicts.

REFERENCES

1. Graham D, Sung J. *Helicobacter pylori* Sleisenger & Fordtran's gastrointestinal and liver disease. In: Feldman M, Friedman LS, Brandt LJ, editors. Pathophysiology, diagnosis, management. 7th edition. Philadelphia: WB Saunders Co; 2006. p. 1049–66.
2. Marshall BJ, Goodwin CS, Warren JR, et al. Prospective double-blind trial of duodenal ulcer relapse after eradication of *Campylobacter pylori*. Lancet 1988; 2(8626–8627):1437–42.
3. Ofman JJ, Etchason J, Fullerton S, et al. Management strategies for *Helicobacter pylori*-seropositive patients with dyspepsia: clinical and economic consequences. Ann Intern Med 1997;126(4):280–91.
4. Furuta T, Futami H, Arai H, et al. Effects of lansoprazole with or without amoxicillin on ulcer healing: relation to eradication of *Helicobacter pylori*. J Clin Gastroenterol 1995;20(Suppl 2):S107–11.
5. Wotherspoon AC. *Helicobacter pylori* infection and gastric lymphoma. Br Med Bull 1998;54(1):79–85.
6. Uemura N, Mukai T, Okamoto S, et al. Effect of *Helicobacter pylori* eradication on subsequent development of cancer after endoscopic resection of early gastric cancer. Cancer Epidemiol Biomarkers Prev 1997;6(8):639–42.
7. Uemura N, Okamoto S, Yamamoto S, et al. *Helicobacter pylori* infection and the development of gastric cancer. N Engl J Med 2001;345(11):784–9.
8. Fukase K, Kato M, Kikuchi S, et al. Effect of eradication of *Helicobacter pylori* on incidence of metachronous gastric carcinoma after endoscopic resection of early gastric cancer: an open-label, randomised controlled trial. Lancet 2008; 372(9636):392–7.
9. Grayson ML, Eliopoulos GM, Ferraro MJ, et al. Effect of varying pH on the susceptibility of *Campylobacter pylori* to antimicrobial agents. Eur J Clin Microbiol Infect Dis 1989;8(10):888–9.
10. Scott D, Weeks D, Melchers K, et al. The life and death of *Helicobacter pylori*. Gut 1998;43(Suppl 1):S56–60.
11. Scott DR, Weeks D, Hong C, et al. The role of internal urease in acid resistance of *Helicobacter pylori*. Gastroenterology 1998;114(1):58–70.
12. Goddard AF, Jessa MJ, Barrett DA, et al. Effect of omeprazole on the distribution of metronidazole, amoxicillin, and clarithromycin in human gastric juice. Gastroenterology 1996;111(2):358–67.
13. Midolo PD, Turnidge JD, Lambert JR, et al. Oxygen concentration influences proton pump inhibitor activity against *Helicobacter pylori* in vitro. Antimicrobial Agents Chemother 1996;40(6):1531–3.
14. Sim SC, Risinger C, Dahl ML, et al. A common novel CYP2C19 gene variant causes ultrarapid drug metabolism relevant for the drug response to proton pump inhibitors and antidepressants. Clin Pharmacol Ther 2006;79(1): 103–13.
15. Kurzawski M, Gawronska-Szklarz B, Wrzesniewska J, et al. Effect of CYP2C19*17 gene variant on *Helicobacter pylori* eradication in peptic ulcer patients. Eur J Clin Pharmacol 2006;62(10):877–80.
16. De Morais SM, Wilkinson GR, Blaisdell J, et al. Identification of a new genetic defect responsible for the polymorphism of (S)-mephenytoin metabolism in Japanese. Mol Pharmacol 1994;46(4):594–8.
17. de Morais SM, Goldstein JA, Xie HG, et al. Genetic analysis of the S-mephenytoin polymorphism in a Chinese population. Clin Pharmacol Ther 1995;58(4):404–11.

18. de Morais SM, Wilkinson GR, Blaisdell J, et al. The major genetic defect responsible for the polymorphism of S- mephenytoin metabolism in humans. J Biol Chem 1994;269(22):15419–22.
19. Xie HG, Kim RB, Stein CM, et al. Genetic polymorphism of (S)-mephenytoin 4'-hydroxylation in populations of African descent. Br J Clin Pharmacol 1999;48(3):402–8.
20. Kubota T, Chiba K, Ishizaki T. Genotyping of S-mephenytoin 4'-hydroxylation in an extended Japanese population. Clin Pharmacol Ther 1996;60(6):661–6.
21. Xie HG, Stein CM, Kim RB, et al. Allelic, genotypic and phenotypic distributions of S-mephenytoin 4'- hydroxylase (CYP2C19) in healthy Caucasian populations of European descent throughout the world. Pharmacogenetics 1999;9(5):539–49.
22. Furuta T, Ohashi K, Kosuge K, et al. CYP2C19 genotype status and effect of omeprazole on intragastric pH in humans. Clin Pharmacol Ther 1999;65(5):552–61.
23. Shirai N, Furuta T, Moriyama Y, et al. Effects of CYP2C19 genotypic differences in the metabolism of omeprazole and rabeprazole on intragastric pH. Aliment Pharmacol Ther 2001;15(12):1929–37.
24. Shirai N, Furuta T, Xiao F, et al. Comparison of lansoprazole and famotidine for gastric acid inhibition during the daytime and night-time in different CYP2C19 genotype groups. Aliment Pharmacol Ther 2002;16(4):837–46.
25. Ferrero JL, Bopp BA, Marsh KC, et al. Metabolism and disposition of clarithromycin in man. Drug Metab Dispos 1990;18(4):441–6.
26. Chang WL, Sheu BS, Cheng HC, et al. Resistance to metronidazole, clarithromycin and levofloxacin of Helicobacter pylori before and after clarithromycin-based therapy in Taiwan. J Gastroenterol Hepatol 2009;24(7):1230–5.
27. Versalovic J, Shortridge D, Kibler K, et al. Mutations in 23S rRNA are associated with clarithromycin resistance in Helicobacter pylori. Antimicrobial Agents Chemother 1996;40(2):477–80.
28. De Francesco V, Margiotta M, Zullo A, et al. Clarithromycin-resistant genotypes and eradication of Helicobacter pylori. Ann Intern Med 2006;144(2):94–100.
29. Furuta T, Ohashi K, Kobayashi K, et al. Effects of clarithromycin on the metabolism of omeprazole in relation to CYP2C19 genotype status in humans. Clin Pharmacol Ther 1999;66(3):265–74.
30. Wakasugi H, Yano I, Ito T, et al. Effect of clarithromycin on renal excretion of digoxin: interaction with P-glycoprotein. Clin Pharmacol Ther 1998;64(1):123–8.
31. Jenks PJ, Edwards DI. Metronidazole resistance in Helicobacter pylori. Int J Antimicrob Agents 2002;19(1):1–7.
32. Romano M, Iovene MR, Russo MI, et al. Failure of first-line eradication treatment significantly increases prevalence of antimicrobial-resistant Helicobacter pylori clinical isolates. J Clin Pathol 2008;61(10):1112–5.
33. Hylek EM. Oral anticoagulants. Pharmacologic issues for use in the elderly. Clin Geriatr Med 2001;17(1):1–13.
34. Wells PS, Holbrook AM, Crowther NR, et al. Interactions of warfarin with drugs and food. Ann Intern Med 1994;121(9):676–83.
35. Miyachi H, Miki I, Aoyama N, et al. Primary levofloxacin resistance and gyrA/B mutations among Helicobacter pylori in Japan. Helicobacter 2006;11(4):243–9.
36. Di Caro S, Franceschi F, Mariani A, et al. Second-line levofloxacin-based triple schemes for Helicobacter pylori eradication. Dig Liver Dis 2009;41(7):480–5.
37. al-Assi MT, Ramirez FC, Lew GM, et al. Clarithromycin, tetracycline, and bismuth: a new non-metronidazole therapy for Helicobacter pylori infection. Am J Gastroenterol 1994;89(8):1203–5.
38. Egan BJ, Marzio L, O'Connor H, et al. Treatment of Helicobacter pylori infection. Helicobacter 2008;13(Suppl 1):35–40.

39. Hassan C, De Francesco V, Zullo A, et al. Sequential treatment for *Helicobacter pylori* eradication in duodenal ulcer patients: improving the cost of pharmacotherapy. Aliment Pharmacol Ther 2003;18(6):641–6.

40. Essa AS, Kramer JR, Graham DY, et al. Meta-analysis: four-drug, three-antibiotic, non-bismuth-containing "concomitant therapy" versus triple therapy for *Helicobacter pylori* eradication. Helicobacter 2009;14(2):109–18.

41. Furuta T, Ohashi K, Kamata T, et al. Effect of genetic differences in omeprazole metabolism on cure rates for *Helicobacter pylori* infection and peptic ulcer. Ann Intern Med 1998;129(12):1027–30.

42. Asaka M, Sugiyama T, Kato M, et al. A multicenter, double-blind study on triple therapy with lansoprazole, amoxicillin and clarithromycin for eradication of *Helicobacter pylori* in Japanese peptic ulcer patients. Helicobacter 2001;6(3):254–61.

43. Andersson T, Miners JO, Veronese ME, et al. Identification of human liver cytochrome P450 isoforms mediating secondary omeprazole metabolism. Br J Clin Pharmacol 1994;37(6):597–604.

44. Rodrigues AD, Roberts EM, Mulford DJ, et al. Oxidative metabolism of clarithromycin in the presence of human liver microsomes. Major role for the cytochrome P4503A (CYP3A) subfamily. Drug Metab Dispos 1997;25(5):623–30.

45. Furuta T, Shirai N, Takashima M, et al. Effect of genotypic differences in CYP2C19 on cure rates for *Helicobacter pylori* infection by triple therapy with a proton pump inhibitor, amoxicillin, and clarithromycin. Clin Pharmacol Ther 2001;69(3):158–68.

46. Dojo M, Azuma T, Saito T, et al. Effects of CYP2C19 gene polymorphism on cure rates for *Helicobacter pylori* infection by triple therapy with proton pump inhibitor (omeprazole or rabeprazole), amoxycillin and clarithromycin in Japan. Dig Liver Dis 2001;33(8):671–5.

47. Inaba T, Mizuno M, Kawai K, et al. Randomized open trial for comparison of proton pump inhibitors in triple therapy for *Helicobacter pylori* infection in relation to CYP2C19 genotype. J Gastroenterol Hepatol 2002;17(7):748–53.

48. Zhao F, Wang J, Yang Y, et al. Effect of CYP2C19 genetic polymorphisms on the efficacy of proton pump inhibitor-based triple therapy for *Helicobacter pylori* eradication: a meta-analysis. Helicobacter 2008;13(6):532–41.

49. Versalovic J, Osato MS, Spakovsky K, et al. Point mutations in the 23S rRNA gene of *Helicobacter pylori* associated with different levels of clarithromycin resistance. J Antimicrob Chemother 1997;40(2):283–6.

50. Stone GG, Shortridge D, Versalovic J, et al. A PCR-oligonucleotide ligation assay to determine the prevalence of 23S rRNA gene mutations in clarithromycin-resistant *Helicobacter pylori*. Antimicrob Agents Chemother 1997;41(3):712–4.

51. Menard A, Santos A, Megraud F, et al. PCR-restriction fragment length polymorphism can also detect point mutation A2142C in the 23S rRNA gene, associated with *Helicobacter pylori* resistance to clarithromycin. Antimicrobial Agents Chemother 2002;46(4):1156–7.

52. Furuta T, Sagehashi Y, Shirai N, et al. Influence of CYP2C19 polymorphism and *Helicobacter pylori* genotype determined from gastric tissue samples on response to triple therapy for *H. pylori* infection. Clin Gastroenterol Hepatol 2005;3(6):564–73.

53. Adamek RJ, Suerbaum S, Pfaffenbach B, et al. Primary and acquired *Helicobacter pylori* resistance to clarithromycin, metronidazole, and amoxicillin—influence on treatment outcome. Am J Gastroenterol 1998;93(3):386–9.

54. Bayerdorffer E, Miehlke S, Mannes GA, et al. Double-blind trial of omeprazole and amoxicillin to cure *Helicobacter pylori* infection in patients with duodenal ulcers. Gastroenterology 1995;108(5):1412–7.

55. Graham DY, Lu H, Yamaoka Y. Therapy for *Helicobacter pylori* infection can be improved: sequential therapy and beyond. Drugs 2008;68(6):725–36.
56. Graham DY, Shiotani A. New concepts of resistance in the treatment of *Helicobacter pylori* infections. Nat Clin Pract Gastroenterol Hepatol 2008;5(6):321–31.
57. Furuta T, Shirai N, Xiao F, et al. High-dose rabeprazole/amoxicillin therapy as the second-line regimen after failure to eradicate *H. pylori* by triple therapy with the usual doses of a proton pump inhibitor, clarithromycin and amoxicillin. Hepatogastroenterology 2003;50(54):2274–8.
58. Furuta T, Shirai N, Takashima M, et al. Effects of genotypic differences in CYP2C19 status on cure rates for *Helicobacter pylori* infection by dual therapy with rabeprazole plus amoxicillin. Pharmacogenetics 2001;11(4):341–8.
59. Julapalli VR, Graham DY. Appropriate use of intravenous proton pump inhibitors in the management of bleeding peptic ulcer. Dig Dis Sci 2005;50(7):1185–93.
60. Hunt RH, Armstrong D, Yaghoobi M, et al. Predictable prolonged suppression of gastric acidity with a novel proton pump inhibitor, AGN 201904-Z. Aliment Pharmacol Ther 2008;28(2):187–99.
61. Tanimura H, Kawano S, Kubo M, et al. Does *Helicobacter pylori* eradication depend on the period of amoxicillin treatment? A retrospective study. J Gastroenterol 1998;33(1):23–6.
62. Furuta T, Shirai N, Kodaira M, et al. Pharmacogenomics-based tailored versus standard therapeutic regimen for eradication of *H. pylori*. Clin Pharmacol Ther 2007;81(4):521–8.
63. Furuta T, Shirai N, Xiao F, et al. Effect of high-dose lansoprazole on intragastic pH in subjects who are homozygous extensive metabolizers of cytochrome P4502C19. Clin Pharmacol Ther 2001;70(5):484–92.
64. Tanigawara Y, Aoyama N, Kita T, et al. CYP2C19 genotype-related efficacy of omeprazole for the treatment of infection caused by *Helicobacter pylori*. Clin Pharmacol Ther 1999;66(5):528–34.
65. Sapone A, Vaira D, Trespidi S, et al. The clinical role of cytochrome p450 genotypes in *Helicobacter pylori* management. Am J Gastroenterol 2003;98(5):1010–5.
66. Shirai N, Sugimoto M, Kodaira C, et al. Dual therapy with high doses of rabeprazole and amoxicillin versus triple therapy with rabeprazole, amoxicillin, and metronidazole as a rescue regimen for *Helicobacter pylori* infection after the standard triple therapy. Eur J Clin Pharmacol 2007;63(8):743–9.
67. Miehlke S, Kirsch C, Schneider-Brachert W, et al. A prospective, randomized study of quadruple therapy and high-dose dual therapy for treatment of *Helicobacter pylori* resistant to both metronidazole and clarithromycin. Helicobacter 2003;8(4):310–9.
68. Graham DY, Javed SU, Keihanian S, et al. Dual proton pump inhibitor plus amoxicillin as an empiric anti-*H. pylori* therapy: studies from the United States. J Gastroenterol 2010;45(8):816–20.

Current Medical Treatments of Dyspepsia and Irritable Bowel Syndrome

Michael Camilleri, MD[a],*, Jan F. Tack, MD[b]

KEYWORDS

• Pharmacology • Pharmacodynamics • Clinical trials
• Serotonergics • Opioids

Functional dyspepsia (FD) and irritable bowel syndrome (IBS) are two of the most common functional gastrointestinal disorders.[1,2] Dyspepsia is increasingly recognized as related to ingestion of food; it is currently considered to consist of two main conditions: epigastric pain syndrome (EPS) and postprandial distress syndrome (PDS), the latter characterized by early satiation and postprandial fullness/discomfort. In addition, symptoms of nausea (and rarely vomiting), bloating, and belching may also be present. A subset of patients with FD may also lose weight. Among tertiary referral patients with FD, approximately 30% of patients have delayed gastric emptying, 10% have accelerated gastric emptying, 40% have impaired gastric accommodation after meals, and 30% have evidence of hypersensitivity to gastric distention.[3,4] Alternatively, among community FD patients, there is little evidence of abnormal gastric sensory or motor physiology, and the predominant associated factor is psychosocial disturbance.[5] In tertiary care dyspeptics, psychosocial disturbance was also identified as the major factor underlying symptom severity.[6]

IBS is characterized by abdominal pain and discomfort in association with altered bowel habits; symptoms are not explained by structural abnormalities using current standard diagnostic tests.[7] The pathophysiology of IBS is still not well understood but is most likely multifactorial. Several factors, such as motor and sensory dysfunction, neuroimmune mechanisms, psychological factors, and changes in the intraluminal milieu seem to play a role (**Fig. 1**).[7,8] Recent imaging-based studies using

[a] Clinical Enteric Neuroscience Translational and Epidemiological Research (CENTER), Mayo Clinic College of Medicine, Charlton 8-110, 200 First Street Southwest, Rochester, MN 55905, USA
[b] Department of Gastroenterology, University Hospitals Leuven, Herestraat 49, Leuven B3000, Belgium
* Corresponding author.
E-mail address: camilleri.michael@mayo.edu

Gastroenterol Clin N Am 39 (2010) 481–493
doi:10.1016/j.gtc.2010.08.005
0889-8553/10/$ – see front matter © 2010 Elsevier Inc. All rights reserved.

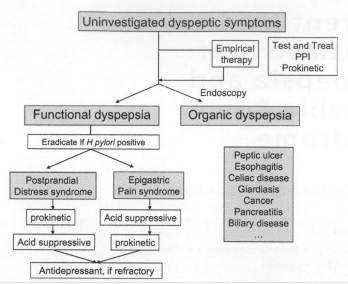

Fig. 1. Treatment algorithm for FD.

radiopaque markers or scintigraphy show that approximately 20% of patients with constipation predominant (IBS-C) and 45% of patients with diarrhea predominant (IBS-D), respectively, have retardation or acceleration of colonic transit.[9,10] The increased release of serotonin in the circulation, especially in the IBS-D group,[11,12,13] and increased serine proteases (derived from mast cells) in the stool of patients with IBS[14] provide evidence for the potential role of neurotransmitters or chemical mediators such as proteases in the disorder.

Changes in mucosal serotonin or mucosal dysfunction, immune activation, or inflammation may contribute to IBS symptoms[15,16,17,18] and, possibly, alterations in colonic bacterial flora. An increased number of activated mast cells in the proximity of colonic nerves in the lamina propria is associated with abdominal pain severity.[19] Mucosal immune activation is associated with systemic evidence for a proinflammatory state (decreased IL-10/IL-12 ratio) in IBS patients[20] and changes in local defense mechanisms in the sigmoid and colonic mucosa in IBS.[21] These provide novel promising targets for future therapies. Studies of colonic mucosal function in vitro suggest there is a barrier function in IBS patients; in vivo measurements have not provided a uniform message.

Traditional IBS therapies (see Fig. 1) are mainly directed at relief of individual symptoms (eg, antidiarrheals for diarrhea, laxatives for constipation, or smooth muscle relaxants for pain). They are often of limited efficacy in addressing the overall symptom complex.

This article reviews the current management of dyspepsia and IBS therapy (Box 1, Fig. 2); pharmacology of medications is reviewed when there is at least phase IIb or phase III evidence of efficacy or approval for use in clinical practice.

DYSPEPSIA: CURRENT TREATMENT

Patient history and physical examination allow distinction of dyspepsia from symptoms that are suggestive of esophageal, pancreatic, or biliary disease in the majority of cases. Specific attention should be given to elicit a history suggestive of heartburn or a word picture that adequately describes the heartburn. The presence of frequent and typical

> **Box 1**
> **Treating Patients with IBS in Clinical Practice**
>
> 1. The most effective treatments of IBS remain those that influence bowel function.
>
> 2. Effective secretagogues, lubiprostone and linaclotide, accelerate small bowel and colonic transit and relieve abdominal symptoms as well as bowel dysfunction in IBS.
>
> 3. Despite meta-analyses of antidepressants in IBS, the pharmacodynamics and clinical trial evidence of efficacy of antidepressants are limited.
>
> 4. Probiotics tend to relieve bloating, flatulence, and, possibly, pain in IBS.
>
> 5. Nonabsorbable antibiotics, such as rifaximin, persist for some weeks after cessation of therapy; efficacy is unrelated to result of sugar substrate–hydrogen breath test.

reflux symptoms should lead to a provisional diagnosis of gastroesophageal reflux disease (GERD) rather than dyspepsia, and patients should initially be managed as patients with reflux disease. In addition, the use of prescription and nonprescription medications should be reviewed, and medications commonly associated with dyspepsia (especially nonsteroidal anti-inflammatory drugs [NSAIDs]) should be discontinued, if possible.[22,23]

Assessing the presence of alarm symptoms is also recommended, although this has not been shown to be helpful in distinguishing functional from organic causes of dyspepsia. Patients with typical dyspeptic symptoms and no alarm symptoms are referred to as having uninvestigated dyspepsia and are managed empirically. Most guidelines advocate prompt endoscopy when there are risk factors, such as NSAID use, age above a threshold (eg, 45–55 years), and alarm symptoms, including unintended weight loss. The finding of organic disease at endoscopy determines further

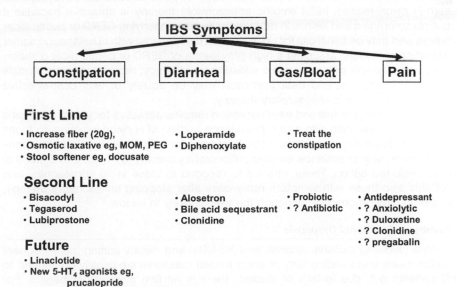

Fig. 2. Current management of IBS and potential role of therapies in pipeline for IBS. (*Reproduced from* Camilleri M, Andresen V. Current and novel therapeutic options for irritable bowel syndrome management. Dig Liver Dis 2009;41[12]:854–62; with permission.)

treatment, but when the endoscopy is negative, which is the case in approximately 70% of patients, a diagnosis of FD is made. Endoscopy is also advocated in patients with uninvestigated dyspepsia who fail to respond favorably to empiric management.[22]

Therapy in Uninvestigated Dyspepsia

The optimal management strategy for uninvestigated dyspepsia is a matter of ongoing debate and is influenced by population prevalence of *Helicobacter pylori* infection, cost of medications, and ease of access to endoscopy. The available options include (1) prompt endoscopy, followed by targeted medical therapy; (2) noninvasive testing for *H pylori* infection, followed by treatment based on the result (test and treat); or (3) empiric antisecretory therapy.[22]

Several randomized controlled trials have compared prompt endoscopy with empiric noninvasive management strategies and none has shown cost-effectiveness of the prompt endoscopy approach.[24,25,26] The available data, therefore, do not support early endoscopy as a cost-effective initial management strategy for all patients with uncomplicated dyspepsia. Nevertheless, most available practice guidelines advocate initial endoscopy in all patients above a certain age threshold, usually 45 to 55 years old, to detect potentially curable upper gastrointestinal malignancies.[27,28]

Because of the involvement of *H pylori* infection in peptic ulcer disease, several consensus panels advocate noninvasive testing for *H pylori* infection in young patients (below 45–55 years) with uninvestigated dyspepsia.[29,30] Patients with a positive test result receive therapy to eradicate *H pylori,* with a frequently advocated regimen containing a proton pump inhibitor (PPI) and two antibiotics, such as amoxicillin and clarithromycin, taken twice daily for 10 to 14 days. In contrast, patients with a negative test result are treated empirically, usually with a PPI. The benefits of this test and treat strategy are the cure of peptic ulcer disease, the prevention of future peptic ulcers, and the cure of a small subset (less than 10%) of patients in whom FD symptoms seem *H pylori* related. Initial empiric antisecretory therapy is attractive because it controls symptoms and lesions in most patients with underlying GERD or peptic ulcer disease and may be beneficial for up to one-third of patients with FD. Although earlier cost-efficacy models, assuming a high prevalence of GERD or peptic ulcer disease, suggested a benefit with the empiric antisecretory therapy, recent economic models suggest that the test and treat approach may be equally or less cost-effective compared with empiric antisecretory therapy.

Taken together, the test and treat approach remains attractive for young dyspeptic patients in a population with a high prevalence (>20%) of *H pylori* infection. In those who are *H pylori* negative, empiric PPI is started for 1 to 2 months. In populations with a low *H pylori* prevalence, empiric antisecretory therapy (a PPI for 1 to 2 months) is the preferred option. Those who fail to respond to these initial approaches, and probably also those with symptom recurrence after stopping antisecretory therapy, should undergo endoscopy, although the yield is likely to be low.[31,32,33]

Therapy in Functional Dyspepsia

Lifestyle (avoiding caffeine, alcohol, and NSAIDs) and dietary (eating more frequent smaller meals and avoiding fatty or spicy meals) measures are usually prescribed to FD patients but, due to lack of studies, there is no firm evidence of benefit. For many patients, pharmacotherapy is considered, but proof of efficacy to date is limited.

Antisecretory therapy

Meta-analyses of antisecretory therapy in FD have demonstrated significant efficacy of H_2 receptor antagonists and PPIs whereas antacids, sucralfate, and misoprostol were not beneficial.[34] A significant benefit was found for H_2 receptor antagonists over placebo with a relative risk reduction of 23% and a number needed to treat of 7, but many of these trials probably included GERD patients in a broad interpretation of the diagnosis of dyspepsia. A meta-analysis of placebo-controlled, randomized trials with PPIs in FD also confirmed efficacy with a number needed to treat of 10 and a relative risk reduction of 13%.[35] These numbers are lower than for H_2 receptor antagonists, but this probably reflects more stringent inclusion of true FD and exclusion of GERD, rather than less efficacy for PPIs. No difference in efficacy was found between half-dose, full-dose, or double-dose PPIs. PPI therapy is most effective in the group with overlapping reflux symptoms, less effective in the epigastric pain group (probably EPS according to Rome III definition), and not superior to placebo in FD with dysmotility symptoms (probably PDS according to Rome III).[22,35]

Helicobacter pylori *eradication therapy*
A Cochrane meta-analysis reported a 10% pooled relative risk reduction compared with placebo at 12 months of follow-up, with a number to treat of 14.[30] The impact of eradication therapy in FD remains limited, partly because of the low yield and the lack of a short-term symptomatic benefit. Moreover, in Western populations, the prevalence of *H pylori* infection is steadily declining, and the prevalence of *H pylori* positivity in FD patients is below 20% in many series.

Prokinetic agents
Gastroprokinetics are a heterogenous class of compounds, which act through different types of receptors to enhance gastric motor activity. Meta-analyses suggest superiority of prokinetics over placebo in FD, with a relative risk reduction of 33% and a number needed to treat of 6, but this is mainly based on studies with domperidone and cisapride, and there is a suggestion of publication bias.[34] Domperidone, a dopamine-2 receptor antagonist, and cisapride, a 5-HT_4 receptor agonist, stimulate gastric motility by facilitating the release of acetylcholine from the enteric nervous system. Cisapride, however, has been withdrawn because of safety concerns and domperidone is not widely available.

More recent studies with other types of prokinetic agents have generally failed to provide substantial symptom relief in FD. Controlled trials in FD have been conducted with newer 5-HT_4 agonists, including mosapride, which failed to show benefit, and tegaserod, with which a small benefit of unlikely clinical significance was found in the phase 3 studies.[36,37] Itopride, a mixed dopamine-2 receptor antagonist/cholinesterase inhibitor, seemed beneficial in a phase 2 study, but this was not confirmed in phase 3 studies.[38,39,40] ABT-229, which is prokinetic acting through agonism at the motilin receptor, actually worsened FD symptoms compared with placebo when administered at high doses.[41]

Psychotropic agents
Although systematic reviews suggest that anxiolytics and antidepressants, especially tryciclic antidepressants, may have some benefit in treating FD (pooled relative risk reduction of 45%), the available trials are small and of poor quality, and publication bias cannot be excluded.[41] The mechanism of action of antidepressants is unclear, because symptomatic relief from these medications seems independent of the presence of depression, and no significant effects of antidepressants on visceral sensitivity have been established in FD.[42] The selective serotonin reuptake inhibitor (SSRI), paroxetine, enhanced gastric accommodation in healthy subjects,[43] but clinical studies evaluating this class of agents in FD are lacking. A large controlled trial with

the SSRI and norepinephrine reuptake inhibitor, venlafaxine, in FD failed to show any benefit.[44]

Psychological therapies

Although clinical trials of psychological interventions (such as hypnotherapy, cognitive behavioral therapy, and relaxation training) for FD claim benefit, these studies suffer from inadequate blinding, biased patient recruitment, and problematic statistical analysis.[45] Moreover, not all patients are motivated for psychological interventions, and it is often difficult to find therapists with experience and interest in this particular area.

Investigational drugs

Novel targets in the treatment of FD are impaired gastric accommodation and visceral hypersensitivity, using fundic relaxants or visceral analgesics. Although nitrates, sildenafil and sumatriptan, can relax the proximal stomach, they seem less suitable for therapeutic application in FD.[46,47,48] Several serotonergic drugs are also able to enhance gastric accommodation, including 5-HT_{1A} receptor agonists and 5-HT_4 receptor agonists.[47,48] A clinical trial with the anxiolytic 5-HT_{1A} receptor agonist, tandospirone, showed significant benefit over placebo, whereas the novel 5-HT_{1A} receptor agonist, R137696, failed to show any symptomatic benefit.[49,50] Z-338 (acotiamide) is a novel compound that enhances acetylcholine release via antagonism of M1 and M2 muscarinic receptors. In a pilot study, acotiamide showed potential to improve FD symptoms and quality of life through a mechanism that may involve enhanced gastric accommodation.[51,52]

Visceral hypersensitivity is another attractive target for drug development. The principal drug classes under evaluation are neurokinin receptor antagonists and peripherally acting κ-opioid receptor agonists. The κ-opioid agonist, fedotozine, showed potential efficacy in FD, but development of this drugs was discontinued.[53] More recently, asimadoline, another κ-opioid receptor agonist, failed to improve symptoms in a small pilot study in FD.[54,55]

Practical management approach

In FD patients with mild or intermittent symptoms, reassurance, and some lifestyle advice may be sufficient. In those who do not respond to these measures, or those with more severe symptoms, drug therapy can be considered.[22,23] Testing for *H pylori* infection is recommended and, if positive, should be followed by eradication therapy. An early impact on symptoms beyond a reassurance and placebo effect is unlikely, and any symptom benefit, if present, is only obtained after several months of follow-up. Both PPIs and prokinetics can be used in initial pharmacotherapy. The symptom pattern may help in determining the most appropriate initial choice, but a change of drug class is advisable in case of insufficient therapeutic response (see **Fig. 1**).

A 4- to 8-week trial of PPI therapy is the first-line approach in all patients with coexisting heartburn and can also be considered in those with EPS (see **Fig. 1**). In the case of symptomatic relief, interruption of treatment should be tried and intermittent or chronic therapy can be used for patients with repeated relapses. In PDS, a prokinetic drug can be considered as the first approach. In cases of insufficient response, a switch between PPI and prokinetic drugs can be considered. Although in theory combinations of PPIs and prokinetics may have additive symptomatic effects, single-drug therapy is preferable. In patients with bothersome symptoms that persist in spite of these initial therapies, a trial of a low-dose tricyclic antidepressant may be considered, even in the absence of overt anxiety or depression, whereas SSRIs and noradrenaline reuptake inhibitors are probably best avoided in FD. Referral to a psychiatrist or psychotherapist can be considered in those with obvious coexisting psychiatric disease or those with a history of abuse or with a debilitating impact of FD symptoms on their daily functioning.

IRRITABLE BOWEL SYNDROME: CURRENT TREATMENT

The diagnosis of IBS is based primarily on the recognition of the constellation of symptoms, typically the concomitant presence of abdominal discomfort or pain in association with alteration of bowel movement frequency, consistency or ease of passage, or completeness of evacuation of bowel movements. Bloating is often present in IBS, and there is overlap with many other functional disorders, including FD and heartburn. The presence of blood passed per rectum, weight loss, or a significant change in the characteristics of the symptoms after a stable pattern over many years constitutes alarm features that necessitate further investigation, including imaging and biopsy of the colon. In the vast majority of patients, a diagnosis of IBS is safe in the absence of alarm features. In a cohort of patients with IBS-D and IBS-C, 46% had accelerated transit, and 20% delayed colonic transit respectively.[55] There is also significant overlap between symptoms of IBS-D and microscopic colitis, which is identifiable with colonic mucosal biopsies and responds well to budesonide treatment. Thus, although it is reasonable to use a symptom-based diagnosis and empiric first-line therapies (such as fiber, osmotic laxatives, or opioids, as needed), when patients first present to a primary care physician, it is important to exclude the other diagnoses or evaluate patients further, if they are not responding to treatment. For example, Voderholzer and colleagues[56] showed that if patients with constipation do not respond to fiber supplementation, they are likely to have medication-induced or slow transit constipation or an evacuation disorder.

In general, IBS therapy follows the approaches in see **Fig. 2**. It is often best to focus on the predominant symptom: diarrhea, constipation, or pain/gas/bloat.

First-Line Therapies

The first-line treatment for diarrhea in IBS is loperamide (2 mg); although the general recommendation is to administer one capsule after each loose bowel movement, this may be insufficient or it may lead to rebound constipation. Because many patients experience bouts of diarrhea lasting days, but it is not consistent every day, or patients may experience postprandial diarrhea, another approach is to administer loperamide (2 mg) on awakening in the morning for periods when patients experience loose movements and 2 mg 15 minutes before meals to try to avoid postprandial diarrhea. The liquid formula provides a convenient way to titrate the dose of loperamide, up to a maximum of 16 mg per day.

Diphenoxylate is an alternative to loperamide; caution is necessary because some preparations also contain atropine, which may result in undesirable anticholinergic side effects. There is no evidence that fiber relieves diarrhea in IBS.

The first-line treatment for constipation in IBS is fiber (12 to 20 g per day) in the form of dietary fiber or supplements. Several studies actually show that fiber aggravates several symptoms of IBS, including bloating.[57,58] For this reason, an alternative first-line therapy for constipation in IBS is the class of osmotic laxatives, such as magnesium salts (typically 1 g up to 4 times per day) or polyethylene glycol (typically 17 g in 240 mL water up to twice per day).

The first-line treatments for abdominal pain or discomfort in IBS, especially if unrelieved after relief of constipation or antidiarrheal treatment, are the anticholinergic antispasmodics. These are typically used on an as-needed basis (eg, dicyclomine [0.125 mg orally or sublingually] or [in Europe] otilonium bromide or mebeverine).

This class of drugs was recently the subject of a meta-analysis[59] that suggested some agents (eg, peppermint oil) are effective, although the trials are small, of low quality, or require replication.

Second-Line Treatments

If loperamide fails to control the diarrhea associated with IBS, and a patient continues to have significant symptoms, bile acid malabsorption should be considered and either screened with serum $7\alpha C4$ measurement or diagnosed with the[75] Se-selenomethionine retention test. If these tests are not available, a therapeutic trial with cholestyramine (12 g per day) or colesevelam (1.875 mg once or twice daily)[60] should be performed. If there is no relief of the diarrhea, the bile acid sequestrant should be stopped and a therapeutic trial with alosetron (0.5 mg once or twice daily)[61] may be considered in accordance with the Food and Drug Administration guidance documents in the United States. This medication is not available in most countries. Patients should be informed about the risk of ischemic colitis and should be advised to inform the physician if there is rectal bleeding.

If first-line treatments for constipation fail, there are two potential approaches. First, use of a simple stimulant laxative, such as bisacodyl, which has been shown effective in stimulating colonic transit[62]; a colonic prokinetic (in Europe, prucalopride is approved for chronic constipation not responsive to laxatives); or an intestinal secretagogue, specifically lubiprostone starting at a dose of 8 µg twice a day.[63] The highest approved dose in chronic constipation is 24 µg twice a day. Approximately 20% of patients experience nausea with lubiprostone. A novel secretagogue that is promising, but not yet approved, is the guanylate cyclase C agonist, linaclotide.[64,65]

Second, if the pain or discomfort does not respond to antispasmodics, many physicians prescribe antidepressants: low-dose tricyclic agents to avoid development or aggravation of constipation or standard doses of SSRIs (**Fig. 3**). There is growing

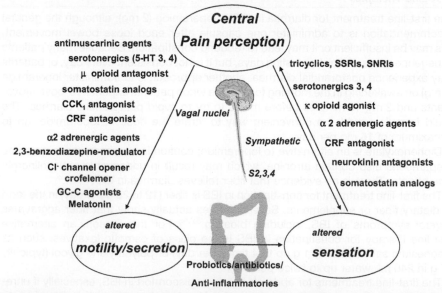

Fig. 3. Current, novel, and experimental treatments for IBS. (*Reproduced from* Camilleri M, Andresen V. Current and novel therapeutic options for irritable bowel syndrome management. Dig Liver Dis 2009;41[12]:854–62; with permission.)

appreciation that the latter medications may not be as innocuous as claimed; because they are frequently associated with sexual dysfunction, such as anorgasmia, at least 30% of men and women experience anorgasmia from antidepressant drugs with serotonin agonist activity,[66] and there is some evidence that they may affect bone density.[67] If a patient's predominant discomfort is bloating, a trial of probiotics (single species or combination) may be indicated. Single trials have been associated with evidence of marked benefit,[68] and meta-analyses are supportive, although this is controversial.[69] There is increasing evidence that the nonabsorbable antibiotic, rifaximin, results in overall IBS relief and relief of bloating in phase IIB trials.[70] In patients with severe abdominal pain, some physicians prescribe antipsychotic medications or pregabalin, although the evidence is based only on open-label or pharmacodynamic trials.[71]

What About Antidepressants in IBS?

Many patients with IBS receive psychoactive agents for comorbid psychiatric illnesses, including anxiety, mood, and somatoform disorders, and for potential effects on visceral sensation (see **Fig. 3**). Some SSRIs accelerate small bowel transit; others have effects on colorectal sensation, compliance, or tone (eg, citalopram and venlafaxine[72,73,74]).

Analyses of efficacy of antidepressants in the treatment of IBS in recent meta-analyses reached different conclusions.[75,76] One analysis estimated a number needed to treat with antidepressant therapy of 4 in order to prevent persistence of IBS symptoms (95% CI, 3–6). Few (typically, small single-center) trials, however, individually show significance; racial or ethnic differences in responses may suggest reasons why efficacy seems greatest in trials conducted in Iran and Germany.[77,78,79] The meta-analyses involved small studies; diverse medications and doses (some as low as 10 mg of amitriptyline),[77] study designs, and endpoints; questionable generalizability (because the majority of trials were in secondary or tertiary care)[75]; surprisingly low placebo response rate[78]; and funnel plot asymmetry, suggesting publication bias. SSRIs were not effective in a study of pediatric IBS patients.[80]

ACKNOWLEDGMENTS

The excellent secretarial support of Cindy Stanislav is gratefully acknowledged.

REFERENCES

1. Drossman DA, Li Z, Andruzzi E, et al. U.S. householder survey of functional gastrointestinal disorders. Prevalence, sociodemography, and health impact. Dig Dis Sci 1993;38:1569–80.
2. Cremonini F, Talley NJ. Irritable bowel syndrome: epidemiology, natural history, health care seeking and emerging risk factors. Gastroenterol Clin North Am 2005;34:189–204.
3. Tack J, Bisschops R, Sarnelli G. Pathophysiology and treatment of functional dyspepsia. Gastroenterology 2004;127:1239–55.
4. Bredenoord AJ, Chial HJ, Camilleri M, et al. Gastric accommodation and emptying in evaluation of patients with upper gastrointestinal symptoms. Clin Gastroenterol Hepatol 2003;1:264–72.
5. Castillo EJ, Camilleri M, Locke GR III, et al. A community based, controlled study of the epidemiology and pathophysiology of dyspepsia. Clin Gastroenterol Hepatol 2004;2:985–96.

6. Van Oudenhove L, Vandenberghe J, Geeraerts B, et al. Determinants of symptoms in functional dyspepsia: gastric sensorimotor function, psychosocial factors or somatisation? Gut 2008;57(12):1666–73.

7. Drossman DA, Camilleri M, Mayer EA, et al. AGA technical review on irritable bowel syndrome. Gastroenterology 2002;123:2108–31.

8. Camilleri M. Mechanisms in IBS: something old, something new, something borrowed. Neurogastroenterol Motil 2005;17:311–6.

9. Sadik R, Stotzer PO, Simrén M, et al. Gastrointestinal transit abnormalities are frequently detected in patients with unexplained GI symptoms at a tertiary centre. Neurogastroenterol Motil 2008;20:197–205.

10. Manabe N, Wong BS, Camilleri M, et al. Lower functional gastrointestinal disorders: evidence of abnormal colonic transit in a 287 patient cohort. Neurogastroenterol Motil 2010;22(3):293.

11. Dunlop SP, Coleman NS, Blackshaw E, et al. Abnormalities of 5-hydroxytryptamine metabolism in irritable bowel syndrome. Clin Gastroenterol Hepatol 2005; 3:349–57.

12. Bearcroft CP, Perrett D, Farthing MJ. Postprandial plasma 5-hydroxytryptamine in diarrhoea predominant irritable bowel syndrome: a pilot study. Gut 1998;42:42–6.

13. Houghton LA, Atkinson W, Whitaker RP, et al. Increased platelet depleted plasma 5-hydroxytryptamine concentration following meal ingestion in symptomatic female subjects with diarrhoea predominant irritable bowel syndrome. Gut 2003;52:663–70.

14. Roka R, Rosztoczy A, Leveque M, et al. A pilot study of fecal serine-protease activity: a pathophysiologic factor in diarrhea-predominant irritable bowel syndrome. Clin Gastroenterol Hepatol 2007;5:550–5.

15. Borman R. Serotonergic modulation and irritable bowel syndrome. Expert Opin Emerg Drugs 2001;6:57–68.

16. Spiller RC. Postinfectious irritable bowel syndrome. Gastroenterology 2003;124: 1662–71.

17. Spiller RC, Jenkins D, Thornley JP, et al. Increased rectal mucosal enteroendocrine cells, T lymphocytes, and increased gut permeability following acute campylobacter enteritis and in post-dysenteric irritable bowel syndrome. Gut 2000;47:804–11.

18. Spiller RC. Infection, immune function, and functional gut disorders. Clin Gastroenterol Hepatol 2004;2:445–55.

19. Barbara G, Stanghellini V, De Giorgio R, et al. Activated mast cells in proximity to colonic nerves correlate with abdominal pain in irritable bowel syndrome. Gastroenterology 2004;126:693–702.

20. O'Mahony L, McCarthy J, Kelly P, et al. Lactobacillus and bifidobacterium in irritable bowel syndrome: symptom responses and relationship to cytokine profiles. Gastroenterology 2005;128:541–51.

21. Aerssens J, Camilleri M, Talloen W, et al. Alterations in mucosal immunity identified in the colon of patients with irritable bowel syndrome. Clin Gastroenterol Hepatol 2008;6:194–205.

22. Tack J, Talley NJ, Camilleri M, et al. Functional gastroduodenal disorders. Gastroenterology 2006;130(5):1466–79.

23. Tack J, Talley NJ. Gastroduodenal disorders. Am J Gastroenterol 2010;105(4): 757–63.

24. Lassen A, Pedersen F, Bytzer P, et al. Helicobacter pylori test-and-eradicate versus prompt endoscopy for management of dyspeptic patients: a randomized trial. Lancet 2000;356:455.

25. Ford AC, Qume M, Moayyedi P, et al. Helicobacter pylori "test and treat" or endoscopy for managing dyspepsia: an individual patient data meta-analysis. Gastroenterology 2005;128(7):1838–44.
26. Delaney B, Ford AC, Forman D, et al. Initial management strategies for dyspepsia. Cochrane Database Syst Rev 2005;4:CD001961.
27. Talley NJ, Vakil N. Practice Parameters Committee of the American College of Gastroenterology. Guidelines for the management of dyspepsia. Am J Gastroenterol 2005;100(10):2324–37.
28. National Institute for Clinical Excellence. Dyspepsia: managing dyspepsia in adults in primary care. London: NICE; 2004.
29. Malfertheiner P, Megraud F, O'Morain C, et al. Current concepts in the management of helicobacter pylori infection: the maastricht iii consensus report. Gut 2007;56(6):772–81.
30. Moayyedi P, Soo S, Deeks J, et al. Eradication of Helicobacter pylori for non-ulcer dyspepsia. Cochrane Database Syst Rev 2006;2:CD002096.
31. Ladabaum U, Chey WD, Scheiman JM, et al. Reappraisal of non-invasive management strategies for uninvestigated dyspepsia: a cost-minimization analysis. Aliment Pharmacol Ther 2002;16:1491–501.
32. Spiegel B, Vakil N, Ofman J. Dyspepsia management in primary care: a decision analysis of competing strategies. Gastroenterology 2002;122:1270.
33. Rabeneck L, Souchek J, Wristers K, et al. A double-blind, randomized, placebo-controlled trial of proton pump inhibitor therapy in patients with uninvestigated dyspepsia. Am J Gastroenterol 2002;97:3045.
34. Moayyedi P, Soo S, Deeks J, et al. Pharmacological interventions for non-ulcer dyspepsia. Cochrane Database Syst Rev 2006;4:CD001960.
35. Moayyedi P, Delaney BC, Vakil N, et al. The efficacy of proton pump inhibitors in nonulcer dyspepsia: a systematic review and economic analysis. Gastroenterology 2004;127(5):1329–37.
36. Hallerbäck BI, Bommelaer G, Bredberg E, et al. Dose finding study of mosapride in functional dyspepsia: a placebo-controlled, randomized study. Aliment Pharmacol Ther 2002;16(5):959–67.
37. Vakil N, Laine L, Talley NJ, et al. Tegaserod treatment for dysmotility-like functional dyspepsia: results of two randomized, controlled trials. Am J Gastroenterol 2008;103(8):1906–19.
38. Holtmann G, Talley NJ, Liebregts T, et al. A placebo-controlled trial of itopride in functional dyspepsia. N Engl J Med 2006;354:832–40.
39. Talley NJ, Tack J, Ptak T, et al. Itopride in functional dyspepsia: results of two phase iii multicenter, randomized, double-blind, placebo-controlled trials. Gut 2008;57(6):740–6.
40. Talley NJ, Verlinden M, Snape W, et al. Failure of a motilin receptor agonist (ABT-229) to relieve the symptoms of functional dyspepsia in patients with and without delayed gastric emptying: a randomized double-blind placebo-controlled trial. Aliment Pharmacol Ther 2000;14(12):1653–61.
41. Hojo M, Miwa H, Yokoyama T, et al. Treatment of functional dyspepsia with antianxiety or antidepressive agents: systematic review. J Gastroenterol 2005;40(11):1036–42.
42. Mertz H, Fass R, Kodner A, et al. Effect of amitriptyline on symptoms, sleep, and visceral perception in patients with functional dyspepsia. Am J Gastroenterol 1998;93(2):160–5.
43. Tack J, Broekaert D, Coulie B, et al. Influence of the selective serotonin re-uptake inhibitor, paroxetine, on gastric sensorimotor function in humans. Aliment Pharmacol Ther 2003;17(4):603–8.

44. van Kerkhoven LA, Laheij RJ, Aparicio N, et al. Effect of the antidepressant venlafaxine in functional dyspepsia: a randomized, double-blind, placebo-controlled trial. Clin Gastroenterol Hepatol 2008;6(7):746–52.

45. Soo S, Moayyedi P, Deeks J, et al. Psychological interventions for non-ulcer dyspepsia. Cochrane Database Syst Rev 2005;2:CD002301.

46. Karamanolis G, Tack J. Promotility medications—now and in the future. Dig Dis 2006;24(3–4):297–307.

47. Kindt S, Tack J. Impaired gastric accommodation and its role in dyspepsia. Gut 2006;55(12):1685–91.

48. Tack J. Prokinetics and fundic relaxants in upper functional GI disorders. Curr Opin Pharmacol 2008;8(6):690–6.

49. Miwa H, Nagahara A, Tominaga K, et al. Efficacy of the 5-HT1A agonist tandospirone citrate in improving symptoms of patients with functional dyspepsia: a randomized controlled trial. Am J Gastroenterol 2009;104(11):2779–87.

50. Tack J, Van Den Elzen B, Tytgat G, et al. A placebo-controlled trial of the 5-HT1A agonist R-137696 on symptoms, visceral hypersensitivity and on impaired accommodation in functional dyspepsia. Neurogastroenterol Motil 2009;21(6):619–26, e23–4.

51. Tack J, Masclee A, Heading RC, et al. A dose-ranging, placebo-controlled pilot trial of acotiamide in patients with functional dyspepsia. Neurogastroenterol Motil 2009;21(3):272–80.

52. Matsueda K, Hongo M, Tack J, et al. Clinical trial: dose-dependent therapeutic efficacy of acotiamide hydrochloride (Z-338) in patients with functional dyspepsia—100 mg t.i.d. is an optimal dosage. Neurogastroenterol Motil 2010;22(6):618.

53. Read NW, Abitbol JL, Bardhan KD, et al. Efficacy and safety of the peripheral kappa agonist fedotozine versus placebo in the treatment of functional dyspepsia. Gut 1997;41(5):664–8.

54. Talley NJ, Choung RS, Camilleri M, et al. Asimadoline, a kappa-opioid agonist, and satiation in functional dyspepsia. Aliment Pharmacol Ther 2008;27(11):1122–31.

55. Camilleri M, McKinzie S, Busciglio I, et al. Prospective study of motor, sensory, psychologic, and autonomic functions in patients with irritable bowel syndrome. Clin Gastroenterol Hepatol 2008;6:772–81.

56. Voderholzer WA, Schatke W, Mühldorfer BE, et al. Clinical response to dietary fiber treatment of chronic constipation. Am J Gastroenterol 1997;92:95–8.

57. Francis CY, Whorwell PJ. Bran and irritable bowel syndrome: time for reappraisal. Lancet 1994;344:39–40.

58. Miller V, Lea R, Agrawal A, et al. Bran and irritable bowel syndrome: the primary-care perspective. Dig Liver Dis 2006;38:737–40.

59. Ford AC, Talley NJ, Spiegel BM, et al. Effect of fibre, antispasmodics, and peppermint oil in the treatment of irritable bowel syndrome: systematic review and meta-analysis. BMJ 2008;337:a2313.

60. Odunsi-Shiyanbade ST, Camilleri M, McKinzie S, et al. Effects of chenodeoxycholate and a bile acid sequestrant, colesevelam, on intestinal transit and bowel function. Clin Gastroenterol Hepatol 2010;8:159–65.

61. Andresen V, Montori VM, Keller J, et al. Effects of 5-hydroxytryptamine (serotonin) type 3 antagonists on symptom relief and constipation in nonconstipated irritable bowel syndrome: a systematic review and meta-analysis of randomized controlled trials. Clin Gastroenterol Hepatol 2008;6:545–55.

62. Manabe N, Cremonini F, Camilleri M, et al. Effects of bisacodyl on ascending colon emptying and overall colonic transit in healthy volunteers. Aliment Pharmacol Ther 2009;30:930–6.

63. Johanson JF, Drossman DA, Panas R, et al. Clinical trial: phase 2 study of lubiprostone for irritable bowel syndrome with constipation. Aliment Pharmacol Ther 2008;27:685–96.

64. Johnston JM, Kurtz CB, Drossman DA, et al. Pilot study on the effect of linaclotide in patients with chronic constipation. Am J Gastroenterol 2009;104:125–32.

65. Lembo AJ, Kurtz CB, Macdougall JE, et al. Efficacy of linaclotide for patients with chronic constipation. Gastroenterology 2010;138:886–95.

66. Stimmel GL, Gutierrez MA. Counseling patients about sexual issues. Pharmacotherapy 2006;26:1608–15.

67. Williams LJ, Pasco JA, Jacka FN, et al. Depression and bone metabolism. A review. Psychother Psychosom 2009;78:16–25.

68. Enck P, Zimmermann K, Menke G, et al. A mixture of Escherichia coli (DSM 17252) and Enterococcus faecalis (DSM 16440) for treatment of the irritable bowel syndrome–a randomized controlled trial with primary care physicians. Neurogastroenterol Motil 2008;20:1103–9.

69. Moayyedi P, Ford AC, Talley NJ, et al. The efficacy of probiotics in the therapy of irritable bowel syndrome: a systematic review. Gut 2010;59:325–32.

70. Pimentel M, Park S, Mirocha J, et al. The effect of a nonabsorbed oral antibiotic (rifaximin) on the symptoms of the irritable bowel syndrome: a randomized trial. Ann Intern Med 2006;145:557–63.

71. Houghton LA, Fell C, Whorwell PJ, et al. Effect of a second-generation alpha2delta ligand (pregabalin) on visceral sensation in hypersensitive patients with irritable bowel syndrome. Gut 2007;56:1218–25.

72. Gorard DA, Libby GW, Farthing MJ. Influence of antidepressants on whole gut and orocaecal transit times in health and irritable bowel syndrome. Aliment Pharmacol Ther 1994;8:159–66.

73. Tack J, Broekaert D, Corsetti M, et al. Influence of acute serotonin reuptake inhibition on colonic sensorimotor function in man. Aliment Pharmacol Ther 2006;23:265–74.

74. Chial HJ, Camilleri M, Ferber I, et al. Effects of venlafaxine, buspirone, and placebo on colonic sensorimotor functions in healthy humans. Clin Gastroenterol Hepatol 2003;1:211–8.

75. Ford AC, Talley NJ, Schoenfeld PS, et al. Efficacy of antidepressants and psychological therapies in irritable bowel syndrome: systematic review and meta-analysis. Gut 2009;58:367–78.

76. Rahimi R, Nikfar S, Rezaie A, et al. Efficacy of tricyclic antidepressants in irritable bowel syndrome: a meta-analysis. World J Gastroenterol 2009;15:1548–53.

77. Vahedi H, Merat S, Rashidioon A, et al. Effect of fluoxetine in patients with pain and constipation-predominant irritable bowel syndrome: a double-blind randomized-controlled study. Aliment Pharmacol Ther 2005;22:381–5.

78. Vahedi H, Merat S, Momtahen S, et al. Clinical trial: effect of amitriptyline in patients with diarrhea-predominant irritable bowel syndrome. Aliment Pharmacol Ther 2008;27:678–84.

79. Bergmann M, Heddergott A, Schlosser T. Die therapie des colon irritabile mit trimaprimin (Herphonal)—eine kontrollierte studie. Z Klin Med 1991;46:1621–8.

80. Saps M, Youssef N, Miranda A, et al. Multicenter, randomized, placebo-controlled trial of amitriptyline in children with functional gastrointestinal disorders. Gastroenterology 2009;137:1261–9.

Pharmacological Management of Diarrhea

Alexandra J. Kent, MBChB[a],
Matthew R. Banks, BSc, MB BS, PhD, FRCP[b],*

KEYWORDS

- Diarrhea • Secretory diarrhea • Secretion
- Enkephalinase inhibitors • Vasoactive intestinal polypeptide
- 5-HT

According to the World Health Organization, there are approximately 2 billion annual cases of diarrhea worldwide. Diarrhea is the leading cause of death in children younger than 5 years and kills 1.5 million children each year. It is especially prevalent in the developing world, where mortality is related to dehydration, electrolyte disturbance, and the resultant acidosis, and in 2001 it accounted for 1.78 million deaths (3.7% of total deaths) in low- and middle-income countries.[1] However, diarrhea is also a common problem in the developed world, with 211 million to 375 million episodes of infectious diarrheal illnesses in the United States annually, resulting in 73 million physician consultations, 1.8 million hospitalizations, and 3100 deaths.[2] Furthermore, 4% to 5% of the Western population suffers from chronic diarrhea.[3] Given the high prevalence of diarrhea, research has been directed at learning more about the cellular mechanisms underlying diarrheal illnesses in order to develop new medications directed at novel cellular targets. These cellular mechanisms and targets are discussed in this article.

MECHANISMS OF DIARRHEA

Ingestion of fluids and secretion of salivary, gastrointestinal, and pancreatic juices result in up to 10 L of fluid passing through the small intestinal lumen daily. A maximum of 16 L/d and 5 L/d can be absorbed in to the small intestine and colon, respectively. Normally, secretion and absorption of fluids are tightly regulated. Diarrhea develops

Funding support: The authors have received no funding support and have no conflict of interests to declare.
a Department of Gastroenterology, John Radcliffe Hospital, Headley Way, Oxford OX3 9DU, UK
b Department of Gastroenterology, University College Hospital, Maples House, 2nd Floor, 25 Grafton Way, London WC1 6DB, UK
* Corresponding author.
E-mail address: matthew.banks@uclh.nhs.uk

Gastroenterol Clin N Am 39 (2010) 495–507
doi:10.1016/j.gtc.2010.08.003
0889-8553/10/$ – see front matter Crown Copyright © 2010 Published by Elsevier Inc. All rights reserved.

when the balance between secretion and absorption is disrupted, and in adults, diarrhea has been defined as a stool output of 200 mL or more per day. Patients typically complain of increased stool frequency, reduced stool consistency, and urgency. Diarrhea can be defined as secretory, osmotic, or due to disordered motility. Secretory diarrhea results from excessive secretion or reduced absorption of water and electrolytes by epithelial cells, usually with little structural damage. Secretory diarrhea is commonly caused by some microbial infections, gastrointestinal hormone–producing tumors, and inflammatory mediators (eg, prostaglandins). Osmotic diarrhea occurs when there is an excessive luminal osmotic load, causing retention of water in the intestinal lumen. Osmotic diarrhea typically occurs in 2 situations: ingestion of a poorly absorbed substrate (eg, laxative use, mannitol, sorbitol) or malabsorption (eg, lactase deficiency, celiac disease). Disordered motility can lead to accelerated transit, reducing the ability of the gastrointestinal tract to absorb water and nutrients. Hyperthyroidism and irritable bowel syndrome can cause diarrhea via this mechanism.

Ion Secretion

Epithelial cells form an impermeable and selective barrier, adjoined to each other by tight junctions that act as selective pores, thus determining the permeability of the membrane. Intestinal fluid secretion results predominantly from the active secretion of chloride and bicarbonate ions. Chloride secretion relies on 4 membrane transport complexes: the apical chloride channel, the basolateral potassium channel, the sodium-potassium pump (Na$^+$,K$^+$-ATPase), and the Na$^+$/K$^+$/2Cl$^-$ cotransporter (**Fig. 1**). The opening of the chloride channels results in the movement of chloride into the intestinal lumen down an electrochemical gradient. Chloride secretion is regulated by a coordinated intracellular and extracellular cascade, involving agonists or antagonists from the intestinal lumen or lamina propria. These agonists or antagonists bind to membrane-bound receptors, for example, vasoactive intestinal polypeptides

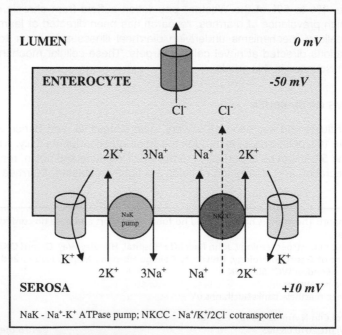

Fig. 1. Sodium and chloride secretion.

(VIP) and muscarinic receptors, initiating an intracellular cascade leading to the production of cyclic nucleotides, which enhance chloride secretion. Calcium is another intracellular messenger that binds to calmodulin. This binding creates a complex that increases adenylate cyclase and guanylate cyclase levels, resulting in elevated levels of cAMP and cGMP, which also occurs across intestinal epithelial cells. Calcium-dependent chloride channels, including the Ca^{2+}-activated channel proteins, have been described in humans,[4] and in vitro studies suggest that these channels mediate chloride conductance in the human intestine.[5] Further studies[6] show that these channels are regulated by Ca^{2+}/calmodulin-dependent protein kinase II, leading to phosphorylation and increased conductance. Inhibition of this kinase has an antidiarrheal effect.[7] Besides inducing chloride secretion, calcium also leads to a decrease in sodium chloride absorption in animal studies.[8] Apical chloride channels have an important role in overall chloride secretion, with the cystic fibrosis transmembrane conductance regulator (CFTR) being the most important. There is evidence to suggest that the interactions between second messenger systems result in greatly enhanced chloride secretion, for example, those activated by cholera toxin.[9]

Epithelial Absorption

Chloride absorption is a passive process and is dependent on concentration gradients and transmural potential differences. Sodium absorption occurs via 3 mechanisms including apical transport proteins: Na^+/H^+ exchange, Na^+ substrate cotransport, and Na^+-PO_4/Na^+-SO_4 cotransport. Sodium and glucose transport by the Na^+-glucose cotransporter (SGLT1) occurs by secondary active transport, with sodium gradients, produced by the Na^+,K^+-ATPase pump, being the driving force. This process is unaffected by pathologic processes inducing secretion. Chloride secretion is also affected by the proabsorptive neurotransmitters, enkephalins.[10] Enkephalinergic nerves extend to the basolateral membrane of enterocytes, and enkephalins bind to opioid δ receptors, inducing a selective increase in chloride absorption.[11] Water transport across the epithelium has been closely coupled with solute movement.

Intestinal secretion and absorption are also regulated by the peptide hormone, somatostatin. Somatostatin inactivates adenylate cyclase or inhibits calcium influx and potassium efflux.[12] It effectively inhibits the release of gastrointestinal hormones, including secretin, gastrin, cholecystokinin, VIP, motilin, gastric inhibitory polypeptide, and enteroglucagon. The overall effects of this inhibition are reduction in gastric emptying, smooth muscle contractions, level of gastric and pancreatic secretions, and level of chloride secretion by epithelial cells. Both somatostatin and enkephalins are potent intestinal absorbagogues, which have been utilized in the development of diarrheal pharmacotherapy.

Intestinal Secretagogues

Serotonin (5-hydroxytryptamine; 5-HT) and prostaglandin E_2 (PGE$_2$) are potent intestinal secretagogues. Enterochromaffin cells are the main reservoirs of 5-HT.[13] Studies have shown 5-HT to induce fluid secretion from human small intestine and colon. It has a key role in the intestinal secretion induced by cholera toxin, and intraluminal 5-HT concentrations correlate with the magnitude of intestinal secretion.[14] However, *Escherichia coli* enterotoxins mediate secretion through a 5-HT–independent pathway,[15] confirming the diversity of pathways in the development of diarrheal illnesses. PGE$_2$ is another potent intestinal secretagogue, with studies showing its administration to cause water and electrolyte secretion.[16] Prostaglandins increase intestinal levels of adenylate cyclase,[17] thereby increasing levels of cAMP, which mediates the secretory effect. The addition of prostaglandins to small intestinal and colonic mucosae mounted in Ussing-type chambers increases short-circuit currents and shifts in sodium and chloride fluxes.[17,18] Studies in patients with cholera have shown indomethacin (a nonselective cyclooxygenase inhibitor) to reduce fluid secretion.[19] Prostaglandins are integral to the development of diarrhea in inflammatory conditions, with the therapeutic effect attributed to inhibition of PGE_2 synthesis.[20] Relevant neurotransmitter secretagogues include VIP and substance P. VIP is a potent stimulator of cAMP in the intestine and subsequently leads to water and electrolyte secretion in the small intestine. VIP also increases pancreatic bicarbonate secretion and induces smooth muscle relaxation and is thought to be a fundamental part of the secretory neuronal reflex. Patients with neuroendocrine tumors with hypersecretion of VIP experience watery diarrhea, with the initial cases succumbing to dehydration and renal failure.[21] Substance P has been shown to change the net chloride absorption to net secretion.[22] σ-Receptors (opioid σ receptor) are found throughout the central nervous system but their function has been more difficult to characterize. Studies have shown the receptors to be densely expressed in the intestinal mucosa and submucosa of guinea pigs,[23] with a functional role in intestinal motility.[24] More recent studies have proposed that σ-receptors are important in water and electrolyte transport.[25,26]

PHARMACOTHERAPY

Various cellular pathways have been described earlier and can be used in the development of pharmacotherapy for diarrhea. Although only a limited number of drugs have been evaluated in clinical trials, there are several drugs underdevelopment with future clinical potential.

Drugs Evaluated in Clinical Trials

Oral rehydration therapy

The greatest complication of acute diarrhea is dehydration; therefore, the priority and mainstay of therapy is oral rehydration therapy (ORT). ORT involves the use of glucose-containing fluids, based on the scientific rationale that glucose promotes intestinal ion absorption.[27] SGLT1 cotransports glucose and sodium, closely followed by water,[27] a process that is largely unaffected by pathologic processes. ORT does not reduce the stool volume or duration of illness and, conversely, may increase fecal fluid loss.[28] An attempt to reduce this complication led to the development of hypo-osmolar solutions. Hypo-osmolar ORT in children with persistent diarrhea reduced stool output by approximately 40% and provided a greater resolution of diarrhea compared with standard ORT.[29] Concerns regarding an increased risk of hyponatremia proved to be unfounded.[30] The addition of nonabsorbable starch to ORT reduces fecal fluid loss and shortens the duration of illness in adolescents and adults.[31] This concept is based on the fact that short-chain fatty acids, which are produced in the colon from nonabsorbed carbohydrates, enhance sodium absorption.

Opiates

This class of drugs includes opiates derived from opium, such as morphine or codeine, and synthetic opiates such as loperamide and diphenoxylate. They bind to opioid μ receptors, inducing the secretion of inhibitory neurotransmitter, γ-aminobutyric acid. The result is complex, with increased tone and contraction of intestinal smooth muscles but overall reduced peristaltic activity. The slowed intestinal transit allows increased time for absorption of luminal contents, and constipation is a well-recognized side effect of these medications. It has also been suggested that the antidiarrheal effect of opiates may be due to an antisecretory effect. This suggestion was based on studies showing that morphine and loperamide inhibit chloride secretion in rabbit ileal mucosa[32,33] and studies in humans showing that loperamide reduced PGE_2-induced intestinal secretion.[34] However, these findings have not been confirmed by further studies.[35] Morphine crosses the blood-brain barrier, binding to cerebral opioid μ receptors, thereby exerting central effects, including sedation and hypotension. Because of these effects, alongside the risk of morphine dependence, loperamide and diphenoxylate are generally considered for first line treatment, given that they do not cross the blood-brain barrier. Codeine, loperamide, and diphenoxylate are effective in the treatment of chronic diarrhea.[36] Studies have also shown loperamide to increase the maximum basal anal sphincter pressure and the rectal volume required to abolish recovery of the rectoanal inhibitory reflex and to reduce rectal compliance.[37] Consequently, loperamide is effective in the treatment of fecal incontinence, alongside treatment of diarrhea caused by chemotherapy,[38] ileocolic disease or resection,[39] or post-vagotomy,[40] and as an adjunct to antibiotics for traveler's diarrhea.[41]

Antibiotics
Antibiotics are considered in first line therapy for infectious diarrhea only during specific circumstances. The increasing incidence of antibiotic-resistant infections,[42] treatment side effects, disruption of normal luminal bacterial flora, and the association with complications limit the safety and efficacy of antimicrobial agents. Antibiotics should specifically be avoided in case of E coli 0157 infection because of the association of the antibiotic treatment with the development of hemolytic uremic syndrome.[43] Guidelines[2] suggest situations in which antibiotic treatment is appropriate, which include the following:

1. Traveler's diarrhea, in which E coli is the likely pathogen, and treatment can shorten the duration of illness[44]
2. Persistent diarrhea, suggestive of giardiasis
3. Febrile diarrheal illnesses consistent with invasive disease
4. Clostridium difficile infection.

Somatostatin
Somatostatin is a potent inhibitor of intestinal secretion and has been used in the development of octreotide, a synthetic analogue with a longer half-life and greater potency than somatostatin. This medication has been most effective in the treatment of neuroendocrine tumors, especially carcinoid tumors, VIPomas, and gastrinomas.[45,46] However, controlled studies have also shown use of octreotide to be an effective therapy for chemotherapy-induced diarrhea[47,48] and diarrhea associated with human immunodeficiency virus or AIDS,[49] postgastrectomy dumping syndrome,[50] radiation-induced diarrhea,[51] and short bowel syndrome.[52] Case reports and series have also suggested that somatostatin analogues can be effective for treating diabetic diarrhea,[53] eosinophilic gastroenteritis,[54] graft-versus-host disease,[55] and amyloidosis,[56,57] although controlled trials are needed to support these clinical applications.

Enkephalinase inhibitors
Enkephalins are endogenous peptides that directly inhibit the production of cAMP by binding to δ-opioid receptors on the enterocyte.[58] The proabsorptive antisecretory potential of enkephalins has been exploited for the pharmacotherapy of diarrhea. Enkephalins are rapidly degraded by the membrane-bound metalloproteinase,

enkephalinase, which is found abundantly in the gastrointestinal tract. An inhibitor of enkephalinase, racecadotril (originally known as acetorphan), has been developed for the treatment of acute diarrhea. In vivo studies showed racecadotril to stop cholera toxin-induced secretion, although having no effect on water and electrolyte absorption.[59] Further studies have shown racecadotril to be effective in the treatment of acute diarrhea in adults,[60,61] with resolution of diarrhea in 92% to 96% of patients. Although efficacy of racecadotril equaled with that of treatment with loperamide, the incidence of reactive constipation was significantly less in the racecadotril group (12.9% vs 29%).[60] Racecadotril has also been effective in treating diarrhea in children, with up to 50% reduction in stool output compared with placebo[62] and also with a reduced duration of illness.[63]

Cholestyramine

The normal enterohepatic circulation of bile salts involves absorption in the distal ileum into the hepatic portal circulation. Diseases that interrupt this process lead to elevated concentrations of bile salts in the colon, where the salts can increase colonic secretion and mucosal permeability and potentially cause mucosal damage.[64] Bile salt malabsorption can be idiopathic; caused by ileal resection, Crohn disease, radiation enteritis, and bacterial overgrowth; or may occur postcholecystectomy. Cholestyramine is a nonabsorbable anion exchanger that binds and neutralizes bile salts, and studies have shown cholestyramine to be an effective antidiarrheal agent for bile salt diarrhea.[65]

5-HT antagonists

5-HT is an obvious pharmacologic target, but studies in humans investigating 5-HT antagonists have produced conflicting results.[66] Antagonists to $5-HT_2$, $5-HT_3$, and $5-HT_4$ receptors can markedly reduce or reverse the cholera toxin–induced secretory state.[67,68] However, this effect is generally observed only when antagonists are given before exposure to the toxin rather than during the illness. More significantly, when used in humans, the $5-HT_3$ antagonist, alosetron, was associated with ischemic colitis and is therefore only available with a restricted label for safety reasons. Cilansetron has been withdrawn from the market.

Calcium-calmodulin antagonists

Calmodulin is involved in calcium-dependent chloride secretion and is a natural target for the development of antidiarrheal medicines. Calmodulin binding has an antidiarrheal effect.[69] Studies that first exploited this pathway used chlorpromazine, a phenothiazine that inhibits calmodulin, adenylate cyclase, and cAMP.[70] Chlorpromazine reduced the duration of diarrhea, frequency of vomiting, and the amount of intravenous fluid required.[71] However, its use is limited by its α-adrenergic receptor–blocking activity, resulting in hypotension and sedation. Zaldaride maleate, a calmodulin antagonist, is an effective antidiarrheal agent but has no superiority over loperamide.[72,73] As a result, further development in these agents was discontinued, especially given the incidence of cardiovascular effects when used at high doses.

Bismuth

Traditionally, bismuth has been used in the treatment of dyspepsia. However, it has also been shown to act as an antidiarrheal agent due to its antisecretory,[74] antiinflammatory,[74] and antimicrobial properties.[75] Bismuth is most effective in the prevention of traveler's diarrhea,[76] more specifically by reducing the incidence of enterotoxigenic E coli.[77] A study showed bismuth to be an effective agent in the treatment of irritable bowel syndrome[78] and microscopic colitis.

Berberine
Berberine is a plant alkaloid with a long history of medicinal use in Chinese and Ayurvedic medicine. It has been shown to have in vitro activity against viruses,[79] parasites,[80] and bacteria.[81] This antimicrobial activity has been translated into the clinical setting, with trials showing berberine to reduce stool volume and stop diarrhea more effectively than placebo in cases of enterotoxigenic *E coli*.[82] There has also been a single pilot placebo-controlled study investigating the use of berberine in patients undergoing abdominal radiotherapy. Berberine significantly reduced the incidence and severity of radiation-induced acute intestinal symptoms (RIAIS) and delayed the occurrence of RIAIS in patients undergoing abdominal or whole pelvic radiotherapy.[83]

Drugs Underdevelopment

Chloride channel antagonists

The chloride channel, CFTR, is a crucial factor in the intestinal secretory process, and research has been directed at the potential of using CFTR as a pharmacologic target. In vitro studies have shown sulfonylureas (glibenclamide[84]) and nonsulfonylurea hypoglycemic drugs[85] to block the CFTR channel and inhibit chloride currents. Disulfonic stilbenes and arylaminobenzoates also block the CFTR, but in vitro studies have shown these compounds, as well as sulfonylureas, to be nonspecific, working at several cellular sites that may indirectly alter the CFTR.[86] Glycine hydrazide and thiazolidinone CFTR inhibitors reduce intestinal fluid losses in animal models of cholera toxin–mediated secretory diarrhea.[87,88] The thiazolidinedione drugs, rosiglitazone and pioglitazone, are peroxisome proliferator-activated receptor γ agonists, which are in widespread clinical use as insulin-sensitizing agents in type 2 diabetes. These drugs reduced cholera toxin–induced intestinal fluid accumulation by 65% in mouse intestinal segments, and these changes were partly attributed to a reduced expression of the CFTR-chloride channel.[89] Traditional antidiarrheal remedies, including cocoa beans,[90] bark latex of the tree *Croton lechleri* (Euphorbiaceae; "sangre de drago"),[91] boiled rice (or more specifically an unidentified rice factor),[92] and hydrolyzable tannin extracted from Chinese gallnut,[93] exert their effect through inhibition of the CFTR channel. Despite in vitro and animal studies suggesting a role for CFTR inhibition in the treatment of diarrhea, the only study in humans investigating CFTR inhibition was with SP-303, a novel investigatory agent derived from *C lechleri*. A placebo-controlled trial showed SP-303 to reduce the duration of traveler's diarrhea by 21%.[94]

σ-Receptor agonists

The function of the σ-receptor has not yet been clearly defined,[95] with the activation of the receptor leading to a variety of physiologic changes, including tachycardia, mydriasis, hypertonia, tachypnea, as well as psychotropic effects such as anti-depressive actions, euphoria, malaise, and anxiety. However, σ-receptor ligands have also been shown to have an antisecretory role in animal studies of bacteria-induced secretory diarrhea.[96,97] A small study investigating igmesine, a σ-receptor ligand, in PGE$_2$-induced intestinal secretion, showed igmesine to inhibit secretion in humans.[98]

VIP antagonists

VIP is a potent intestinal secretagogue, and a study on VIP antagonists has confirmed the role of VIP in fluid and electrolyte secretion induced by heat-labile toxins of cholera and *E coli*.[99] In cholera toxin–induced secretion in the rat jejunum, the VIP antagonist, [4Cl-*D*-Phe6, Leu17]-VIP, reduced intestinal secretion to normal levels.[100] Ultimately, VIP antagonists can inhibit the secretory responses to electric stimulation of mucosal neurons and effectively attenuate the secretory response both before and after luminal application of cholera and *E coli* enterotoxins.[99,100] The use of VIP antagonists has not yet been studied in humans.

Substance P antagonists

Animal studies have shown substance P antagonists to reduce electrolyte and water secretion caused by cholera toxin[101] and *C difficile* toxin A[102] but not by *E coli* enterotoxin.[101] The exact role of substance P in the development of diarrhea has not been clarified, and consequently, the importance of substance P antagonists in human disease is unknown. Studies have not been performed in humans, and it is unlikely these antagonists will have a major role as antidiarrheal agents.

SUMMARY

The pharmacotherapy of diarrhea remains limited, with opiates and ORT remaining the mainstay of therapy. This scenario is disappointing given the mortality and morbidity associated with both acute and chronic diarrhea across the world. Advances in the understanding of the cellular mechanisms causing diarrhea have identified novel cellular targets that can be used in drug development. Drug targets showing potential include enkephalinase inhibitors, CFTR antagonists, σ-receptor agonists, and VIP antagonists. The enkephalinase inhibitor, racecadotril, is licensed for use in a limited number of countries in the developing world and its availability is likely to increase. However, most of these new drugs need larger studies in humans before they can be used in clinical practice. However, it is questionable whether these drugs will show superiority over well-established medications, such as synthetic opiates (eg, loperamide).

REFERENCES

1. Lopez AD, Mathers CD, Ezzati M, et al. Global and regional burden of disease and risk factors, 2001: systematic analysis of population health data. Lancet 2006;367(9524):1747–57.
2. Guerrant RL, Van Gilder T, Steiner TS, et al. Practice guidelines for the management of infectious diarrhea. Clin Infect Dis 2001;32(3):331–51.
3. Fine KD, Schiller LR. AGA technical review on the evaluation and management of chronic diarrhea. Gastroenterology 1999;116(6):1464–86.
4. Gruber AD, Elble RC, Ji HL, et al. Genomic cloning, molecular characterization, and functional analysis of human CLCA1, the first human member of the family of Ca2+-activated Cl- channel proteins. Genomics 1998;54(2):200–14.
5. Fuller CM, Benos DJ. Electrophysiological characteristics of the Ca2+-activated Cl- channel family of anion transport proteins. Clin Exp Pharmacol Physiol 2000; 27(11):906–10.
6. Fuller CM, Ismailov II, Keeton DA, et al. Phosphorylation and activation of a - bovine tracheal anion channel by Ca2+/calmodulin-dependent protein kinase II. J Biol Chem 1994;269(43):26642–50.
7. Shook JE, Burks TF, Wasley JW, et al. Novel calmodulin antagonist CGS 9343B inhibits secretory diarrhea. J Pharmacol Exp Ther 1989;251(1):247–52.
8. Bolton JE, Field M. Ca ionophore-stimulated ion secretion in rabbit ileal mucosa: relation to actions of cyclic 3',5'-AMP and carbamylcholine. J Membr Biol 1977; 35(2):159–73.
9. Banks MR, Golder M, Farthing MJ, et al. Intracellular potentiation between two second messenger systems may contribute to cholera toxin induced intestinal secretion in humans. Gut 2004;53(1):50–7.

10. Turvill J, Farthing M. Enkephalins and enkephalinase inhibitors in intestinal fluid and electrolyte transport. Eur J Gastroenterol Hepatol 1997;9(9):877–80.
11. Farthing MJ. Novel targets for the control of secretory diarrhoea. Gut 2002; 50(Suppl 3):III15–8.
12. Szilagyi A, Shrier I. Systematic review: the use of somatostatin or octreotide in refractory diarrhoea. Aliment Pharmacol Ther 2001;15(12):1889–97.
13. Penttila A, Lempinen M. Enterochromaffin cells and 5-hydroxytryptamine in the human intestinal tract. Gastroenterology 1968;54(3):375–81.
14. Bearcroft CP, Perrett D, Farthing MJ. 5-hydroxytryptamine release into human jejunum by cholera toxin. Gut 1996;39(4):528–31.
15. Mourad FH, O'Donnell LJ, Dias JA, et al. Role of 5-hydroxytryptamine type 3 receptors in rat intestinal fluid and electrolyte secretion induced by cholera and *Escherichia coli* enterotoxins. Gut 1995;37(3):340–5.
16. Matuchansky C, Mary JY, Bernier JJ. Further studies on prostaglandin E1-induced jejunal secretion of water and electrolytes in man, with special reference to the influence of ethacrynic acid, furosemide, and aspirin. Gastroenterology 1976;71(2):274–81.
17. Kimberg DV, Field M, Johnson J, et al. Stimulation of intestinal mucosal adenyl cyclase by cholera enterotoxin and prostaglandins. J Clin Invest 1971;50(6): 1218–30.
18. Bukhave K, Rask-Madsen J. Saturation kinetics applied to in vitro effects of low prostaglandin E2 and F 2 alpha concentrations on ion transport across human jejunal mucosa. Gastroenterology 1980;78(1):32–42.
19. Van Loon FP, Rabbani GH, Bukhave K, et al. Indomethacin decreases jejunal fluid secretion in addition to luminal release of prostaglandin E2 in patients with acute cholera. Gut 1992;33(5):643–5.
20. Sharon P, Ligumsky M, Rachmilewitz D, et al. Role of prostaglandins in ulcerative colitis. Enhanced production during active disease and inhibition by sulfasalazine. Gastroenterology 1978;75(4):638–40.
21. Verner JV, Morrison AB. Islet cell tumor and a syndrome of refractory watery diarrhea and hypokalemia. Am J Med 1958;25(3):374–80.
22. Walling MW, Brasitus TA, Kimberg DV. Effects of calcitonin and substance P on the transport of Ca, Na and Cl across rat ileum in vitro. Gastroenterology 1977; 73(1):89–94.
23. Roman F, Pascaud X, Chomette G, et al. Autoradiographic localization of sigma opioid receptors in the gastrointestinal tract of the guinea pig. Gastroenterology 1989;97(1):76–82.
24. Campbell BG, Scherz MW, Keana JF, et al. Sigma receptors regulate contractions of the guinea pig ileum longitudinal muscle/myenteric plexus preparation elicited by both electrical stimulation and exogenous serotonin. J Neurosci 1989;9(10):3380–91.
25. Pascaud XB, Chovet M, Roze C, et al. Neuropeptide Y and sigma receptor agonists act through a common pathway to stimulate duodenal alkaline secretion in rats. Eur J Pharmacol 1993;231(3):389–94.
26. Riviere PJ, Pascaud X, Junien JL, et al. Neuropeptide Y and JO 1784, a selective sigma ligand, alter intestinal ion transport through a common, haloperidol-sensitive site. Eur J Pharmacol 1990;187(3):557–9.
27. Fisher RB. The absorption of water and of some small solute molecules from the isolated small intestine of the rat. J Physiol 1955;130(3):655–64.
28. Meeuwisse GW. High sugar worse than high sodium in oral rehydration solutions. Acta Paediatr Scand 1983;72(2):161–6.

29. Sarker SA, Mahalanabis D, Alam NH, et al. Reduced osmolarity oral rehydration solution for persistent diarrhea in infants: a randomized controlled clinical trial. J Pediatr 2001;138(4):532–8.

30. Alam NH, Yunus M, Faruque AS, et al. Symptomatic hyponatremia during treatment of dehydrating diarrheal disease with reduced osmolarity oral rehydration solution. JAMA 2006;296(5):567–73.

31. Ramakrishna BS, Venkataraman S, Srinivasan P, et al. Amylase-resistant starch plus oral rehydration solution for cholera. N Engl J Med 2000;342(5):308–13.

32. Hughes S, Higgs NB, Turnberg LA. Antidiarrhoeal activity of loperamide: studies of its influence on ion transport across rabbit ileal mucosa in vitro. Gut 1982; 23(11):974–9.

33. McKay JS, Linaker BD, Higgs NB, et al. Studies of the antisecretory activity of morphine in rabbit ileum in vitro. Gastroenterology 1982;82(2):243–7.

34. Hughes S, Higgs NB, Turnberg LA. Loperamide has antisecretory activity in the human jejunum in vivo. Gut 1984;25(9):931–5.

35. Schiller LR, Santa Ana CA, Morawski SG, et al. Mechanism of the antidiarrheal effect of loperamide. Gastroenterology 1984;86(6):1475–80.

36. Palmer KR, Corbett CL, Holdsworth CD. Double-blind cross-over study comparing loperamide, codeine and diphenoxylate in the treatment of chronic diarrhea. Gastroenterology 1980;79(6):1272–5.

37. Read M, Read NW, Barber DC, et al. Effects of loperamide on anal sphincter function in patients complaining of chronic diarrhea with fecal incontinence and urgency. Dig Dis Sci 1982;27(9):807–14.

38. Cascinu S, Bichisao E, Amadori D, et al. High-dose loperamide in the treatment of 5-fluorouracil-induced diarrhea in colorectal cancer patients. Support Care Cancer 2000;8(1):65–7.

39. Mainguet P, Fiasse R. Double-blind placebo-controlled study of loperamide (Imodium) in chronic diarrhoea caused by ileocolic disease or resection. Gut 1977;18(7):575–9.

40. O'Brien JD, Thompson DG, McIntyre A, et al. Effect of codeine and loperamide on upper intestinal transit and absorption in normal subjects and patients with postvagotomy diarrhoea. Gut 1988;29(3):312–8.

41. Riddle MS, Arnold S, Tribble DR. Effect of adjunctive loperamide in combination with antibiotics on treatment outcomes in traveler's diarrhea: a systematic review and meta-analysis. Clin Infect Dis 2008;47(8):1007–14.

42. White DG, Zhao S, Simjee S, et al. Antimicrobial resistance of foodborne pathogens. Microbes Infect 2002;4(4):405–12.

43. Wong CS, Jelacic S, Habeeb RL, et al. The risk of the hemolytic-uremic syndrome after antibiotic treatment of Escherichia coli O157:H7 infections. N Engl J Med 2000;342(26):1930–6.

44. Hill DR, Ericsson CD, Pearson RD, et al. The practice of travel medicine: guidelines by the Infectious Diseases Society of America. Clin Infect Dis 2006;43(12): 1499–539.

45. Vinik AI, Tsai ST, Moattari AR, et al. Somatostatin analogue (SMS 201-995) in the management of gastroenteropancreatic tumors and diarrhea syndromes. Am J Med 1986;81(6B):23–40.

46. Dharmsathaphorn K, Sherwin RS, Cataland S, et al. Somatostatin inhibits diarrhea in the carcinoid syndrome. Ann Intern Med 1980;92(1):68–9.

47. Cascinu S, Fedeli A, Fedeli SL, et al. Octreotide versus loperamide in the treatment of fluorouracil-induced diarrhea: a randomized trial. J Clin Oncol 1993; 11(1):148–51.

48. Cascinu S, Fedeli A, Fedeli SL, et al. Control of chemotherapy-induced diarrhea with octreotide. A randomized trial with placebo in patients receiving cisplatin. Oncology 1994;51(1):70–3.

49. Cello JP, Grendell JH, Basuk P, et al. Effect of octreotide on refractory AIDS-associated diarrhea. A prospective, multicenter clinical trial. Ann Intern Med 1991;115(9):705–10.

50. Geer RJ, Richards WO, O'Dorisio TM, et al. Efficacy of octreotide acetate in treatment of severe postgastrectomy dumping syndrome. Ann Surg 1990; 212(6):678–87.

51. Yavuz MN, Yavuz AA, Aydin F, et al. The efficacy of octreotide in the therapy of acute radiation-induced diarrhea: a randomized controlled study. Int J Radiat Oncol Biol Phys 2002;54(1):195–202.

52. Ladefoged K, Christensen KC, Hegnhoj J, et al. Effect of a long acting somatostatin analogue SMS 201-995 on jejunostomy effluents in patients with severe short bowel syndrome. Gut 1989;30(7):943–9.

53. Nakabayashi H, Fujii S, Miwa U, et al. Marked improvement of diabetic diarrhea with the somatostatin analogue octreotide. Arch Intern Med 1994;154(16):1863–7.

54. Rausch T, Gyr K, Wegmann W, et al. [Symptomatic therapy of severe diarrhea in eosinophilic gastroenteritis with the somatostatin analog octreotide (Sandostatin)]. Schweiz Med Wochenschr Suppl 1997;89:9S–13S [in German].

55. Crouch MA, Restino MS, Cruz JM, et al. Octreotide acetate in refractory bone marrow transplant-associated diarrhea. Ann Pharmacother 1996;30(4):331–6.

56. Yam LT, Oroplla SB. Octreotide for diarrhea in amyloidosis. Ann Intern Med 1991;115(7):577.

57. O'Connor CR, O'Dorisio TM. Amyloidosis, diarrhea, and a somatostatin analogue. Ann Intern Med 1989;110(8):665–6.

58. Nano JL, Fournel S, Rampal P. Characterization of delta-opioid receptors and effect of enkephalins on IRD 98 rat epithelial intestinal cell line. Pflugers Arch 2000;439(5):547–54.

59. Hinterleitner TA, Petritsch W, Dimsity G, et al. Acetorphan prevents cholera-toxin-induced water and electrolyte secretion in the human jejunum. Eur J Gastroenterol Hepatol 1997;9(9):887–91.

60. Wang HH, Shieh MJ, Liao KF. A blind, randomized comparison of racecadotril and loperamide for stopping acute diarrhea in adults. World J Gastroenterol 2005;11(10):1540–3.

61. Prado D. A multinational comparison of racecadotril and loperamide in the treatment of acute watery diarrhoea in adults. Scand J Gastroenterol 2002;37(6): 656–61.

62. Cezard JP, Duhamel JF, Meyer M, et al. Efficacy and tolerability of racecadotril in acute diarrhea in children. Gastroenterology 2001;120(4):799–805.

63. Szajewska H, Ruszczynski M, Chmielewska A, et al. Systematic review: racecadotril in the treatment of acute diarrhoea in children. Aliment Pharmacol Ther 2007;26(6):807–13.

64. Robb BW, Matthews JB. Bile salt diarrhea. Curr Gastroenterol Rep 2005;7(5): 379–83.

65. Hofmann AF, Poley JR. Cholestyramine treatment of diarrhea associated with ileal resection. N Engl J Med 1969;281(8):397–402.

66. Farthing MJ. Antisecretory drugs for diarrheal disease. Dig Dis 2006;24(1–2): 47–58.

67. Beubler E, Horina G. 5-HT2 and 5-HT3 receptor subtypes mediate cholera toxin-induced intestinal fluid secretion in the rat. Gastroenterology 1990;99(1):83–9.

68. Sjoqvist A, Cassuto J, Jodal M, et al. Actions of serotonin antagonists on cholera-toxin-induced intestinal fluid secretion. Acta Physiol Scand 1992; 145(3):229–37.
69. Zavecz JH, Jackson TE, Limp GL, et al. Relationship between anti-diarrheal activity and binding to calmodulin. Eur J Pharmacol 1982;78(3):375–7.
70. Palmer GC, Pajer KA, Manian AA. Comparison of inhibitory actions of chlorpromazine or its 7,8-dihydroxy and 7,8-dioxo-didesmethyl analogs on DA-sensitive adenylate cyclase and calmodulin activation of phosphodiesterase in rat striatum. Arch Int Pharmacodyn Ther 1985;273(2):202–11.
71. Rabbani GH, Greenough WB 3rd, Holmgren J, et al. Controlled trial of chlorpromazine as antisecretory agent in patients with cholera hydrated intravenously. Br Med J (Clin Res Ed) 1982;284(6326):1361–4.
72. Silberschmidt G, Schick MT, Steffen R, et al. Treatment of travellers' diarrhoea: zaldaride compared with loperamide and placebo. Eur J Gastroenterol Hepatol 1995;7(9):871–5.
73. Okhuysen PC, DuPont HL, Ericsson CD, et al. Zaldaride maleate (a new calmodulin antagonist) versus loperamide in the treatment of traveler's diarrhea: randomized, placebo-controlled trial. Clin Infect Dis 1995;21(2):341–4.
74. Ericsson CD, Tannenbaum C, Charles TT. Antisecretory and antiinflammatory properties of bismuth subsalicylate. Rev Infect Dis 1990;12(Suppl 1):S16–20.
75. Sox TE, Olson CA. Binding and killing of bacteria by bismuth subsalicylate. Antimicrob Agents Chemother 1989;33(12):2075–82.
76. DuPont HL, Ericsson CD, Johnson PC, et al. Prevention of travelers' diarrhea by the tablet formulation of bismuth subsalicylate. JAMA 1987;257(10):1347–50.
77. Graham DY, Estes MK, Gentry LO. Double-blind comparison of bismuth subsalicylate and placebo in the prevention and treatment of enterotoxigenic *Escherichia coli*-induced diarrhea in volunteers. Gastroenterology 1983;85(5):1017–22.
78. Iakovenko EP, Agafonova NA, Pokhal'skaia O, et al. [The use of bismuth tripotassium dicitrate (De-Nol), a promising line of pathogenetic therapy for irritated bowel syndrome with diarrhea]. Klin Med (Mosk) 2008;86(10):47–52 [in Russian].
79. Hayashi K, Minoda K, Nagaoka Y, et al. Antiviral activity of berberine and related compounds against human cytomegalovirus. Bioorg Med Chem Lett 2007; 17(6):1562–4.
80. Kaneda Y, Torii M, Tanaka T, et al. In vitro effects of berberine sulphate on the growth and structure of *Entamoeba histolytica*, *Giardia lamblia* and *Trichomonas vaginalis*. Ann Trop Med Parasitol 1991;85(4):417–25.
81. Freile ML, Giannini F, Pucci G, et al. Antimicrobial activity of aqueous extracts and of berberine isolated from *Berberis heterophylla*. Fitoterapia 2003; 74(7–8):702–5.
82. Rabbani GH, Butler T, Knight J, et al. Randomized controlled trial of berberine sulfate therapy for diarrhea due to enterotoxigenic *Escherichia coli* and *Vibrio cholerae*. J Infect Dis 1987;155(5):979–84.
83. Li GH, Wang DL, Hu YD, et al. Berberine inhibits acute radiation intestinal syndrome in human with abdomen radiotherapy. Med Oncol 2010;27(3): 919–25.
84. Schultz BD, DeRoos AD, Venglarik CJ, et al. Glibenclamide blockade of CFTR chloride channels. Am J Physiol 1996;271(2 Pt 1):L192–200.
85. Cai Z, Lansdell KA, Sheppard DN. Inhibition of heterologously expressed cystic fibrosis transmembrane conductance regulator Cl- channels by non-sulphonylurea hypoglycaemic agents. Br J Pharmacol 1999;128(1):108–18.

86. Schultz BD, Singh AK, Devor DC, et al. Pharmacology of CFTR chloride channel activity. Physiol Rev 1999;79(Suppl 1):S109–44.
87. Sonawane ND, Hu J, Muanprasat C, et al. Luminally active, nonabsorbable CFTR inhibitors as potential therapy to reduce intestinal fluid loss in cholera. FASEB J 2006;20(1):130–2.
88. Ma T, Thiagarajah JR, Yang H, et al. Thiazolidinone CFTR inhibitor identified by high-throughput screening blocks cholera toxin-induced intestinal fluid secretion. J Clin Invest 2002;110(11):1651–8.
89. Bajwa PJ, Lee JW, Straus DS, et al. Activation of PPARgamma by rosiglitazone attenuates intestinal Cl- secretion. Am J Physiol Gastrointest Liver Physiol 2009; 297(1):G82–9.
90. Schuier M, Sies H, Illek B, et al. Cocoa-related flavonoids inhibit CFTR-mediated chloride transport across T84 human colon epithelia. J Nutr 2005;135(10): 2320–5.
91. Fischer H, Machen TE, Widdicombe JH, et al. A novel extract SB-300 from the stem bark latex of *Croton lechleri* inhibits CFTR-mediated chloride secretion in human colonic epithelial cells. J Ethnopharmacol 2004;93(2–3):351–7.
92. Mathews CJ, MacLeod RJ, Zheng SX, et al. Characterization of the inhibitory effect of boiled rice on intestinal chloride secretion in guinea pig crypt cells. Gastroenterology 1999;116(6):1342–7.
93. Wongsamitkul N, Sirianant L, Muanprasat C, et al. A plant-derived hydrolysable tannin inhibits CFTR chloride channel: a potential treatment of diarrhea. Pharm Res 2010;27(3):490–7.
94. DiCesare D, DuPont HL, Mathewson JJ, et al. A double blind, randomized, placebo-controlled study of SP-303 (Provir) in the symptomatic treatment of acute diarrhea among travelers to Jamaica and Mexico. Am J Gastroenterol 2002;97(10):2585–8.
95. Leonard BE. Sigma receptors and sigma ligands: background to a pharmaco-logical enigma. Pharmacopsychiatry 2004;37(Suppl 3):S166–70.
96. Theodorou V, Chovet M, Eutamene H, et al. Antidiarrhoeal properties of a novel sigma ligand (JO 2871) on toxigenic diarrhoea in mice: mechanisms of action. Gut 2002;51(4):522–8.
97. Turvill JL, Kasapidis P, Farthing MJ. The sigma ligand, igmesine, inhibits cholera toxin and *Escherichia coli* enterotoxin induced jejunal secretion in the rat. Gut 1999;45(4):564–9.
98. Roze C, Bruley Des Varannes S, Shi G, et al. Inhibition of prostaglandin-induced intestinal secretion by igmesine in healthy volunteers. Gastroenterology 1998; 115(3):591–6.
99. Banks MR, Farthing MJ, Robberecht P, et al. Antisecretory actions of a novel vasoactive intestinal polypeptide (VIP) antagonist in human and rat small intestine. Br J Pharmacol 2005;144(7):994–1001.
100. Mourad FH, Nassar CF. Effect of vasoactive intestinal polypeptide (VIP) antagonism on rat jejunal fluid and electrolyte secretion induced by cholera and *Escherichia coli* enterotoxins. Gut 2000;47(3):382–6.
101. Turvill JL, Connor P, Farthing MJ. Neurokinin 1 and 2 receptors mediate cholera toxin secretion in rat jejunum. Gastroenterology 2000;119(4):1037–44.
102. Pothoulakis C, Castagliuolo I, LaMont JT, et al. CP-96,345, a substance P antagonist, inhibits rat intestinal responses to *Clostridium difficile* toxin A but not cholera toxin. Proc Natl Acad Sci U S A 1994;91(3):947–51.

Pharmacologic Management of Chronic Constipation

Siddharth Singh, MD, Satish S.C. Rao, MD, PhD, FRCP (Lon)*

KEYWORDS

- Chronic constipation • Medical management • Laxatives
- Lubiprostone • Linaclotide • Methylnaltrexone
- Alvimopan • Prucalopride

Chronic constipation (CC) affects 20% of the population,[1] has a significant effect on quality of life and use of health care resources including drug therapy,[2] and causes significant psychological distress.[3] Almost 85% of physician visits for constipation result in a prescription for laxatives,[2] and $821 million is spent annually on over-the-counter laxatives.[3]

Constipation comprises many symptoms such as hard stools, excessive straining, infrequent bowel movement, feeling of incomplete evacuation, and abdominal bloating; its treatment largely encompasses relieving these symptoms and restoring a normal bowel habit. An essential component of management of CC is identification and management of secondary causes such as drug-induced constipation, for example opioid-induced constipation or an obstructive lesion in the colon, the management of which usually results in resolution of constipation.

If excluded, primary constipation consists of 3 overlapping subtypes[3,4]: (1) slow transit constipation, characterized by prolonged transit through the colon owing to a primary dysfunction of colonic smooth muscle (myopathy) or its nerve innervations (neuropathy)—this usually requires aggressive medical management but may need surgical intervention[3]; (2) dyssynergic defecation, a disorder of impaired abdominal, rectoanal, and pelvic floor muscle coordination that requires both medical management and biofeedback treatment[3]; (3) constipation-predominant irritable bowel syndrome (IBS-C), seen in patients in whom abdominal pain or discomfort is the predominant symptom with usually normal colonic transit and pelvic floor function, and thought to be a result of an interaction of genetic, environmental, social, biologic,

Conflict of interest: None.

Division of Gastroenterology/Hepatology, Department of Internal Medicine, University of Iowa Carver College of Medicine, University of Iowa Hospitals and Clinics, 4612 JCP, Iowa City, IA 52242, USA

* Corresponding author.

E-mail address: Satish-rao@uiowa.edu

and psychological factors.[3] IBS-C is managed medically, using a wide variety of medications.

The treatment of constipation should be customized for each individual considering the cause of constipation, patient's age, comorbid conditions, underlying pathophysiology, and the patient's concerns and expectations. Lifestyle changes such as an adequate fluid intake, increased dietary fiber intake, regular nonstrenuous exercise, and dedicated time for passing bowel movements can be useful, but there is limited evidence to support these measures.[3] This article focuses on the pharmacologic management of constipation, not related to IBS, with special emphasis on newer agents.

PRESENT TREATMENT OPTIONS FOR CHRONIC CONSTIPATION

Several over-the-counter laxatives are available for the management of CC. However, studies using conventional laxatives were not well designed and have been summarized previously.[5–7]

Bulk (Fiber) Laxatives

Bulking agents are organic polymers that increase the weight and water-absorbent properties of stool. The efficacy and side effects of bulking agents are shown in **Table 1**.

Stool Softeners or Wetting Agents

Stool softeners are surface-acting agents that function primarily as detergents, that is, they allow water to interact more effectively with solid stool, thereby softening the stool, and include dioctyl sodium sulfosuccinate/docusate sodium (Colace) and docusate calcium (Surfak). The efficacy and side effects are shown in **Table 1**.

Stimulant Laxatives

Stimulant laxatives increase intestinal motility by stimulating the colonic myenteric plexus on their contact with the colonic mucosa, and by inhibiting water absorption. Both bisacodyl and sodium picosulfate (SPS) are prodrugs that are converted in the gut into the same active metabolite, bis-(p-hydroxyphenyl)-pyridyl-2-methane, which causes the desired laxative effect. There is limited evidence to support their use. In a recent 4-week, double-blind, placebo-controlled trial using SPS, there was a significant increase in number of complete spontaneous bowel movements (CSBMs) per week (SPS: 0.9 ± 0.1 to 3.4 ± 0.2; placebo: 1.1 ± 0.1 to 1.7 ± 0.1; $P<.0001$), constipation-related symptoms, and quality of life.[8] These agents have often been used as rescue therapy in many constipation and IBS-C trials, and their chronic use may induce tolerance. Abdominal discomfort and cramps are well-known side effects. Senna may cause melanosis coli or hepatotoxicity.

Osmotic Laxatives

Osmotic laxatives contain poorly absorbed ions or molecules, which create an osmotic gradient within the intestinal lumen, thereby retaining water in the lumen, leading to softer stools and improved propulsion. Polyethylene glycol (PEG) is a nonabsorbable, nonmetabolized osmotic agent. Electrolyte-free PEG has been used for the management of constipation. In 5 high-quality, placebo-controlled trials, PEG consistently increased stool frequency and improved stool consistency.[5] PEG was shown to be more effective than tegaserod, with a favorable adverse effect profile.[9] An open-labeled study of PEG, 17 g/d for 12 months, demonstrated that it was safe and

Table 1
Summary of the pharmacologic properties of conventional laxatives used in the treatment of constipation and evidence-based medicine recommendation

Laxative Class	Medications	Mechanism of Action	Side Effects	Level of Evidence	Grade of Recommendation
Bulk (fiber) laxatives	Psyllium, calcium polycarbophil, methylcellulose, bran	Retaining water in stool, increasing stool bulk, and improving consistency	Flatulence, bloating, abdominal distension, rarely causing mechanical obstruction of esophagus and colon	Psyllium II; Others III	B/C
Stool softeners or wetting agents	Docusate sodium, docusate calcium	Promoting luminal water binding by detergent-like action, increasing stool bulk	Intestinal cramping, irritation of throat (liquid formulation)	III	C
Stimulant laxatives	Senna, aloe, bisacodyl, sodium picosulfate	Increasing intestinal peristalsis by acting on myenteric nerve plexus; decreasing large intestinal water absorption	Abdominal discomfort, rarely electrolytes disturbance, melanosis coli	Sodium picosulfate II; Others III	A/C
Osmotic laxatives	PEG, lactulose, sorbitol, milk of magnesia, magnesium citrate	Osmotic water binding	Bloating, flatulence, abdominal cramping, in rare instances, electrolytes disturbances	PEG I; Lactulose I; Sorbitol/Milk of Magnesia III	A; A; B/C
Mixed laxatives	Dried plums	Stool bulking and osmotic action	Flatulence, bloating	II	B

Level of Evidence - Level I (Good evidence): consistent evidence from well-designed, well-conducted studies; Level II (Fair evidence): results show benefit, but strength is limited by the number, quality or consistency of the individual studies; Level III (Poor evidence): insufficient because of limited number or power of studies, flaws in their design or conduct; Grade of Recommendation - Grade A: good evidence in support of use of a modality in the treatment of constipation, Grade B: moderate evidence in support of use of a modality in the treatment of constipation, Grade C: poor evidence in support of use of a modality in the treatment of constipation.

Abbreviation: PEG, polyethylene glycol.

effective for adults and elderly patients with CC.[10] PEG may be associated with diarrhea, nausea, abdominal bloating, cramping, and flatulence, especially in nursing home residents. Rarely, electrolyte abnormalities may occur. A decision analysis model suggests that PEG is more cost-effective than lactulose.[11] Three placebo-controlled randomized controlled trials (RCTs) have demonstrated that lactulose is safe and effective.[5] Magnesium hydroxide and other similar salts (magnesium citrate, magnesium sulfate, sodium phosphate) act as osmotic agents. Hypermagnesemia has been reported in patients with renal impairment.

Dried plums and prune juice have been traditionally used for the treatment of constipation. Their effects may be caused by fiber, sorbitol, and phenolic compounds. In a recent 8-week, randomized crossover trial, dried plums was more efficacious than psyllium, with significant improvement in the number of CSBMs per week and stool consistency.[12]

The aforementioned approaches are usually the first-line agents used in the management of constipation, owing to their low cost and wide availability. However, 50% of CC patients report dissatisfaction with these therapies and concerns include unpredictability (71%–75%), bloating (52%–67%), poor symptom relief (44%–50%), or inability to improve quality of life (44%–68%).[13] Hence, several new pharmacologic classes of medications have been developed that are reviewed later (**Tables 2 and 3**).

CHLORIDE CHANNEL ACTIVATORS

Chloride channels are voltage-gated anion channels, which allow the transport of chloride ions across cell membranes and play a critical role in fluid transport, maintenance of cell volume, and intracellular pH [148]. Lubiprostone (Amitiza), approved by the US Food and Drug Administration (FDA) for the treatment of chronic-idiopathic constipation, is an oral bicyclic fatty acid that selectively activates type 2 chloride channels in the apical membrane of the intestinal epithelial cells. This activity stimulates chloride secretion, along with passive secretion of sodium and water,[14] and is mediated by a protein kinase-A independent, as well as the cystic fibrosis transmembrane regulator (CFTR)-mediated pathway.[15,16] The fluid-induced bowel distention secondarily induces peristalsis and causes laxation, but lubiprostone has no direct stimulatory effect on gastrointestinal smooth muscle.[14] Lubiprostone has low systemic bioavailability after oral administration, and is extensively metabolized in the stomach and jejunum by microsomal carbonyl transferase to form an active metabolite, M3; the cytochrome P450 system is not involved. Lubiprostone has a rapid onset of action with a half-life of 3 hours.[14]

Clinical Efficacy

Lubiprostone, 24 μg twice a day was shown to be effective in the treatment of chronic idiopathic constipation in 2 RCTs,[17,18] as well as 3 large open-label trials.[19] There was a significant increase in SBM frequency, improvement of straining effort, stool consistency, constipation severity, and global satisfaction with bowel function.

Adverse Effects and Safety

Nausea (31%), diarrhea (12%), and headache (11%) were the most common side effects. Abdominal distension, pain, and flatulence occurred in more than 5% patients who received lubiprostone. No electrolyte changes were observed up to 48 weeks.[14]

GUANYLATE CYCLASE C ACTIVATORS

Activation of guanylate cyclase C (GC-C) receptor, a heat-stable enterotoxin receptor found on the apical surface of the intestinal epithelium, promotes intracellular cyclic guanosine monophosphate (cGMP) production, and subsequent activation of the CFTR. Linaclotide is a novel 14-amino-acid peptide GC-C agonist; it activates the luminal GC-C receptor on intestinal enterocytes, with an increase in intracellular as well as extracellular cGMP. The former activates CFTR, with an increase in luminal chloride and bicarbonate secretion, resulting in increased fluid secretion and acceleration of intestinal transit.[20] The extracellular cGMP, however, helps to ameliorate visceral hypersensitivity by a direct action on afferent nerve endings in the gut.[21] Guanilib is an orally available synthetic analogue of uroguanylin, with very low systemic absorption, and is presently in early-phase trials.

Clinical Efficacy

In 2 recent phase 3 RCTs of 1200 patients, linaclotide, 150 to 300 μg/d increased the number of CSBMs per week,[20] and improved bloating, discomfort, stool consistency, straining, and constipation severity, as well as quality of life measures.

Adverse Effects and Safety

Dose-dependent diarrhea was the most common side effect, and was usually rated mild to moderate; the rate of discontinuation from side effects was 2.4%.[20]

OPIOID ANTAGONISTS

Opiate-induced constipation and postoperative ileus impose significant costs on the health care system and are mediated by the activation of enteric μ-receptors that cause inhibition of enteric nerve activity.[22] The peripherally acting μ-receptor antagonists, methylnaltrexone and alvimopan, are a new class of medications designed to reverse opioid-induced gastrointestinal side effects without compromising pain relief.[23]

Methylnaltrexone

Methylnaltrexone is a quaternary derivative of the μ-opioid receptor antagonist naltrexone. The N-terminal methylation of the uncharged naltrexone molecule results in increased polarity and reduced lipid solubility. This process prevents the drug from crossing the blood-brain barrier and affects the central μ-opioid receptor,[24] but antagonizes the peripheral gastrointestinal μ-opioid receptor. The reversal of opioid-induced inhibition of enteric nerve activity increases propulsion and secretory activity.[24] In healthy volunteers, methylnaltrexone decreases the opioid-induced delay in gastric and orocecal transit time without affecting analgesia.[24] Methylnaltrexone is approved by the FDA for opioid-induced constipation.

Methylnaltrexone's metabolism is species-dependent; in primates, including humans, it is not demethylated spontaneously.[24] Methylnaltrexone is very specific for the μ-opioid receptor. It is approved for use subcutaneously, and reaches peak concentration in 0.5 hours with a half-life of 2.9 hours.[24]

Clinical efficacy

Several trials have shown efficacy in reversing opioid-induced gastrointestinal problems, including an increased rate of CSBMs, rapid onset of first bowel movement, improvement in constipation severity scores, as well as improved overall health-related quality of life.[24,25] In a systematic review of 4 studies, methylnaltrexone

Table 2

Summary of the major newer classes of medications for CC including their indications, doses, mechanism of action, side effects, and EBM recommendations

Pharmacologic Class	Drug	Mechanism of Action	Indication	Usual Dose and Route of Administration	Dose Adjustment	Side Effects	Special Populations	Cost	Level of Evidence	Grade of Recommendations
Chloride channel activators	Lubiprostone (Amitiza)	Selective activation of intestinal epithelial chloride channel 2, increasing chloride secretion	Chronic idiopathic constipation, IBS-C	24 µg BID, orally	Not studied in hepatic and renal disease	Nausea, diarrhea, headache	Pregnancy Class C, avoid during breast feeding	$178/month	I	A
Guanylate cyclase C activators	Linaclotide	Activation of GC-C receptor on enterocytes, increasing cGMP, activating CFTR, increasing luminal chloride/bicarbonate secretion; ameliorating visceral hypersensitivity	Chronic idiopathic constipation, IBS-C	75–600 µg/d, orally	Not studied in hepatic and renal disease	Diarrhea	Class C, not studied in breast feeding	?	I	A
Opioid receptor antagonists	Methylnal-trexone (Relistor)	Enteric opioid receptor antagonism, with minimal absorption and not crossing blood-brain barrier	Opiate-induced constipation, postoperative ileus, chronic methadone users	8–12 mg (0.15–0.3 mg/kg) every other day as needed, subcutaneously	Half dose in severe renal and hepatic impairment	Abdominal cramping, flatulence, nausea	Class B, use with caution during breast feeding	$40/injection	I	A
	Alvimopan (Entereg)		Postoperative ileus, opiate-induced constipation	6–12 mg BID, 30–300 min before surgery, then BID for 7 d	Avoid in severe renal and hepatic impairment	Nausea, vomiting	Class B: avoid during breast feeding	$700 per Tx course	I	A

| Serotonergic agonists | Prucalopride (Resolor), Tegaserod, TD-5108, ATI-7505 | Selective 5-HT$_4$ receptor activation with enhancement of gut motility by contraction of proximal smooth muscles and relaxation of distal smooth muscles; cAMP mediated colonic chloride secretion | Chronic idiopathic constipation, IBS-C | Prucalopride: 2 mg daily, Tegaserod: 2–6 mg BD | Dose adjustment in severe renal and hepatic impairment | Headache, nausea, diarrhea, abdominal pain, tegaserod with unfounded concerns for ischemic colitis | Class C, avoid during breast feeding | Prucalopride (?), Tegaserod: $100–199 per month | I | A |

Abbreviations: BID, twice a day; cAMP, cyclic adenosine monophosphate; CFTR, cystic fibrosis transmembrane regulator; cGMP, cyclic guanosine monophosphate; GC-C, guanylate cyclase C; IBS-C, constipation-predominant irritable bowel syndrome.

Table 3
Summary of major clinical trials evaluating the efficacy of newer agents in the treatment of CC and other constipation-related symptoms

| | Study Type | | Patients | | | | |
	Design	Duration	N	Mean Age	Females (%)	Interventions	Key Results
Lubiprostone							
Johanson et al[17]	Randomized, double-blind, placebo-controlled, multicenter, phase 3 trial	4 wk	242	48.6	90	Group 1: Lubiprostone 24 µg BID; Group 2: Placebo, BID	1. Increased SBMs/wk (Group 1 vs Group 2; 5.69 vs 3.46; P<.001); 2. SBM within 24 and 48 h (Group 1 vs Group 2; 56.7% vs 36.9%, 80.0% vs 60.7%; P<.01); 3. Improved symptom scores for stool consistency, straining, constipation scores, abdominal bloating, and discomfort
Johanson et al[19]	3 open-label, long-term trials	24–48 wk	880 (308 + 248 + 324)	N/A	N/A	Lubiprostone 24 µg BID	Significant and persistent improvement in constipation severity [29% at 24 wk (n = 512); 28% at 48 wk (n = 281)], bloating [20% at 48 wk], abdominal discomfort [17% at 48 wk]

Linaclotide

| Lembo et al[47] | Randomized, double-blind, placebo-controlled, multicenter, phase 2b trial | 4 wk | 310 | 47.3 | 92 | Group 1: Placebo; Group 2–5: Linaclotide 75 μg/d, 150 μg/d, 300 μg/d, 600 μg/d, respectively | 1. Increased mean weekly CSBM frequency with increases of 1.5, 1.6, 1.8, and 2.3 for groups 2–5, compared with 0.5 for placebo (*P*<.01); 2. Higher rate of SBM within 24 h (Groups 2–5 vs group 1: 14.3%–35.5% vs 7.4%; *P*<.05); 3. Improved symptom scores for stool consistency, straining, constipation scores, abdominal bloating and discomfort, and quality of life |

Prucalopride

| Camilleri et al[37] | Randomized, double-blind, placebo-controlled, multicenter, phase 3 trial | 12 wk | 620 | 48.3 | 87.9 | Group 1: Placebo; Group 2/3: Prucalopride 2 mg/4 mg QID | 1. Increased proportion of patients with ≥3 CSBMs/wk (Group 1 vs Group 2/3: 12.0% vs 28.4%–30.9%; *P*<.001); 2. Higher proportion of patients with improved symptom scores for straining and stool consistency; 3. Improved patient perceived satisfaction with bowel function and constipation symptoms |

(continued on next page)

Table 3
(continued)

	Study Type	Patients				
	Design	Duration	N	Mean Age	Females (%)	Interventions	Key Results

	Design	Duration	N	Mean Age	Females (%)	Interventions	Key Results
Quigley et al[38]	Randomized, double-blind, placebo-controlled, multicenter, phase 3 trial	12 wk	641	47.9	86.6	Group 1: Placebo; Group 2/3: Prucalopride 2 mg/4 mg QID	1. Increased proportion of patients with ≥3 CSBMs/wk (Group 1 vs Group 2/3: 12.1% vs 23.5–23.9%; $P<.01$); 2. Increased proportion of patients with increase from baseline of ≥1 CSBM/wk (Group 1 vs Group 2/3: 27.5% vs 42.6–46.6%; $P<.001$); 3. Improved patient perceived satisfaction as well as quality of life assessment
TD-5108 (Velusetrag)							
Theravance press release	Randomized, double-blind, placebo-controlled, phase 2 trial	4 wk	400	N/A	N/A	Group 1: Placebo; Group 2–4: TD-5108 15/30/50 mg QID	1. Increased proportion of patients with ≥3 CSBMs/wk (Group 1 vs Group 2–4: 22% vs 42%–61%; $P<.001$); 2. Significant reduction in time to first SBM

Methylnaltrexone

Study	Design	Duration	Patients			Intervention	Outcomes
Thomas et al[25]	Randomized, double-blind, placebo-controlled, multicenter, phase 3 trial	2 wk	133 (on opiates for ≥2 wk and on stable dose of opiates and laxatives for ≥3 d with no benefit)	71	57	Group 1: Placebo; Group 2: 0.15 mg/kg methylnaltrexone, SC, every other day, for 2 wk	1. Higher likelihood of laxation within 4 h of first dose (Group 1 vs Group 2; 15% vs 48%; $P<.01$); 2. Short median time to laxation (Group 1 vs Group 2; >48 h vs 6.3 h; $P<.001$); 3. Improved scores on stool consistency, constipation distress scores; 4. Stable pain scores and no symptoms of opioid withdrawal

Alvimopan

Study	Design	Duration	Patients			Intervention	Outcomes
Büchler et al[29]	Randomized, double-blind, placebo-controlled, multicenter, phase 3 trial	7 d	911 (undergoing small or large bowel resection)	64	45	Group 1: Oral Placebo; Group 2/3: Alvimopan 6/12 mg BID administered 2 h before surgery, then BID until discharge or for 7 d; opiates administered for pain via PCA or boluses	1. Quicker time to recovery of gastrointestinal function (Group 1 vs Group 2 vs Group 3: 92.6 h vs 84.2 h vs 87.8 h; $P<.05$ for group 2 vs 1); 2. In post hoc analysis of patients who received PCA, significantly quicker time to recovery for groups 2/3 as compared with group 1; 3. No reversal of analgesia

(continued on next page)

Table 3
(continued)

	Study Type		Patients			Interventions	Key Results
	Design	Duration	N	Mean Age	Females (%)		
Ludwig et al[30]	Randomized, double-blind, placebo-controlled, multicenter, phase 3 trial	7 d	654 (undergoing laparotomy for partial small- or large-bowel resection, with IV PCA opiates	59	50	Group 1: Oral placebo; Group 2: Alvimopan 12 mg BID PO administered 30–90 min before surgery, then BID until discharge or for 7 d	1. Hazard ratio of time to gastrointestinal recovery compared with group 1: 1.5 (1.29–1.82) [*P*<.001]; 2. Mean postoperative LOS 1 d less for group 2 vs group 1 (5.2 d vs 6.2 d; *P*<.001)
NKTR-118							
Webster et al[32]	Randomized, double-blind, placebo-controlled, multicenter, phase 2 trial	4 wk	208 (being treated for moderate to severe pain with 30–1000 morphine equivalent units)	N/A	N/A	Group 1: Placebo; Group 2: NKTR-118 5 mg PO QID Group 3: NKTR-118 25 mg PO QID; Group 4: NKTR-118 50 mg PO QID	1. Mean increase in the mean number of SBMs/wk as compared with baseline (Group 1 vs Group 3: 1.9 vs 3.6, *P*<.005; Group 1 vs Group 4: 1.9 vs 4.4, *P*<.001); 2. Shorter median time to first BM (Group 1 vs Group 3: 48.6 h vs 6.6 h, *P* = .001; Group 1 vs Group 4: 44.9 h vs 2.9 h, *P*<.002); 3. No reversal of opioid-mediated analgesia

Neurotrophin-3

| Parkman et al[42] | Randomized, double-blind, placebo-controlled, dose- and dose-interval ranging study, multicenter, phase 2 trial | 4 wk | 107 | 43.5 | 91 | Group 1: Placebo TTW; Group 2: NT-3 3 mg QW; Group 3: NT-3 3 mg TTW; Group 4: NT-3 9 mg QW; Group 5: NT-3 9 mg TTW; Group 6: NT-3 9 mg TTW × 1 wk followed by 9 mg QW × 3 wk | 1. Significant increase in mean weekly CSBM frequency in a dose-dependent manner, with increase of 5.7 CSBMs/ wk with group 5; 2. Trend toward improvement (softening) of stool form, ease of stool passage, and in other constipation-related symptoms, as well as in colonic transit |

Abbreviations: BID, twice a day; (C)SBM, (complete) spontaneous bowel movements; IV, intravenous; LOS, length of stay; N/A, not available; PCA, patient-controlled analgesia; PO, by mouth; QID, every day; QW, once a week; TTW, 3 times per week.

reduced the gastrointestinal transit time by approximately 52 minutes (95% confidence interval, −73 to −32 minutes), compared with placebo, without affecting the centrally mediated effects of analgesia.[26] Recent cost-effective analysis suggests that methylnaltrexone is cost-effective.[27] Early phase 2 trials of methylnaltrexone in the prevention of postoperative ileus have also shown promising results with an accelerated time to first bowel movement (methylnaltrexone, 0.3 mg/kg intravenously vs placebo; 1.1 hours vs 3.0 hours; $P<.01$) and discharge eligibility (119 hours vs 149 hours, respectively; $P<.05$).[23]

Adverse effects and safety

The most common adverse effects are abdominal cramping (approximately 28%), flatulence (approximately13%), nausea (approximately 11%), and dizziness (approximately 7%). At plasma concentrations greater than 1400 ng/mL, methylnaltrexone can cause transient and self-limited orthostatic hypotension; this is seldom seen at the usual therapeutic dose of 0.3 mg/kg subcutaneously.[24] The long-term use of methylnaltrexone has not been evaluated.

Alvimopan

Alvimopan is a quaternary μ-opioid receptor antagonist that exists in the zwitterion form, and this polarity restricts gastrointestinal absorption and prevents the drug from crossing the blood-brain barrier. Hence, like methylnaltrexone, it reverses the μ-opioid receptor-mediated inhibition of orocecal transit, without affecting centrally mediated effects such as analgesia or pupillary constriction.[28] Alvimopan accelerates colonic transit in healthy individuals, suggestive of a prokinetic effect. Alvimopan has a poor oral bioavailability of only 6%, resulting in predominantly gut-limited activity. As compared with methylnaltrexone, alvimopan has a higher binding affinity for human μ-opioid receptors and is more potent. Also, unlike methylnaltrexone, alvimopan undergoes enteric flora mediated amide hydrolysis, with an active metabolite, ADL-08-0011, which seems to be absorbed systemically, and in vitro is equipotent to alvimopan, but its contribution to clinical effectiveness in vivo is not known.[28] The major route of excretion is fecal, and there does not seem to be any relationship between renal function and alvimopan.

Clinical efficacy

Several studies in opiate-induced bowel dysfunction have shown that alvimopan decreases the median time to first bowel movement, increases mean weekly bowel movements, and reduces hard stools and the need for severe straining without compromising patient analgesia.[28] Multiple RCTs in patients undergoing bowel resection or total abdominal hysterectomy, and receiving opioid-based patient-controlled analgesia (PCA), have shown that alvimopan 6 or 12 mg orally, given 30 to 300 minutes before surgery, followed by twice-daily administration for 7 days or until hospital discharge, reduced the time to pass flatus and to discharge without pain and with improved tolerance to food and passage of bowel movements.[28–30] In a systematic review of 5 RCTs assessing 2225 patients at risk for postoperative ileus, alvimopan resulted in a 4% absolute risk reduction.[26] Cost-effective analysis has shown that alvimopan use reduces the mean length of hospital stay by 1 day compared with placebo, resulting in hospital cost savings of $879 to $977 per patient.[31]

Adverse effects and safety

The most common side effects include nausea and vomiting.[26] There was concern that alvimopan might increase cardiovascular adverse events; these were noted in patients with established coronary artery disease, but were not dose-related.[28]

Alvimopan is approved for the management of postoperative ileus, with a risk evaluation and mitigation strategy, that is, restricted to inpatient use only.

NKTR-118 is an investigational orally acting peripheral opioid antagonist that is being studied in opiate-induced constipation. Early studies show an increase in the number of SBMs per week, with no reversal of opioid-induced analgesia.[32]

SEROTONERGIC ENTEROKINETIC AGENTS

Serotonin (5-hydroxytryptamine; 5-HT) is produced from gastrointestinal mucosal enterochromaffin (EC) cells.[33] Of the 14 subtypes of the 5-HT receptor family, $5\text{-}HT_3$ and $5\text{-}HT_4$ are the most extensively studied.[33] The $5\text{-}HT_4$ receptors are G-protein coupled receptors found on smooth muscle cells, EC cells, myenteric plexus neurons, and intrinsic pathway primary afferent neurons, and they alter gut motility. Activation of these receptors augments peristalsis by stimulating secondary messengers (acetylcholine and calcitonin gene-related peptide), enhancing proximal smooth muscle contraction, and relaxing distal smooth muscles resulting in effective peristalsis.[33] These receptors also modulate cyclic adenosine monophosphate–mediated chloride secretion and visceral sensitivity.[33] The $5\text{-}HT_3$ is a ligand-gated ion channel. Antagonism of $5\text{-}HT_3$ receptors decreases postprandial colonic motility and delays colonic transit.[33]

5-HT₄ Receptor Agonists

Three $5\text{-}HT_4$ receptor agonists have been tested for constipation: indoles (eg, tegaserod), substituted benzamides (eg, cisapride, mosapride, renzapride), and dihydrobenzofurancarboxamide (eg, prucalopride).

Tegaserod is a selective $5\text{-}HT_4$ agonist. Several RCTs have shown that tegaserod is effective in the treatment of CC, by improving CSBM per week, decreasing straining, bloating, and abdominal distension, at doses of 2 to 6 mg twice a day, orally.[34] Common side effects included transient diarrhea, abdominal pain, headache, and nasopharyngitis. Because of a numerically higher incidence of ischemic cardiovascular adverse events, tegaserod was withdrawn in March 2007.[35] At present, tegaserod is available only on a restricted basis for use in IBS-C and CC in women younger than 55 years who are not at risk for cardiovascular events.

Prucalopride, a dihydrobenzofurancarboxamide, is a highly selective, high-affinity $5\text{-}HT_4$ receptor agonist, with minimal activity at other 5-HT receptors.[36] Prucalopride has a 90% bioavailability after oral ingestion, with a half-life of 24 to 30 hours. Unlike cisapride and erythromycin, it does not undergo CYP3A4 metabolism, and hence has low potential for drug-drug interactions.[36] Three large phase 3 RCTs have demonstrated efficacy in relieving all aspects of constipation (see **Table 2**).[37,38] During an open-label continuation for approximately 12 to 24 months, patients' satisfaction with tegaserod was maintained. No incremental benefit was noted with the 4-mg dose.[36] The drug is well tolerated; the most common side effects are headache, nausea, abdominal pain, and diarrhea. Of importance, no clinical cardiovascular side effects have been noted.

TD-5108 (Velusetrag) and ATI-7505 (Norcisapride) are orally active, selective $5\text{-}HT_4$ receptor agonists under development for the management of CC. An early phase 2 study of TD-5108 in patients with CC identified a dose-dependent increase in colonic and orocecal transit and a significant efficacy in the management of constipation.[39] ATI-7505 is more selective than cisapride, with minimal activity on the hERG channel. Early phase 2 trials have demonstrated efficacy at a dose of 80 mg twice a day with an increase in the frequency of SBMs, without serious side effects.[40]

NEUROTROPHIN-3

Neurotrophin-3 (NT-3) belongs to a family of protein growth factors, neurotrophins that play an important role in the development and maintenance of the central, peripheral, autonomic, and enteric nervous systems.[41] NT-3 increases or decreases absorption, rather than serving as a promotility agent.[41] After trials demonstrated an increase in the frequency of SBMs as well as scintigraphically proven acceleration of gastrointestinal transit, a multicenter RCT showed that NT-3, at a dose of 9 mg subcutaneously 3 times per week, significantly increased SBMs, softened stool and ease of passage, improved constipation-related symptoms, and decreased colonic transit time.[42] The drug can be administered only by a subcutaneous injection. Minor injection site reactions (approximately 33%) were the most common adverse events. After 4 weeks of therapy, approximately 50% of patients developed anti-NT3 antibodies.[42]

COLCHICINE

Colchicine is a plant alkaloid regularly used to treat acute gouty arthritis and familial Mediterranean fever. Colchicine's side effect of diarrhea forms the basis for its use for constipation. Colchicine may increase prostaglandin synthesis, induce intestinal secretion, and alter gastrointestinal motility.[43] Data from 2 small RCTs of colchicine, 1 mg/d to 0.6 mg 3 times a day, demonstrated an increase in the number of SBMs and reduced colonic transit time as compared with baseline and placebo.[43–45] Oral colchicine was found to be effective in treating refractory constipation in developmentally challenged patients. Long-term therapy with colchicine delivered by mouth is safe, and has very few adverse effects. The most common side effects are diarrhea; nausea, vomiting, and abdominal pain. Neuropathy and myopathy are rare side effects.[43]

MOTILIN AGONISTS

Motilin is a 22-amino-acid peptide, secreted from EC cells, that stimulates gut motility through activation of a G-protein–coupled motilin receptor found in the enteric nervous system and intestinal smooth muscle.[45] Recently a nonantibiotic, orally active motilin agonist, Mitemcinal, has been developed and is in phase 2 trials for IBS and gastroparesis, and is also being considered for CC.[46]

PROBIOTICS AND PREBIOTICS

Probiotics are defined as live organisms that when ingested in adequate amounts exert a health benefit to the host (eg, lactic acid bacteria, Lactobacillus species, and nonpathogenic yeasts). Prebiotics are defined as nondigestible, but fermentable, foods that beneficially affect the host by selectively stimulating the growth and activity of one species or a limited number of species of bacteria in the colon. Synbiotics are defined as a combination of a probiotic and a prebiotic, aiming to increase the survival and activity of proven probiotics in vivo and stimulating indigenous bifidobacteria and lactobacilli.[6] Data on their effect on CC are lacking. Bifidobacterium animalis has been shown to accelerate colonic transit in healthy individuals and patients with IBS, suggesting a direct effect on colonic motility. Two RCTs have shown a positive benefit for the probiotics Lactobacillus casei and Bifidobacterium lactis DN-173,010.[6]

SUMMARY

In conclusion, with the increasing awareness of a high prevalence and effect on health-related quality of life and the large unmet therapeutic needs, there is a new-found interest in developing novel and effective therapeutic agents for CC. The development of novel agents directed at correcting the underlying pathophysiology together with well-designed rigorous clinical trials should improve the management of patients with CC.

REFERENCES

1. Higgins PD, Johanson JF. Epidemiology of constipation in North America: a systematic review. Am J Gastroenterol 2004;99:750–9.
2. Dennison C, Prasad M, Lloyd A, et al. The health-related quality of life and economic burden of constipation. Pharmacoeconomics 2005;23:461–76.
3. Rao SS. Constipation: evaluation and treatment of colonic and anorectal motility disorders. Gastroenterol Clin North Am 2007;36:687–711.
4. Lembo A, Camilleri M. Chronic constipation. N Engl J Med 2003;349:1360–8.
5. Ramkumar D, Rao SS. Efficacy and safety of traditional medical therapies for chronic constipation: systematic review. Am J Gastroenterol 2005;100:936–71.
6. Emmanuel AV, Tack J, Quigley EM, et al. Pharmacological management of constipation. Neurogastroenterol Motil 2009;21:41–54.
7. Tramonte S, Brand M, Mulrow C, et al. The treatment of chronic constipation in adults. A systematic review. J Gen Intern Med 1997;12:15–24.
8. Mueller-Lissner S, Kamm MA, Wald A, et al. Multicenter, 4-week, double-blind, randomized, placebo-controlled trial of sodium picosulfate in patients with chronic constipation. Am J Gastroenterol 2010;105:897–903.
9. Dipalma JA, Cleveland MV, McGowan J, et al. A randomized, multicenter, placebo-controlled trial of polyethylene glycol laxative for chronic treatment of chronic constipation. Am J Gastroenterol 2007;102:1436–41.
10. Di Palma JA, Cleveland MV, McGowan J, et al. An open-label study of chronic polyethylene glycol laxative use in chronic constipation. Aliment Pharmacol Ther 2007;25:703–8.
11. Guest JF, Clegg JP, Helter MT. Cost-effectiveness of macrogol 4000 compared to lactulose in the treatment of chronic functional constipation in the UK. Curr Med Res Opin 2008;24:1841–52.
12. Rao SS, Paulson J, Donahue R, et al. Investigation of dried plums in constipation—a randomized controlled trial. Am J Gastroenterol 2009;104:S496.
13. Johanson JF, Kralstein J. Chronic constipation: a survey of the patient perspective. Aliment Pharmacol Ther 2007;25:599–608.
14. Lacy BE, Levy LC. Lubiprostone: a novel treatment for chronic constipation. Clin Interv Aging 2008;3:357–64.
15. MacDonald KD, McKenzie KR, Henderson MJ, et al. Lubiprostone activates non-CFTR-dependent respiratory epithelial chloride secretion in cystic fibrosis mice. Am J Physiol Lung Cell Mol Physiol 2008;295:L933–40.
16. Bijvelds MJ, Bot AG, Escher JC, et al. Activation of intestinal Cl– secretion by lubiprostone requires the cystic fibrosis transmembrane conductance regulator. Gastroenterology 2009;137:976–85.
17. Johanson JF, Morton D, Geenen J, et al. Multicenter, 4-week, double-blind, randomized, placebo-controlled trial of lubiprostone, a locally-acting type-2 chloride channel activator, in patients with chronic constipation. Am J Gastroenterol 2008;103:170–7.

18. Barish CF, Drossman D, Johanson JF, et al. Efficacy and safety of lubiprostone in patients with chronic constipation. Dig Dis Sci 2010;55:1090–7.

19. Johanson JF, Panas R, Holland PC, et al. Long-term efficacy of lubiprostone for the treatment of chronic constipation. Gastroenterology 2006;130:A317.

20. Lembo A, Schneier H, Lavins BJ, et al. Efficacy and safety of once daily linaclotide administered orally for 12-weeks in patients with chronic constipation: results from 2 randomized, double-blind, placebo-controlled phase 3 trials. Gastroenterology 2010;138:S53–4.

21. Bueno C, Beaufraud C, Mahajan-Miklos S. Anti-nociceptive actions of MD-1100, a novel therapeutic agent for C-IBS, in animal models of visceral pain. Am J Gastroenterol 2004;99:A283.

22. De Schepper HU, Cremonini F, Park MI, et al. Opioids and the gut: pharmacology and current clinical experience. Neurogastroenterol Motil 2004;16:383–94.

23. Becker G, Blum HE. Novel opioid antagonists for opioid-induced bowel dysfunction and postoperative ileus. Lancet 2009;373:1198–206.

24. Yuan CS, Israel RJ. Methylnaltrexone, a novel peripheral opioid receptor antagonist for the treatment of opioid side effects. Expert Opin Investig Drugs 2006;15:541–52.

25. Thomas J, Karver S, Cooney GA, et al. Methylnaltrexone for opioid-induced constipation in advanced illness. N Engl J Med 2008;358:2332–43.

26. McNicol ED, Boyce D, Schumann R, et al. Mu-opioid antagonists for opioid-induced bowel dysfunction. Cochrane Database Syst Rev 2008;2:CD006332.

27. Earnshaw SR, Klok RM, Iyer S, et al. Review article: methylnaltrexone bromide for the treatment of opioid-induced constipation in patients with advanced illness—a cost-effectiveness analysis. Aliment Pharmacol Ther 2010;31:911–21.

28. Bream-Rouwenhorst HR, Cantrell MA. Alvimopan for postoperative ileus. Am J Health Syst Pharm 2009;66:1267–77.

29. Büchler MW, Seiler CM, Monson JR, et al. Clinical trial: alvimopan for the management of post-operative ileus after abdominal surgery: results of an international randomized, double-blind, multicentre, placebo-controlled clinical study. Aliment Pharmacol Ther 2008;28:312–25.

30. Ludwig K, Enker WE, Delaney CP, et al. Gastrointestinal tract recovery in patients undergoing bowel resection: results of a randomized trial of alvimopan and placebo with a standardized accelerated postoperative care pathway. Arch Surg 2008;143:1098–105.

31. Bell TJ, Poston SA, Kraft MD, et al. Economic analysis of alvimopan in North American Phase III efficacy trials. Am J Health Syst Pharm 2009;66:1362–8.

32. Webster L, Blonsky ER, Matz P, et al. Efficacy, safety and pharmacokinetics of oral NKTR-118 in patients with opioid-induced constipation: results of a randomized, double-blind, placebo-controlled phase 2 study. Am J Gastroenterol 2009;104:S174.

33. Cash BD, Chey WD. Review article: the role of serotonergic agents in the treatment of patients with primary chronic constipation. Aliment Pharmacol Ther 2005;22:1047–60.

34. Johanson JF, Wald A, Tougas G, et al. Effect of tegaserod in chronic constipation: a randomized, double-blind, controlled trial. Clin Gastroenterol Hepatol 2004;2:796–805.

35. Thompson CA. Novartis suspends tegaserod sales at FDA's request. Am J Health Syst Pharm 2007;64:1020.

36. Camilleri M, Deiteren A. Prucalopride for constipation. Expert Opin Pharmacother 2010;11:451–61.

37. Camilleri M, Kerstens R, Rykx A, et al. A placebo-controlled trial of prucalopride for severe chronic constipation. N Engl J Med 2008;358:2344–54.
38. Quigley EM, Vandeplassche L, Kerstens R, et al. Clinical trial: the efficacy, impact on quality of life, and safety and tolerability of prucalopride in severe chronic constipation—a 12-week, randomized, double-blind, placebo-controlled study. Aliment Pharmacol Ther 2009;29:315–28.
39. Manini ML, Camilleri M, Goldberg M, et al. Effects of Velusetrag (TD-5108) on gastrointestinal transit and bowel function in health and pharmacokinetics in health and constipation. Neurogastroenterol Motil 2010;22:42–9.
40. Aryx Web site. Available at: http://www.aryx.com/wt/page/ati7505. Accessed April 15, 2010.
41. Coulie B, Szarka LA, Camilleri M, et al. Recombinant human neurotrophic factors accelerate colonic transit and relieve constipation in humans. Gastroenterology 2000;119:41–50.
42. Parkman HP, Rao SS, Reynolds JC, et al, Functional Constipation Study Investigators. Neurotrophin-3 improves functional constipation. Am J Gastroenterol 2003;98:1338–47.
43. Verne GN, Davis RH, Robinson ME, et al. Treatment of chronic constipation with colchicine: randomized, double-blind, placebo-controlled, crossover trial. Am J Gastroenterol 2003;98:1112–6.
44. Taghavi SA, Shabani S, Mehramiri A, et al. Colchicine is effective for short-term treatment of slow transit constipation: a double-blind placebo-controlled clinical trial. Int J Colorectal Dis 2010;25:389–94.
45. Feighner SD, Tan CP, McKee KK, et al. Receptor for motilin identified in the human gastrointestinal system. Science 1999;284:2184–8.
46. Peeters TL. GM-611 (Chugai Pharmaceutical). Curr Opin Investig Drugs 2001;2:555–7.
47. Lembo AJ, Kurtz CB, Macdougall JE, et al. Efficacy of linaclotide for patients with chronic constipation. Gastroenterology 2010;138:886–95.

The Safety of Drugs Used in Acid-related Disorders and Functional Gastrointestinal Disorders

Neehar Parikh, MD, Colin W. Howden, MD*

KEYWORDS

- Acid-related disorders • Functional gastrointestinal disorders
- Proton pump inhibitors • H$_2$-receptor antagonists
- Prokinetic agents • Serotonergic agents

Acid-related disorders and functional gastrointestinal disorders (FGIDs) are associated with morbidity and impairment of quality of life. However, with the exception of complicated peptic ulcer disease, these disorders do not have appreciable mortality. Treatments for these disorders have consequently been held to a high standard of safety and tolerability by regulatory authorities. Some agents for FGIDs have been withdrawn or restricted based on assessments and perceptions of unfavorable risk/benefit profiles. For most of the agents discussed in this article, the risk of serious toxicity is low. However, even low risks must be weighed against potential benefit. There is no justification for continuing any treatment that is not having an appreciable positive effect on a patient's symptoms; in the absence of discernable benefit, any risk is unacceptable.

Financial disclosure information: Dr Neehar Parikh has no relationships to disclose. Dr Colin W. Howden has, at various times, been a paid consultant for Takeda Pharmaceuticals North America, Takeda Global Research and Development, Santarus Inc, Novartis Consumer Health, Novartis Oncology, Tercica, Procter & Gamble, Merck/Schering-Plough Healthcare, Xenoport, KV Pharmaceuticals, and Otsuka. In the past 3 years, Dr Howden has received speaking honoraria from Takeda Pharmaceuticals North America, Santarus, AstraZeneca, and Otsuka. Dr Howden has received research support from AstraZeneca for an investigator-initiated project.

Division of Gastroenterology, Northwestern University Feinberg School of Medicine, 676 North Saint Clair Street, Suite 1400, Chicago, IL 60611, USA
* Corresponding author.
E-mail address: c-howden@northwestern.edu

Gastroenterol Clin N Am 39 (2010) 529–542
doi:10.1016/j.gtc.2010.08.009
0889-8553/10/$ – see front matter © 2010 Elsevier Inc. All rights reserved.

PROTON PUMP INHIBITORS

These drugs have been successful both clinically and commercially for the treatment of various acid-related disorders; mainly gastroesophageal reflux disease (GERD). Other indicated uses of proton pump inhibitors (PPIs) include the treatment and prevention of upper gastrointestinal (GI) tract ulcers from nonsteroidal antiinflammatory drugs (NSAIDs), as part of therapeutic regimens for eradication of *Helicobacter pylori* infection, and in the management of patients with bleeding peptic ulcer. These applications are considered elsewhere in this issue. PPIs have also been used in the management of functional dyspepsia (one of the FGIDs), albeit with limited success. Although generally safe, some possible adverse consequences of long-term PPI use deserve further consideration.

Drug-drug Interactions

After systemic absorption and initial wide distribution within the body, the liver rapidly metabolizes PPIs via the cytochrome P450 enzyme system.[1–6] The principal isoenzymes involved are 2C19 and, to a lesser extent, 3A4. The potential for individual PPIs to influence P450 enzyme activity has raised concerns about possible drug-drug interactions (DDIs). However, there is little, if any, clinical significance to PPI interactions with other medicines; those commonly included in package inserts with PPIs as having the potential for P450-related interactions include warfarin, diazepam, tacrolimus, cyclosporine, and theophylline.[1–6] However, dose adjustments are not routinely required in patients taking PPIs and other medications metabolized by the cytochrome P450 system.

Most medicines with which at least some PPIs have been proposed to interact have wide therapeutic indices. That is, their steady-state plasma concentrations associated with toxicity are much higher than those associated with the desired therapeutic effect. A perfect example is diazepam. Although omeprazole interacts with diazepam to slow its metabolism and raise its steady-state plasma concentration, this is not associated with any measurable pharmacodynamic effect. Some drugs (notably warfarin, phenytoin, and theophylline) have much narrower therapeutic indices, so plasma concentrations associated with toxicity are close to those normally associated with their desired therapeutic effects. Theoretically, slowing of the hepatic metabolism of any of these drugs by the concomitant use of a P450 inhibitor (such as a PPI) might increase steady-state plasma concentrations to toxic levels. However, DDIs reported to the United States Food and Drug Administration (FDA) with omeprazole, lansoprazole, and pantoprazole included estimated frequencies of less than 1 per million prescriptions, with no discernable differences among them.[7] The American Gastroenterological Association Institute published a technical review on GERD in 2008, which included an overview of various potential safety concerns with the PPIs, including possible DDIs.[8] They endorsed the view that clinically significant DDIs occurred with a frequency of less than 1 per million prescriptions.

There are a few DDIs common to all the PPIs with respect to their inhibition of gastric acid secretion. All PPIs may reduce the absorption of the antiretroviral agent atazanavir. This reduction may potentially lead to subtherapeutic blood levels of that agent, with risks of treatment failure against human immunodeficiency virus (HIV) infection or the emergence of resistant strains of HIV. All PPIs may increase the bioavailability of digoxin by around 10%, which is unlikely to be clinically relevant.

PPIs and Clopidogrel

Clopidogrel is a prodrug that must be activated in the liver to exert its desired antiplatelet effect. This effect is accomplished in a multistep process that includes cytochrome P450 2C19, the isoenzyme most closely connected with PPI metabolism. Some in vitro studies suggested that omeprazole, and perhaps other PPIs, reduces the rate of conversion of clopidogrel to its active metabolite when used concomitantly.[9] Clopidogrel is generally administered with aspirin, and this combination puts some patients at risk of upper GI hemorrhage. PPI cotherapy is advised for patients with identifiable risk factors such as advanced age, a past history of ulcer or bleeding, or concomitant NSAID or anticoagulant use.[10] Some retrospective studies reported worse cardiovascular outcomes among patients on clopidogrel and a PPI compared with those on clopidogrel alone.[11,12] However, these were prone to bias; for example, in both studies cited, patients taking a PPI and clopidogrel had worse cardiovascular risk profiles and more comorbidity than those not on a PPI. Because these were not randomized trials, it may be that patients with worse disease, and at presumed greater risk of GI bleeding, were more likely to have been given PPI cotherapy. As of March 2010, there were no published, peer-reviewed data from prospective, randomized trials. However, O'Donoghue and colleagues[13] did make a post hoc analysis of prospectively collected data from the Trial to Assess Improvement in Therapeutic Outcomes by Optimizing Platelet Inhibition with Prasugrel-Thrombolysis in Myocardial Infarction (TRITON-TIMI) 38 trial, which had randomized more than 13,000 patients with acute coronary syndrome (ACS) to clopidogrel or prasugrel. Although TRITON-TIMI 38 was not a randomized comparison of PPI cotherapy with no cotherapy in patients receiving clopidogrel, a large number of patients in the trial had been on PPI cotherapy. O'Donoghue and colleagues[13] did not identify any adverse cardiovascular outcomes in the patients treated with clopidogrel who had received PPI cotherapy compared with those who had not. Furthermore, they identified a small but statistically significant reduction in all-cause mortality among the patients treated with clopidogrel on PPI cotherapy. To date, Clopidogrel and the Optimization of Gastrointestinal Events Trial (COGENT) is the only randomized study to have compared PPI cotherapy with no cotherapy in patients taking clopidogrel. However, this trial was terminated prematurely for financial reasons and, at the time of writing, had not been reported in full. It randomized patients to a fixed-dose combination of clopidogrel and omeprazole or to clopidogrel alone after a myocardial infarction, other ACS, or coronary stent placement.[14] Patients who had received the combination of omeprazole and clopidogrel in COGENT did not have demonstrably worse cardiovascular outcomes than those who received clopidogrel alone. The patients who had received omeprazole had a significantly lower rate of adverse GI outcomes than those who did not.

As of March 2010, there is no definitive clinical evidence that PPI cotherapy with clopidogrel is a risk factor for adverse cardiovascular outcomes.[15] Patients taking clopidogrel who have additional risk factors for GI bleeding should receive PPI cotherapy.[10] However, in November 2009, the FDA announced its analysis of some pharmacodynamic and pharmacokinetic studies conducted by the manufacturers of clopidogrel.[16] These showed that omeprazole cotherapy was associated with reduced serum levels of clopidogrel's active metabolite and with a reduction in clopidogrel's in vitro antiplatelet effect. Based on these studies, the FDA recommended that omeprazole (and esomeprazole) be avoided among patients taking clopidogrel. Similar studies are currently being conducted with other PPIs.

Clostridium difficile and Other Enteric Infections

Clostridium difficile is a spore-forming bacterium; its nosocomial acquisition is associated with significant morbidity and it is also emerging as an important community-acquired pathogen.[17,18] Several published studies have investigated the association between PPI use and *C difficile* infection. The proposed mechanism for the increased risk is that gastric acid suppression allows ingested spore survival in the upper GI tract and eventual proliferation in the colon.[19] There is also some evidence that PPIs cause leukocyte inhibition, which may contribute to an increase in various enteric infections, including *C difficile*.[20]

Aseeri and colleagues[21] published a retrospective case-control study of 94 patients with nosocomial *C difficile* infection. Multivariate analysis in which factors such as antibiotic use, sex, and age were controlled for, determined an odds ratio (OR) for PPI use and *C difficile* infection of 3.6 (95% confidence interval [CI] 1.7–5.3). In another case-control study, Yearsley and colleagues[22] investigated 155 patients with nosocomial *C difficile* infection. There was an increased risk of *C difficile* infection with PPI therapy (OR 1.9; 95% CI 1.1–3.3).[22] To determine the effects of PPIs on community-acquired *C difficile*, Dial and colleagues[19] conducted a population-based case-control study of 1233 patients and found an adjusted rate ratio of 2.9 (95% CI 2.4–3.4) for *C difficile* infection among patients using PPIs. Based on the available data, there seems to be a weak association between PPI use and *C difficile* infection, both nosocomial and community-acquired, although causality has not been established.

Similarly, diminished gastric acid secretion is postulated to increase the risk of other enteric infections. Garcia Rodriguez and colleagues[23] studied a retrospective cohort of 6414 patients with age- and sex-matched controls to investigate the risk of culture-positive bacterial enteric infections with PPI use. They found a dose-dependent relationship with a relative risk (RR) of 2.9 (95% CI 2.5–3.5) between gastroenteritis and PPI use. A meta-analysis evaluating 6 observational studies comprising 11,280 patients found a significant association between PPI use and bacterial enteric infection (OR 2.55; 95% CI 1.53 and 4.26).[24] The investigators also found a quantitatively smaller association between use of H_2-receptor antagonists (H_2RAs) and bacterial enteric infection. Taken together, these observations suggest an association between acid suppression and enteric bacterial infections. H_2RAs are associated with a lower risk than PPIs, so there may be some degree of dose response. However, the magnitude of the increased risk is small. In general, when estimates of effect sizes from observational studies are small, they should not be interpreted as proving causation; they imply an association and might be considered to generate hypotheses.

Pneumonia

Gastric acid suppression has also been associated with the development of both community-acquired and nosocomial pneumonia. The proposed mechanism of infection is through the ability of bacteria to colonize the upper GI tract because of the increase in gastric pH with PPI therapy.[25] The association between PPI use and leukocyte inhibition may also play a role.[20] In a population-based cohort study of 364,683 individuals, Laheij and colleagues[26] reported that PPI use was associated with community-acquired pneumonia (CAP) (RR 1.89; 95% CI 1.36–2.62). This association was dose-dependent, with patients on higher doses of PPI having a higher risk of developing CAP.[26] However, there were significant confounders in this study, which did not control for the presence of GERD or chronic obstructive pulmonary disease in their cohort. Sarkar and colleagues[27] subsequently conducted a nested case-control study of 80,066 patients, in which those who were started on a PPI within the 30 days preceding the diagnosis of CAP had a higher risk than those who had been on long-term PPI treatment. The highest risk of CAP was seen within the first 2 days of PPI therapy (OR 6.53; 95% CI 3.95–10.80). The association between CAP and short-term, but not long-term, PPI use may be an example of protopathic bias, in which patients presenting to their health care providers with certain symptoms were inappropriately prescribed a PPI.

Herzig and colleagues[28] investigated the risk of nosocomial pneumonia and PPI use in a prospective cohort of 63,878 patients who were not ventilated and who were hospitalized for at least 72 hours. The OR for developing nosocomial pneumonia for patients on PPIs was 1.3 (95% CI 1.1–1.4) in a multivariate analysis and the association was strongest with aspiration than for nonaspiration pneumonia.

Based on these studies, there may be a slightly increased risk of both CAP and nosocomial pneumonia associated with PPI use. However, the magnitude of the observed effect is small and at least some of the studies were prone to confounding.

Rebound Hypersecretion

One of the consequences of acid suppression with a PPI is hypergastrinemia, which in turn causes enterochromaffinlike cell hyperplasia and may, ultimately, lead to parietal cell hyperplasia. Thus, the potential exists for increased gastric acid secretory capacity compared with that which existed before the introduction of the PPI. This potential has led to concern about the possibility of rebound acid hypersecretion when stopping PPIs after prolonged use.[29,30]

Reimer and colleagues[31] conducted a randomized, double-blind, placebo-controlled study in 120 asymptomatic individuals to investigate the possibility of new upper GI symptoms, possibly related to rebound acid hypersecretion, after 8 weeks of therapy with esomeprazole. They found that heartburn and dyspeptic symptoms were statistically significantly increased among the subjects who had discontinued esomeprazole compared with those who had discontinued placebo, with onset approximately 2 to 4 weeks after stopping the PPI. This study claimed that some previously asymptomatic individuals temporarily develop upper GI symptoms (possibly caused by rebound acid hypersecretion, which was not measured) after withdrawal of a PPI. However, these symptoms were temporary and of a minor nature and should not dissuade physicians from prescribing a PPI to patients with legitimate symptoms expected to respond to acid suppression. At least 1 further study has reported similar findings to Reimer and colleagues.[31] Niklasson and colleagues[32] reported more severe symptoms after PPI withdrawal, but these were also more transient than those detected by Reimer and colleagues. The clinical significance of these findings has been questioned.[33]

Bone Health

In 2006, Yang and colleagues[34] published a nested case-control study investigating the risk of hip fracture with PPI use. They identified 13,566 patients with hip fractures and found that greater than 1 year of PPI use was associated with an adjusted OR of 1.44 (95% CI 1.30–1.59). This risk appeared to increase with PPI dose and with duration of treatment. One theoretic mechanism for the increase in hip fractures was that gastric acid suppression decreases dietary calcium absorption and, in time, this may lead to relative demineralization of bone, osteopenia, osteoporosis, and an increased fracture risk.[35] A retrospective matched cohort study of 15,792 patients found that PPI use was only associated with hip fracture after more than 6 years of exposure (adjusted OR 1.92; 95% CI 1.16–3.18).[36] Corley[37] conducted a retrospective case-control study using the Kaiser Permanente database for Northern California. He matched more than 33,000 individuals with hip fracture with more than 130,000 controls. Greater than 2 years of PPI use was associated with a 30% increase in the rate of hip fracture (OR 1.30; 95% CI 1.21–1.39). In addition, greater than 2 years of H_2RA use was also associated with a slightly increased risk (OR 1.18; 95% CI

1.08–1.28). Corley[37] was able to demonstrate a positive dose-response relationship between PPI use and hip fracture but did not identify any duration-response relationship.

However, a recent study by Targownik and colleagues[38] conducted both a cross-sectional and longitudinal analysis investigating bone mineral density in 2193 and 2549 patients, respectively. The longitudinal study investigated change in bone mineral density in a 1- to 3-year span. The cross-sectional study found no significant relationship between bone density and PPI use. Similarly, PPI use did not have a significant effect on bone mineral density in patients in the longitudinal analysis. Another nested case-control study by Kaye and Jick[39] found no association between PPI use and hip fracture in 1098 patients.

There are slightly inconsistent results among the different retrospective studies of PPI use and fractures. However, most studies suggest a weak positive association, and some criteria for causation are also fulfilled, notably a dose-response relationship and, at least in most of the studies, a duration-response relationship. Although there was a once-plausible biologic rationale to explain the association, the recent findings by Targownik and colleagues[38] call this into question. Patients who have a genuine requirement for PPI treatment should receive it in the lowest effective dose. At this time, there is no recommendation to provide patients with additional bone mineral density monitoring or more than routine calcium and vitamin D supplementation.[8]

B$_{12}$ Deficiency

Vitamin B$_{12}$ deficiency, if left untreated or undetected, has potentially serious and irreversible systemic consequences.[40] An early report of a possible association between B$_{12}$ deficiency and PPI use (>1 year), was made by Valuck and Ruscin[41] in their case-control study of 53 patients greater than 65 years old and 212 age- and sex-matched controls. However, this association has been questioned based on a cross-sectional study published by den Elzen and colleagues,[42] which recruited 125 patients more than 65 years of age on PPI therapy for greater than 3 years and used their partners who were not on PPI therapy as the control group. The study patients had serum B$_{12}$ levels measured and compared with those of their partners. Multivariate analysis, controlling for age, sex, H pylori status, and C-reactive protein, showed no statistical difference in B$_{12}$ levels between patients and their partners. Based on these data, there is no evidence of a discernable association with PPI use and the development of B$_{12}$ deficiency.[43]

Side Effects, Anaphylaxis, and Allergy

As a class, PPIs are well tolerated with few reported side effects,[44–46] the most common being headache, constipation, diarrhea, dizziness, and rash.[1–6] There have been several case reports and series of anaphylactic and allergic reactions to PPI therapy. The largest published case series described 9 patients with adverse reaction to omeprazole: urticaria/angioedema in 7 and anaphylaxis in 2.[47] Most of these patients had positive pin-prick tests suggesting immunoglobulin E–mediated allergy. Four patients also had a positive pin-prick test to pantoprazole. However, lansoprazole was well tolerated, suggesting a lack of a class effect with anaphylactic reactions.

Another reported adverse reaction to PPI therapy is acute interstitial nephritis (AIN). In a systematic review, Sierra and colleagues[48] identified 64 cases of PPI-associated AIN, 59 of which were proven by biopsy. All of the PPIs, except for dexlansoprazole (which was not available at that time), were implicated, suggesting a class effect. In addition, there was improvement in renal function by a mean of 35.5 weeks after withdrawal of PPI therapy, but creatinine levels did not return to baseline.[48] Evidence for causality in the cases reviewed was often poor; in general, patients have not been challenged with reintroduction of the suspected PPI, for obvious reasons. However, these adverse effects are tempered by the extremely low overall rate of adverse reactions, estimated at 0.01% in one case series.[49]

Pregnancy

Given the widespread use of PPIs, there is concern about their possible effects on the developing fetus. Omeprazole is listed by the FDA as a pregnancy class C medication, whereas all other currently available PPIs are class B, which still denotes a possible serious risk to the fetus.[1–6] Gill and colleagues[50] recently published a systematic review evaluating the risk of PPI use in pregnancy. Among 1530 PPI-exposed subjects compared with 133,410 controls, they found no association between major fetal malformations, spontaneous abortions, or pre-term delivery. This lack of association was also apparent when omeprazole alone was investigated.

However, there is some suggestion that acid suppression alone may have an adverse affect on an exposed fetus. In a recent, large, case-control study investigating children with asthma, Dehlink and colleagues[51] found a relationship between maternal gastric acid suppression with a PPI or H_2RA and the development of childhood asthma (OR 1.43; 95% CI 1.29–1.59). The postulated mechanism, based on animal model data, is that acid suppression increases type 2 helper cell bias in their offspring, thus predisposing to increased atopy.[51] Based on these data, the immediate fetal developmental risk of PPIs may be negligible. However, possible risks to the fetus that may only become manifest in childhood require further study.

A summary containing our assessment of the clinical relevance of the various proposed adverse effects of PPIs is given in **Table 1**.

H_2RAS

Cimetidine, ranitidine, famotidine, and nizatidine are commonly used and widely available medications used to treat acid-related disorders. They are generally well tolerated and have a low incidence of side effects,[52–54] with the most commonly ascribed being diarrhea, dizziness, and headache. The estimated incidence of drug-related side effects is 5% to 8%.[52,53] However, in a pooled analysis the side effects were no greater than placebo treatment for ranitidine and famotidine.[52]

Table 1
Potential safety issues associated with PPI use

Safety Issue	Clinical Significance
Cytochrome P450 interaction	Negligible
Clopidogrel interaction	Unclear
Clostridium difficile infection	Probable
Other enteric infections	Probable
Pneumonia	Probable
Rebound hypersecretion	Negligible
Fractures	Negligible
Idiosyncratic reactions (AIN, hepatitis)	Rare
Anaphylaxis	Rare
Pregnancy risk	Likely negligible

The H_2RA with the most reported DDIs is cimetidine, because it is the most potent inhibitor of the cytochrome P450 system and the H_2RA that has been in clinical use for the longest time. The potential exists for interactions with medications that are extensively metabolized by cytochrome P450 and have a narrow therapeutic index, such as warfarin, theophylline, and phenytoin. However, the incidence of clinically relevant DDIs with cimetidine is extremely low, and all the H_2RAs, including cimetidine, are now widely available for purchase without a prescription. The affinity of ranitidine for the cytochrome P450 system is approximately one-sixth that for cimetidine, whereas famotidine and nizatidine have no apparent cytochrome P450 interaction.[55]

In the study by Yu and colleagues,[56] neither the cross-sectional bone mineral density cohort nor the prospective fracture cohort showed any relationship between H_2RA use and bone health.

Transient rebound hypersecretion has been shown after stopping H_2RAs, although the mechanism of this remains unclear.[57]

The association between H_2RA use and CAP was studied in the case-control study by Laheij and colleagues[26] in 475 subjects and 4690 controls. The association had an adjusted OR of 1.43 (95% CI 1.14–2.23). However, Rodriguez and colleagues[58] investigated the relationship between CAP and H_2RA use in 278 patients and 241 controls and found no significant relationship between rates of pneumonia and H_2RA use within the prior 31 days. Herzig and colleagues[28] found no association between hospital-acquired pneumonia and H_2RA use in their prospective cohort of 5686 subjects and 30,956 controls.

H_2RAs have also been implicated in the development of community-acquired C difficile infection, by Dial and colleagues[19] in their case-control study of 83 subjects and 367 controls (adjusted OR 2.0; 95% CI 1.6–2.7). However, there was no evidence of increased risk of other enteric infections in the study by Rodriguez and colleagues,[23] although the systematic review and meta-analysis by Leonard and colleagues[24] did suggest a slight increase in risk.

For many of the suspected adverse effects preliminarily attributed to H_2RA use and ascribed to an acid-suppressing effect, the estimates of effect size are small and generally lower than those found with PPIs. This suggests that pharmacologic acid suppression is associated with slight increases in the rates of these events. H_2RAs suppress acid to a lesser extent than PPIs and are associated with even lower degrees of risk. However the H_2RAs have been available since the late 1970s and have had an excellent record of safety and tolerability. It would be surprising if data showing any serious unintended consequence of H_2RA use were to emerge now or in the future.

Uncommon reported reactions to H_2RAs include AIN and hepatotoxicity. There have been 41 reported cases of H_2RA-induced AIN in the literature, with 28 being proven by biopsy.[59] The patients usually presented with fever and fatigue and were found to have sterile pyuria, proteinuria, and increased erythrocyte sedimentation rate. All the patients described in the series rapidly improved after withdrawal of the medication. H_2RA-related hepatotoxicity and hepatitis have also been rarely reported, with an estimated rate of 0.06%. Ranitidine has been the most commonly implicated, with rates up to 1% of all exposed patients. Normalization of liver function tests typically occurred 1 to 6 weeks after withdrawal of therapy.[59,60]

H_2RAs are commonly used in pregnancy to control reflux symptoms and seem to have no adverse effects on the fetus.[61,62] Magee and colleagues[61] investigated H_2RA use among 178 women and matched controls in the first trimester of pregnancy and found no difference in adverse fetal outcomes. Ruigomez and colleagues[62] analyzed a large population-based cohort of pregnant women who were exposed to cimetidine or ranitidine (or omeprazole) during the first trimester and found no increase in nongenetic congenital malformations with exposure to any of these medicines.

MISCELLANEOUS MEDICINES FOR ACID-RELATED DISORDERS

Sucralfate, magaldrate, and calcium carbonate are commonly used medicines to treat acid-related disorders and are generally safe with few reported side effects. Sucralfate's main side effects are constipation, the potential for aluminum toxicity in patients with impaired renal function, and the possibility of DDIs by decreasing the bioavailability of several other medicines, including fluoroquinolones, H_2RAs, and phenytoin.[63] The only significant reported side effect with magaldrate has been mild, self-limiting diarrhea, estimated at 2% in one small series of patients.[64] Calcium carbonate is a generally benign drug, with only isolated reports of increased total body calcium levels in patients with renal insufficiency, typically with dosages greater than 6 g per day.[65]

SAFETY OF DRUGS USED TO TREAT FGIDS

In the United States, lubiprostone is currently the only FDA-approved medicine to treat irritable bowel syndrome (IBS). It is used in constipation-predominant IBS (IBS-C) and is also approved for the management of chronic constipation. The major side effects in the phase 3 clinical trials of 1171 patients with IBS-C were GI-related (nausea, diarrhea, and abdominal distention) with an incidence of 19% versus 14% in the placebo arm.[66] The rates of drug discontinuation because of adverse effects were similar between the lubiprostone and placebo arms (25% vs 23%, respectively).[66]

Antispasmodics are frequently used to treat many GI complaints presumed to be related to disturbed motility or smooth muscle spasm (typically, IBS). Dicyclomine and hyoscyamine are commonly used in IBS; although the package inserts note numerous side effects related to their anticholinergic properties, there are no published studies of serious adverse effects.[67,68]

Loperamide is commonly used for self-treatment of diarrhea. In 2 separate studies conducted in adults and children, there were no differences in rates of adverse events between groups given loperamide or placebo.[69,70]

Alosetron is a selective 5-hydroxytryptamine type 3 (5-HT$_3$) antagonist used to treat IBS with diarrhea that is unresponsive to other therapeutic approaches.[71] Constipation was the most common adverse event seen in clinical trials, with a frequency of 20% to 29%; this appeared to be dose-dependent.[71] The drug was temporarily removed from the market in 2000 because of rare cases of severe constipation and resultant mucosal ischemia requiring surgery.[72,73] The drug was subsequently reintroduced with prescription and dosage restrictions because of these safety concerns.[74] In a randomized, placebo-controlled trial of 705 patients, there was a dose-dependent 9% to 19% incidence of constipation with alosetron use, and 1 episode of ischemic colitis.[75]

Prokinetic Agents

Metoclopramide is a proximal gut prokinetic that induces acetylcholine release by activating 5-hydroxytryptamine type 4 (5HT$_4$) receptors while also acting as an antagonist for dopamine D$_2$ receptors centrally.[76] Common safety concerns with metoclopramide result from its antidopaminergic effects. Acute dystonic reactions have been reported in 0.2% to 6% of patients, typically within 48 hours of initiating therapy.[76] The incidence of (sometimes irreversible) tardive dyskinesia has been estimated as between 1% and 15%, typically occurring after more than 3 months of continuous use.[76,77] Prolonged treatment can also result in a Parkinson–like syndrome, which typically subsides within 2 to 3 months of discontinuation.[76,77]

Domperidone is a D_2 receptor antagonist that primarily acts to increase motility in the upper gut.[78] QT prolongation has been a concern with domperidone administration, although there are few data on the incidence of ventricular arrhythmias.[78]

Renzapride is a recently developed prokinetic that is primarily used for IBS with constipation. Lembo and colleagues[79] evaluated its efficacy in a placebo-controlled, double-blind, randomized trial of 1798 patients. The most common side effects possibly related to renzapride were diarrhea, abdominal pain, nausea, and flatulence, although the incidences were not significantly greater than with placebo. However, in a long-term (>12 weeks) arm of the study of 971 patients, 3 patients on renzapride developed ischemic colitis.[79]

Tegaserod is a selective $5HT_4$ agonist that was developed for IBS-C, chronic constipation, and functional dyspepsia. Its use was suspended in 2007 because of concerns about an increase in ischemic cardiovascular events based on a review of phase III clinical trial data. However, subsequent data from a case-control study of 2603 tegaserod users found no increase in cardiac events.[80] Chey and colleagues[81] evaluated the safety and efficacy of tegaserod in 780 patients in separate 1-year extension studies. The most commonly reported adverse event was diarrhea, with an incidence of approximately 10%, which was generally moderate and led to discontinuation in only 5.9% of patients. Adverse cardiovascular events that were potentially drug related had an incidence of less than 1%.

SUMMARY

Most of the drugs reviewed here have low risks of serious adverse events. At the time of writing, concerns about the interaction between PPIs and clopidogrel were foremost in the minds of prescribers. Other possible consequences of long-term PPI use have also been discussed in detail because these drugs are extremely widely used and because some of the proposed adverse effects can have serious consequences. Clinicians need to be aware of the safety profiles of the drugs they frequently prescribe in their practices. All prescribing decisions are essentially based on a risk-benefit analysis, whether conscious or subconscious. Evidence of benefit is essential, and this must be balanced with an understanding of (even very low) levels of risk.

REFERENCES

1. Pantoprazole [package insert]. Philadelphia: Wyeth Pharmaceuticals; 2007.
2. Omeprazole [package insert]. Wilmington, DE: AstraZeneca LP; 2008.
3. Esomeprazole [package insert]. Wilmington, DE: AstraZeneca LP; 2008.
4. Lansoprazole [package insert]. Lake Forest, IL: Takeda Pharmaceuticals America Inc; 2009.
5. Rabeprazole [package insert]. Titusville, NJ: Eisai Co Ltd; 2009.
6. Dexlansoprazole [package insert]. Deerfield, IL: Takeda Pharmaceuticals America Inc; 2009.
7. Labenz J, Petersen KU, Rösch W, et al. A summary of Food and Drug Administration-reported adverse events and drug interactions occurring during therapy with omeprazole, lansoprazole and pantoprazole. Aliment Pharmacol Ther 2003;17(8):1015–9.
8. Kahrilas PJ, Shaheen NJ, Vaezi MF. American Gastroenterological Association Institute technical review on the management of gastroesophageal reflux disease. Gastroenterology 2008;135(4):1392–413, e1–5.

9. Norgard NB, Mathews KD, Wall GC. Drug-drug interaction between clopidogrel and the proton pump inhibitors. Ann Pharmacother 2009;43(7):1266-74.

10. Bhatt DL, Scheiman J, Abraham NS, et al. ACCF/ACG/AHA 2008 expert consensus document on reducing the gastrointestinal risks of antiplatelet therapy and NSAID use: a report of the American College of Cardiology Foundation Task Force on Clinical Expert Consensus Documents. Circulation 2008;118(18): 1894-909.

11. Juurlink DN, Gomes T, Ko DT, et al. A population-based study of the drug interaction between proton pump inhibitors and clopidogrel. CMAJ 2009;180(7): 713-8.

12. Ho PM, Maddox TM, Wang L, et al. Risk of adverse outcomes associated with concomitant use of clopidogrel and proton pump inhibitors following acute coronary syndrome. JAMA 2009;301(9):937-44.

13. O'Donoghue ML, Braunwald E, Antman EM, et al. Pharmacodynamic effect and clinical efficacy of clopidogrel and prasugrel with or without a proton-pump inhibitor: an analysis of two randomised trials. Lancet 2009;374(9694):989-97.

14. Wood S. COGENT: No CV events but significant GI benefits of PPI omeprazole. Available at: http://www.theheart.org/article/1007145.do. Accessed August 6, 2010.

15. Laine L, Hennekens C. Proton pump inhibitor and clopidogrel interaction: fact or fiction? Am J Gastroenterol 2010;105(1):34-41.

16. FDA announces new warning on Plavix: avoid use with Prilosec/Prilosec OTC. Available at: http://www.fda.gov/NewsEvents/Newsroom/PressAnnouncements/ 2009/ucm191169.htm. Accessed February 4, 2010.

17. Dawson LF, Valiente E, Wren BW. Clostridium difficile-a continually evolving and problematic pathogen. Infect Genet Evol 2009;9.1410-7.

18. Kuijper EJ, van Dissel JT, Wilcox MH. Clostridium difficile: changing epidemiology and new treatment options. Curr Opin Infect Dis 2007;20:376-83.

19. Dial S, Delaney JA, Barkun AN, et al. Use of gastric acid-suppressive agents and the risk of community-acquired Clostridium difficile-associated disease. JAMA 2005;294:2989-95.

20. Capodicasa E, Cornacchione P, Natalini B, et al. Omeprazole induces apoptosis in normal human polymorphonuclear leucocytes. Int J Immunopathol Pharmacol 2008;21(1):73-85.

21. Aseeri M, Schroeder T, Kramer J, et al. Gastric acid suppression by proton pump inhibitors as a risk factor for Clostridium difficile-associated diarrhea in hospitalized patients. Am J Gastroenterol 2008;103:2308-13.

22. Yearsley KA, Gilby LJ, Ramadas AV, et al. Proton pump inhibitor therapy is a risk factor for clostridium difficile-associated diarrhoea. Aliment Pharmacol Ther 2006;24(4):613-9.

23. Garcia Rodriguez LA, Ruigomez A, Panes J. Use of acid-suppressing drugs and the risk of bacterial gastroenteritis. Clin Gastroenterol Hepatol 2007;5(12): 1418-23.

24. Leonard J, Marshall JK, Moayyedi P. Systematic review of the risk of enteric infection in patients taking acid suppression. Am J Gastroenterol 2007;102(9): 2047-56, quiz 2057.

25. Thorens J, Froehlich F, Schwizer W, et al. Bacterial overgrowth during treatment with omeprazole compared with cimetidine: a prospective randomised double blind study. Gut 1996;39(1):54-9.

26. Laheij RJF, Sturkenboom MC, Hassing RJ, et al. Risk of community-acquired pneumonia and use of gastric acid-suppressive drugs. JAMA 2004;292:1955-60.

27. Sarkar M, Hennessy S, Yang Y-X. Proton pump inhibitor use and the risk for community-acquired pneumonia. Ann Intern Med 2008;149:391–8.

28. Herzig SJ, Howell MD, Ngo LH, et al. Acid-suppressive medication use and the risk for hospital-acquired pneumonia. JAMA 2009;301:2120–8.

29. Waldum HL, Sandvik AK, Brenna E, et al. Gastrin-histamine sequence in the regulation of gastric acid secretion. Gut 1991;32(6):698–701.

30. Waldum HL, Arnestad JS, Brenna E, et al. Marked increase in gastric acid secretory capacity after omeprazole treatment. Gut 1996;39:649–53.

31. Reimer C, Sondergaard B, Hilsted L, et al. Proton pump inhibitor therapy induces acid-related symptoms in healthy volunteers after withdrawal of therapy. Gastroenterology 2009;137:80–7.

32. Niklasson A, Lindström L, Simrén M, et al. Dyspeptic symptoms development after discontinuation of a proton pump inhibitor: a double-blind placebo-controlled trial. Am J Gastroenterol 2010;105(7):1531–7.

33. Howden CW, Kahrilas PJ. Just how "difficult" is it to withdraw PPI treatment? Am J Gastroenterol 2010;105(7):1538–40.

34. Yang Y-X, Lewis JD, Epstein S, et al. Long-term proton pump inhibitor therapy and risk of hip fracture. JAMA 2006;296:2947–53.

35. Chonan O, Takahashi R, Yasui H, et al. Effect of L-lactic acid on the absorption of calcium in gastrectomized rats. J Nutr Sci Vitaminol (Tokyo) 1998;44(6):869–75.

36. Targownik LE, Lix LM, Metge CJ, et al. Use of proton pump inhibitors and risk of osteoporosis-related fractures. CMAJ 2008;179(4):319–26.

37. Corley D. Proton pump inhibitors, H2 antagonists, and risk of hip fracture: a large, population-based study [abstract]. Gastroenterology 2009;136(Suppl 1):414.

38. Targownik LE, Lix LM, Leung S, et al. Proton pump inhibitor use is not associated with osteoporosis or accelerated bone mineral density loss. Gastroenterology 2010;138:896–904.

39. Kaye JA, Jick H. Proton pump inhibitor use and risk of hip fractures in patients without major risk factors. Pharmacotherapy 2008;28:951–9.

40. Andres E, Loukili NH, Noel E, et al. Vitamin B12 (cobalamin) deficiency in elderly patients. CMAJ 2004;171(3):251–9.

41. Valuck RJ, Ruscin JM. A case-control study on adverse effects: H2 blocker or proton pump inhibitor use and risk of vitamin B12 deficiency in older adults. J Clin Epidemiol 2004;57:422–8.

42. den Elzen WPJ, Groeneveld Y, de Ruijter W, et al. Long-term use of proton pump inhibitors and vitamin B12 status in elderly individuals. Aliment Pharmacol Ther 2008;27:491–7.

43. Howden CW. Vitamin B12 levels during prolonged treatment with proton pump inhibitors. J Clin Gastroenterol 2000;30(1):29–33.

44. Calabrese C, Fabbri A, Di Febo G. Long-term management of GERD in the elderly with pantoprazole. Clin Interv Aging 2007;2(1):85–92.

45. Katz PO, Zavala S. Proton pump inhibitors in the management of GERD. J Gastrointest Surg 2010;14:S62–6.

46. Miyamoto M, Haruma K, Kuwabara M, et al. Long-term gastroesophageal reflux disease therapy improves reflux symptoms in elderly patients: five-year prospective study in community medicine. J Gastroenterol Hepatol 2007;22(5):639–44.

47. Lobera T, Navarro B, Del Pozo MD, et al. Nine cases of omeprazole allergy: cross-reactivity between proton pump inhibitors. J Investig Allergol Clin Immunol 2009; 19:57–60.

48. Sierra F, Suarez M, Rey M, et al. Systematic review: proton pump inhibitor-associated acute interstitial nephritis. Aliment Pharmacol Ther 2007;26(4):545–53.

49. Demirkan K, Bozkurt B, Karakaya G, et al. Anaphylactic reaction to drugs commonly used for gastrointestinal system diseases: 3 case reports and review of the literature. J Investig Allergol Clin Immunol 2006;16:203–9.
50. Gill SK, O'Brien L, Einarson TR, et al. The safety of proton pump inhibitors (PPIs) in pregnancy: a meta-analysis. Am J Gastroenterol 2009;104:1541–5 quiz 1540, 1546.
51. Dehlink E, Yen E, Leichtner AM, et al. First evidence of a possible association between gastric acid suppression during pregnancy and childhood asthma: a population-based register study. Clin Exp Allergy 2009;39:246–53.
52. Howden CW, Tytgat GN. The tolerability and safety profile of famotidine. Clin Ther 1996;18:36–54 [discussion: 35].
53. Lewis JH. Safety profile of long-term H2-antagonist therapy. Aliment Pharmacol Ther 1991;5:49–57.
54. Sabesin SM. Safety issues relating to long-term treatment with histamine H2-receptor antagonists. Aliment Pharmacol Ther 1993;7:35–40.
55. Reynolds JC. The clinical importance of drug interactions with antiulcer therapy. J Clin Gastroenterol 1990;12(Suppl 2):S54–63.
56. Yu EW, Blackwell T, Ensrud KE, et al. Acid-suppressive medications and risk of bone loss and fracture in older adults. Calcif Tissue Int 2008;83:251–9.
57. Gillen D, McColl KE. Problems related to acid rebound and tachyphylaxis. Best Pract Res Clin Gastroenterol 2001;15:487–95.
58. Rodríguez LAG, Ruigómez A, Wallander MA, et al. Acid-suppressive drugs and community-acquired pneumonia. Epidemiology 2009;20:800–6.
59. Fisher AA, Le Couteur DG. Nephrotoxicity and hepatotoxicity of histamine H2 receptor antagonists. Drug Saf 2001;24:39–57.
60. Dobbs JH, Muir JG, Smith RN. H2-antagonists and hepatitis. Ann Intern Med 1986;105(5):803.
61. Magee LA, Inocencion G, Kamboj L, et al. Safety of first trimester exposure to histamine H2 blockers. A prospective cohort study. Dig Dis Sci 1996;41(6):1145–9.
62. Ruigomez A, García Rodríguez LA, Cattaruzzi C, et al. Use of cimetidine, omeprazole, and ranitidine in pregnant women and pregnancy outcomes. Am J Epidemiol 1999;150(5):476–81.
63. Marks IN. Sucralfate–safety and side effects. Scand J Gastroenterol Suppl 1991; 185:36–42.
64. Estruch R, Pedrol E, Castells A, et al. Prophylaxis of gastrointestinal tract bleeding with magaldrate in patients admitted to a general hospital ward. Scand J Gastroenterol 1991;26(8):819–26.
65. Malberti F, Surian M, Poggio F, et al. Efficacy and safety of long-term treatment with calcium carbonate as a phosphate binder. Am J Kidney Dis 1988;12(6):487–91.
66. Drossman DA, Chey WD, Johanson JF, et al. Clinical trial: lubiprostone in patients with constipation-associated irritable bowel syndrome–results of two randomized, placebo-controlled studies. Aliment Pharmacol Ther 2009;29:329–41.
67. Dicyclomine [package insert]. Birmingham, AL: Axcan Pharma US Inc; 2008.
68. Hyoscyamine sulfate [package insert]. St. Louis, MO: Ethex Corporation; 2006.
69. Kaplan MA, Prior MJ, Ash RR, et al. Loperamide-simethicone vs loperamide alone, simethicone alone, and placebo in the treatment of acute diarrhea with gas-related abdominal discomfort. A randomized controlled trial. Arch Fam Med 1999;8:243–8.
70. Kaplan MA, Prior MJ, McKonly KI, et al. A multicenter randomized controlled trial of a liquid loperamide product versus placebo in the treatment of acute diarrhea in children. Clin Pediatr (Phila) 1999;38:579–91.

71. Camilleri M. Pharmacology and clinical experience with alosetron. Expert Opin Investig Drugs 2000;9:147–59.
72. Mayer EA, Bradesi S. Alosetron and irritable bowel syndrome. Expert Opin Pharmacother 2003;4:2089–98.
73. Miller DP, Alfredson T, Cook SF, et al. Incidence of colonic ischemia, hospitalized complications of constipation, and bowel surgery in relation to use of alosetron hydrochloride. Am J Gastroenterol 2003;98:1117–22.
74. Andresen V, Hollerbach S. Reassessing the benefits and risks of alosetron: what is its place in the treatment of irritable bowel syndrome? Drug Saf 2004;27: 283–92.
75. Krause R, Ameen V, Gordon SH, et al. A randomized, double-blind, placebo-controlled study to assess efficacy and safety of 0.5 mg and 1 mg alosetron in women with severe diarrhea-predominant IBS. Am J Gastroenterol 2007;102: 1709–19.
76. Parkman HP, Hasler WL, Fisher RS, et al. American Gastroenterological Association technical review on the diagnosis and treatment of gastroparesis. Gastroenterology 2004;127:1592–622.
77. Ganzini L, Casey DE, Hoffman WF, et al. The prevalence of metoclopramide-induced tardive dyskinesia and acute extrapyramidal movement disorders. Arch Intern Med 1993;153:1469–75.
78. Reddymasu SC, Soykan I, McCallum RW. Domperidone: review of pharmacology and clinical applications in gastroenterology. Am J Gastroenterol 2007;102: 2036–45.
79. Lembo AJ, Cremonini F, Meyers N, et al. Clinical trial: renzapride treatment of women with irritable bowel syndrome and constipation - a double-blind, randomized, placebo-controlled, study. Aliment Pharmacol Ther 2010;31:979–90.
80. Anderson JL, May HT, Bair TL, et al. Lack of association of tegaserod with adverse cardiovascular outcomes in a matched case-control study. J Cardiovasc Pharmacol Ther 2009;14:170–5.
81. Chey WD, Howden CW, Tack J, et al. Long-term tegaserod treatment for dysmotility-like functional dyspepsia: results of two identical 1-year cohort studies. Dig Dis Sci 2010;55:684–97.

Tumor Necrosis Factor-α Monoclonal Antibodies in the Treatment of Inflammatory Bowel Disease: Clinical Practice Pharmacology

Thomas W. Lee, MBBS, FRACP, Richard N. Fedorak, MD, FRCPC*

KEYWORDS

- Tumor necrosis factor-α • Infliximab • Adalimumab
- Certolizumab pegol • Crohn disease • Ulcerative colitis

Inflammatory bowel diseases are characterized by a dysfunctional intestinal immune system, associated with the imbalanced upregulation of helper T cells (Th), leukocyte trafficking, chemokines, and tissue repair molecules.[1] As with some other autoimmune diseases the overproduction of tumor necrosis factor (TNF)-α, by monocytes and macrophages is prevalent in the inflamed tissues. In patients with Crohn's disease (CD), the inflamed intestinal tissues have unusually high levels of TNF-α in the deeper layers of the lamina propria and the submucosa[2] whereas ulcerative colitis (UC) patients have high levels of TNF-α in the subepithelium and the upper layers of the lamina propria. The persistent association of unusually high levels of proinflammatory TNF-α in the diseased tissues made this cytokine an obvious target for therapeutic intervention.

TNF-α, a 51 kDa trimer, mediates intercellular communication and plays a central role in the inflammatory response. TNF-α is found on cell surfaces or in solution following enzymatic cleavage by TNF-α converting enzyme (TACE). Transmembrane TNF-α, but not soluble TNF-α, is characterized as "bipolar" because it transmits

The authors have nothing to disclose.
Division of Gastroenterology, University of Alberta, 2-14A Zeidler Building, Edmonton, AB T6G 2X8, Canada
* Corresponding author.
E-mail address: richard.fedorak@ualberta.ca

Gastroenterol Clin N Am 39 (2010) 543–557
doi:10.1016/j.gtc.2010.08.018
0889-8553/10/$ – see front matter © 2010 Elsevier Inc. All rights reserved.

signals as both a ligand and a receptor in cell-to-cell contact.[3] Both membrane and soluble forms of TNF-α can bind to one of two TNF receptors and initiate the signaling cascade.[4] The TNF signal transduction pathway is also involved in cellular metabolism, thrombosis, apoptosis, and fibrinolysis pathways, resulting in granuloma formation.[5] In CD and UC, TNF-α is believed to affect the intestinal barrier by inducing apoptosis in the villi, inducing epithelial cells to secrete chemokines, and increase production of adhesion molecules such as E-selectin.[6] Mucosal T cells are also triggered to increase production of interferon (IFN)-γ, enhancing the immune response.

Recombinant monoclonal antibody technology was used to develop the first generation of anti-inflammatory biologic agents directed at "neutralizing" TNF-α. In 1998, the US Food and Drug Administration (FDA) approved the use of infliximab for the treatment of CD (**Table 1**). The success of anti–TNF-α agents in CD and other autoimmune-mediated inflammatory diseases, such as rheumatoid and psoriatic arthritis, psoriasis, and ankylosing spondylitis, is evidenced by the successive development of other monoclonal antibodies, such as adalimumab and certolizumab pegol. Compared with traditional therapeutic compounds, monoclonal antibodies are less expensive to develop but more expensive to produce en masse; annual prescription costs for inflammatory bowel disease are approximately US$20,000 per patient.[6] Nevertheless, these drugs are much needed and many have been approved for use worldwide. For example, as of January 2010, adalimumab (Humira) has been approved for use in 82 countries and used to treat 420,000 patients. By 2016, global sales forecasts expect adalimumab to be the top-selling pharmaceutical, closely followed by infliximab (Remicade) (**Fig. 1**).[7]

In light of the recent developments and success of monoclonal antibody therapies for the treatment of inflammatory bowel diseases, the focus of this article is to characterize the clinical pharmacology of the available anti–TNF-α agents for use by clinicians on a daily basis. The 3 approved therapies for treatment of CD and UC in North America are infliximab, adalimumab, and certolizumab pegol (see **Table 1**). Trials testing the efficacy of these biologics for use for nonapproved indications are ongoing. Examples are the use of infliximab for pediatric UC[8,9] or CD patients directly following intestinal surgery, although at a lower dosage (3 mg/kg instead of 5 mg/kg).[10] Moreover, a phase IV trial has investigated the efficacy of certolizumab pegol in perianal fistulizing CD.[11]

Table 1
Overview of anti–TNF-α agents approved for the treatment of inflammatory bowel disease in North America

	Infliximab	Adalimumab	Certolizumab
Crohn's disease	Adults and children (>6 y of age)[a] including fistulizing disease	Adults	Adults
Ulcerative colitis	Adults[a]		
Company	Centocor Ortho Biotech Inc	Abbott Laboratories	UCB
Brand name	Remicade	Humira	Cimzia
Commercial age as of April 2010[7]	11.7 y	7.3 y	2.0 y

[a] As of June 2010, approved for use by the US Food and Drug Administration but not in Canada.

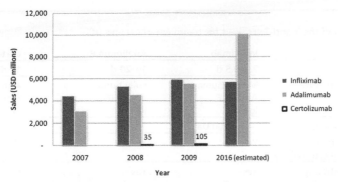

Fig. 1. Worldwide sales of approved anti–TNF-α agents.[7]

Of note, initial trials with etanercept for the treatment of CD proved to be ineffective and were discontinued, although it has been successful in the treatment of other immune-mediated diseases such as rheumatoid arthritis. This suggests the mechanism of action of anti–TNF-α agents for CD is not entirely related to the simple suppression of TNF-α. Etanercept is a fusion protein produced using recombinant DNA, where the DNA "construct" is engineered to link the human gene for soluble TNF receptor 2 to the gene for the Fc component of human immunoglobulin G1 (IgG1).

ANTI–TNF-α MONOCLONAL ANTIBODY STRUCTURE

Infliximab (Remicade) is a chimeric mouse-human recombinant monoclonal antibody comprising a 25% variable murine Fab′ region linked by disulfide bonds to the 75% human IgG1:κ Fc constant region (**Table 2**).[2]

Adalimumab (Humira) is also a recombinant monoclonal antibody like infliximab, but is fully humanized (a controversial topic), containing human-derived variable regions and a human IgG1:κ constant region.[2]

Certolizumab pegol (Cimzia) contains the Fab′ fragment of a humanized anti-TNF monoclonal antibody. To increase the plasma half-life, the Fab′ was attached to a poly-ethylene glycol moiety, consisting of 2 branches of 20 kDa, at a free cysteine residue far removed from the antigen-binding site, to prevent interference.[12]

MECHANISM OF ACTION

Clinical trials involving infliximab, adalimumab and certolizumab have provided insight into how the different agents interrupt the dysfunctional immune system (see **Table 2**). The binding of transmembrane TNF-α has received much attention, as infliximab, adalimumab, and certolizumab each appears to exert different effects.[3] In addition to their direct TNF-α inhibitory effects, some monoclonal antibodies targeting TNF-α have been implicated to have direct cytotoxicity and apoptotic action.

Each of the 3 anti-TNFs binds specifically to free and membrane-bound TNF-α, preventing it from binding to one of two possible receptors, TNF-R1 or TNF-R2.[12] Infliximab and adalimumab do not bind TNF-β, lymphotoxin. The affinities, avidities, and complement activation of infliximab and adalimumab are very similar; certolizumab data are unavailable.[4] The 3 antagonists are known to reduce levels of TNF-α, while infliximab and adalimumab also decrease serum interleukin (IL)-6 and acute-phase reactants, such as C-reactive protein. The clinical practice is aiming for healing. As

Table 2
Comparison of the 3 anti-TNFs used for treatment of CD and UC

	Infliximab	Adalimumab	Certolizumab
Half-life	7.7–9.5 d	10–20 d	14 d
Molecular structure	Mouse-human Anti-TNF IgG1	Fully human Anti-TNF IgG1	Anti-TNF Fab' fragment PEG
Molecular weight	~149,100 Da		~91,000 Da
Mediates complement-dependent cytotoxicity	Yes	Yes	No
Mediates antibody-dependent cell-mediated cytotoxicity	Yes	Yes	No
Increases ratio of apoptotic cells	Yes	Yes	No
Route of administration	Intravenous infusions over 2 h[a]	Subcutaneous injections	Subcutaneous injections
Induction dose and schedule (wk)	5 mg/kg 0, 2, and 6	160 mg at 0 wk 80 mg at 2 wk	400 mg 0, 2, and 4
Maintenance dose and schedule	5 mg/kg Every 8 wk	40 mg Every 2 wk	400 mg Every 4 wk
Loss of response?	Can increase dosage to a maximum of 10 mg/kg and/or decrease infusion frequency (< every 8 wk)[63]		Can add a single extra dose or repeat the induction schedule[64]
Pivotal RCTs in CD: Induction Maintenance	ACCENT I,[65] SONIC[42] ACCENT II[66]	CLASSIC I[67] CLASSIC II[68], CHARM[69]	PRECISE 1[70] PRECISE 2[71]
Pivotal RCTs in UC: Induction Maintenance	ACT 1[72] ACT 2[72]		

Abbreviations: IgG, immunoglobulin G; PEG, polyethylene glycol; RCT, randomized controlled trial; TNF, tumor necrosis factor.
[a] Infusion time can be reduced to 1 h to prevent adverse reactions.[73]

mucosal healing as the gold standard for remission and treatment success, this is certainly achievable with infliximab, adalimumab, and certolizumab pegol.[13] Similarly, infliximab has now been demonstrated to decrease intestinal hyperpermeability in CD patients and colitis-induced animals.[14]

It is interesting that all 3 anti–TNF-α agents can inhibit production of the cytokine, IL-1β, in response to stimulation with lipopolysaccharide.[12] This finding ties in well with the current tenet that inflammatory bowel disease is the result of the combination of environmental stimuli in genetically susceptible individuals with dysfunctional immune systems. Thus, the lipopolysaccharide layer of bacteria resident in the intestinal lumen can elicit an immune response leading to enhanced cytokine production by cells in the intestinal epithelial, endothelial, and submucosal layers.[12] However, the exact mechanisms by which this can be accomplished are the focus of current studies. It should be noted that the observed restoration of the dysregulated expression of antimicrobial peptides in intestinal mucosa of CD and UC patients following infliximab therapy is a consequence of reduced inflammation; anti-TNFs do not exert a direct effect on these proteins.[15]

Infliximab treatment efficacy has now been linked with ameliorating a potential systemic adaptation to active CD. Several cell types release neutrophil gelatinase–associated lipocalin (NGAL), a stress protein, in response to injury. Elevated levels of NGAL have been found in kidney disease as well as CD and UC. The effectiveness of a single infliximab treatment was mirrored by a 62% reduction in NGAL.[16] Moreover, cytogenetic studies in CD patients have found high rates of sister chromatid exchanges in comparison with healthy controls, indicating chromosomal instability. Infliximab induction therapy reduces the rates of these exchanges.[17]

The human IgG1 Fc regions in infliximab and adalimumab have a role in mediating apoptosis in cells expressing TNF-α.[12] This was considered to be an important factor in the therapeutic success of anti-TNFs, however, the success of certolizumab pegol, which lacks this region and substantial apoptosis, suggests that apoptosis is not critical to the therapeutic success of antibodies to TNF-α. As an aside, the TNF-α antagonist etanercept, which possesses the human IgG1 Fc region, is ineffective in treating CD but has been very successful in the treatment of rheumatoid arthritis,[12] suggesting that the mechanism of action of anti-TNFs is inflammatory disease specific.

Infliximab treatment for rheumatoid arthritis is the focus of mechanistic studies with results routinely extrapolated to CD and UC, although not all results are wholly transferable. Nevertheless, results of any research in this area further the understanding of the effect and drug activity in disease, and thus are important and merit inclusion. For example, rheumatoid arthritis patients who respond favorably to infliximab therapy experience an increase in circulating CD4+CD25+ regulatory T cells.[18] However, measures in CD patients before and after infliximab induction therapy found a nearly uniform level of circulating regulatory T cells and no measurable level of "defective" cells, such as CD 62L T regulatory cells, as in rheumatoid arthritis. Recently, infliximab has been demonstrated to redistribute Forkhead box protein3 T-regulatory cells (Foxp3Treg) in CD and UC patients.[19] Specifically, peripheral blood levels of Foxp3-Treg experience a sustained increase in response to infliximab therapy, in contrast to the downregulation of mucosal mRNA and protein levels of Foxp3Treg, effects seen only in patients responding to infliximab treatment.

Infliximab treatment in rheumatoid arthritis appears to inhibit the expression of IL-33R in neutrophils.[20] In turn, neutrophils do not migrate to inflamed tissues in response to the chemotactic activity of IL-33, thereby dampening the immune response and allowing the tissues to recover. Likewise, in UC patients, mucosal IL-33 levels increase in relation to increased disease severity, while serum levels of the cleaved IL-33 are similarly elevated in both CD and UC patients.[21] IL-33 and the IL-1 receptor-related protein, ST2, are known to be regulated by TNF-α. As IL-33 is a potent inducer of IL-5, IL-6, and IL-17 from mucosal immune cells, it is an agent that promotes and maintains tissue inflammation. Infliximab treatment in a murine inflammatory bowel disease model alters the expression of IL-33, causing circulating levels to decrease with a corresponding increase in soluble ST2.

As mentioned earlier, infliximab binding to the transmembrane TNF-α has the potential to evoke many changes in the TNF signal transduction pathway due to its bipolar capabilities. In CD, high levels of circulating IL-15 are associated with disease and inflammation. The IL-15 receptor α, produced by intestinal epithelial cells, binds to IL-15 thereby neutralizing its effects. Infliximab therapy has been shown to increase production of the IL-15 receptor, resulting in decreased circulating levels of IL-15 and elevation in the number of receptor-bound complexes. Bouchaud and colleagues[22] propose that infliximab binding to the transmembrane TNF-α leads to reverse signaling, resulting in the dampening of the inflammatory cascade by including the release of IL-15 receptor α.

In vitro studies with peritoneal macrophages from the TNFαR1 knockout mouse showed significantly reduced downstream expression of inflammatory mediators (inducible nitric oxide synthase and cyclooxygenase-2) and actions (eg, phosphorylation) when exposed to lipopolysaccharides.[23] Incubation with infliximab showed a similar concentration-dependent inhibition of inflammation. The results confirm that infliximab interference with binding of TNF-α with the TNFR1 reduces the inflammatory response when exposed to "foreign" bacterial lipopolysaccharides.

In UC, infliximab has been shown to downregulate the expression of TNF-α and IFN-γ mRNA in inflamed colonic mucosa but not in IL-10 and IL-4 mRNA.[24] Furthermore, UC patients, homozygous for IL23R variants, were twice as likely to respond to infliximab therapy as noncarriers.[25] As such, the therapeutic effect of infliximab binding to TNF-α is amplified by the IL23R gene.

Infliximab pharmacology has been mimicked by wormwood (Artemsia absinthium) extract. A clinical trial of CD patients with active disease receiving the extracts confirmed TNF-α and other interleukins suppression.[26] This result provides another avenue of investigation for future drug development.

In rheumatoid arthritis, adalimumab alters the intracellular signal transduction by exerting effects on T-cell signal transducer and activator of transcription STAT.[27] Specifically, adalimumab increases Th2-associated STAT6 phosphorylation and restores the Th-1-associated activation-induced STAT4 phosphorylation to normal levels seen in healthy individuals.

PHARMACOKINETICS

Significant tissue or serum accumulation of anti–TNF-α agents has been reported in clinical trials to date (see **Table 2**). By contrast, antibody development to the anti–TNF-α agents negatively impacts serum trough levels affecting pharmacokinetics. As both adalimumab and certolizumab pegol are injected subcutaneously, the bioavailability of the active compounds will differ between patients, and trough levels are more susceptible to the presence of antibodies.

Infliximab

The clinical response of CD to infliximab is strongly correlated with the serum infliximab level.[28] Infliximab has a low clearance rate, which appears to be independent of typical drug-metabolizing enzymes and is most likely caused by nonspecific proteases. However, antibody formation to infliximab decreases serum levels to non-detectable levels. In UC patients, infliximab pharmacokinetics has not been associated with either creatinine clearance or aspartate aminotransferase. However, there is evidence pointing to an association between baseline serum albumin and median serum infliximab level, which may be used to predict infliximab pharmacokinetic outcomes and improve screening; patients with low baseline serum albumin are anticipated to have lower infliximab response rates[29] Unlike rheumatoid arthritis, the pharmacokinetics of infliximab in UC were unaffected by concurrent use of either immunomodulators or corticosteroids.[30]

Adalimumab

There are limited data regarding serum adalimumab levels and their relationship to efficacy because serum adalimumab levels were not collected in the pivotal regulatory trials. Adalimumab bioavailability averaged from 3 studies of a single 40 mg/kg dose to healthy human volunteers was 64%. Pharmacokinetics were linear over the dose range.[31]

Certolizumab Pegol

Certolizumab pegol has a long absorption phase and slow elimination rate, due to the covalently linked PEG-moiety. The large molecular weight polyethylene glycol (PEG) moiety is processed similarly to that of other PEGylated drugs, with no indication of toxicity.[12]

IMMUNOGENICITY

Antibodies to anti-TNFs may arise in genetically susceptible patients in response to the IgG1 human components.[32] As previously described, the presence of antidrug antibodies can impede the patient's clinical response to therapy by affecting bioavailability and/or pharmacokinetics, or pharmacodynamics.[32] In some cases, the antagonists' clinical efficacy may be unaffected if the antidrug antibodies have either a low affinity or fail to interact with the drug. Concomitant immunosuppressor therapy, such as azathioprine or methotrexate, has been shown to increase serum trough levels of the active anti–TNF-α agents and reduce antibody formation, although the exact mechanism is not clearly understood.

Infliximab

The variable murine region of infliximab is thought to be the antigenic component that causes the formation of "antibody to infliximab." Antibody formation to infliximab is associated with a lower serum infliximab level and loss of clinical response. As such, practice guidelines recommend the use of regularly scheduled induction and maintenance treatments instead of episodic or on-demand therapy.[33–35] Concomitant use of immunosuppressive agents to reduce antibody formation is also recommended. Techniques are being developed to measure serum infliximab levels in CD patients using fluid-phase enzyme immunoassays.[36] Such measures will allow for adjustment of either dosing amount or dosing frequency in respect of antibody development to infliximab. Another consideration is that rheumatoid arthritis patients with anti-infliximab antibodies who switch to adalimumab are twice as likely to develop anti-adalimumab antibodies in comparison with patients naïve to infliximab therapy.[37] A current barrier to understanding immunogenicity and treatment is the absence of a standard reporting approach, making it impossible to draw conclusions from multiple clinical trial data.[38]

Adalimumab

Adalimumab, similar to infliximab, can lead to the formation of antibodies to adalimumab in some CD patients. Because most of the clinical trials with adalimumab did not report antibody to adalimumab values, this rate is less well described than that for infliximab. Nevertheless, it is believed to be similar to that of infliximab and affected by similar factors. Indeed, one study investigating adalimumab for maintenance found that 9.2% of patients had antibodies against adalimumab therapy, and this was associated with low serum adalimumab trough levels.[39] Additional clinically relevant data from 3 rheumatoid arthritis studies show that approximately 5% of patients developed low titer antibodies that subsequently neutralized the in vitro adalimumab. Patients receiving concomitant methotrexate therapy had a lower rate of antibody formation than those receiving monotherapy (1% vs 12%).[2]

Certolizumab Pegol

Certolizumab pegol therapy was shown to invoke antibody development in 12.3% of CD patients, of whom 37.5% were receiving concomitant immunomodulator therapy.[40] Of note, the presence of antidrug antibodies did not appear to affect drug efficacy at week 12 of the trial. Certolizumab pegol therapy interruption leads to antibody formation, thereby reinforcing the importance of maintenance therapy in CD patients.[41]

COMBINATION THERAPY

Infliximab, adalimumab, and certolizumab have been used in combination with mesalamine, corticosteroids, and immunosuppressors such as azathioprine and methotrexate. Specifically, there has been much interest in the role of immunosuppressor therapy in combination with infliximab to reduce the extent of antibody formation.[32] Recently, the CD clinical trial abbreviated as SONIC found that infliximab in combination with azathioprine therapy yielded the highest corticosteroid-free remission and mucosal healing rates in comparison with either the infliximab or azathioprine monotherapy groups.[42] Analysis of remission rates for the infliximab and azathioprine monotherapy groups suggests the presence of a synergistic effect. Adverse events were not significantly higher in the dual therapy than in the monotherapy infliximab treatment groups.

The concomitant use of methotrexate with infliximab for the induction and maintenance of remission in active CD has recently been shown to significantly reduce the antibody to infliximab rate from 20.4% in those patients not using methotrexate to 4.0% in those patients on concomitant methotrexate with the infliximab.[43] Of interest, this reduction in antibodies to infliximab did not correlate with an increased clinical efficacy at the end of the 1-year study, implying nonantibody-related synergistic effects of concomitant therapy. These results reverse conclusions from the earlier analyses of the effects of immunomodulators and infliximab in the ACCENT trials I and II.[44] Also, a retrospective patient chart review concluded that concomitant immunomodulator therapy with infliximab yielded a nonsignificant trend for improved outcomes compared with infliximab monotherapy.[45] The study differences may be ascribed to improved patient selection parameters and a parallel study design specific for assessing azathioprine in the SONIC trial.

The synergistic therapeutic effect of concomitant immunosuppressive therapy will need to be balanced against adverse events. The concomitant use of immunosuppressors and infliximab has been implicated in the development of a very rare, often lethal cancer, hepatosplenic T-cell lymphoma, occurring in young CD patients (age range: 12–40 years; median age; 22 years).[46] This observation along with the previously identified risk of non-Hodgkin lymphoma with anti–TNF-α therapy resulted in warning statements for all marketed TNF blockers in June 2009, acknowledging that these pharmaceuticals increase the risk for development of lymphomas.[7]

SUCCESSIVE TNF-α ANTAGONIST THERAPY

Patients who do not respond to or lose response to infliximab, adalimumab, or certolizumab may be successfully treated with another. Of importance, antibodies developed against one of the anti–TNF-α agents are very specific and do not affect the bioavailability of the next antagonist.[32] As an aside, data from rheumatoid arthritis indicate that the risk for adalimumab antibody formation is higher in patients who previously developed antibodies to infliximab.[37] Evidence suggests that this does not apply to patients with CD and UC.

Adalimumab was administered to CD patients classified as nonresponders to infliximab of whom two-thirds were successfully treated for a mean follow-up period of 2 years.[39] In all, only 9.2% of the patients developed antibodies against adalimumab. In a pediatric cohort of patients who had failed, lost response to, or were intolerant of infliximab or simply preferred a different administration route, adalimumab therapy was well tolerated and successful for nearly two-thirds of the cohort over a mean duration of 1 year.[47] UC patients who have lost response to or become intolerant to infliximab can be successfully treated with adalimumab for induction followed by a lengthy maintenance phase.[48]

Certolizumab pegol has been used successfully for treatment of CD patients who have ceased infliximab therapy for a variety of reasons.[49,50] However, response rates were lower in patients who switched than in those who were TNF-α naïve.[49]

Adalimumab or certolizumab pegol, used as a third biologic, is a therapeutic possibility for CD patients as the agents do not interact. In a small retrospective study of patients who had developed antibodies to infliximab and either adalimumab or certolizumab, 50% of the cohort achieved a "favorable" clinical response with the third TNF-α antagonist and remained in remission for 20 weeks.[51] Although possibly perceived as extreme, the successive use of these biologic agents confirms their unique mechanisms in the treatment of inflammatory bowel disease.

SAFETY

The 3 monoclonal antibodies to TNF-α have been associated with a range of adverse events, most notably infections, either opportunistic or latent (**Table 3**). In healthy individuals, TNF-α is responsible for controlling mycobacteria and other granulomatous pathogens.[52] In patients receiving TNF antagonists, latent infections of *Mycobacterium tuberculosis* are often reactivated within the first year of treatment, after which incidence rates are attributed to new infections.[52]

It is essential that patients are tested as outlined in practice guidelines for tuberculosis and hepatitis B before treatment initiation, and are closely monitored throughout treatment for viral reactivation. Similarly, vaccinations with live organisms should be received in advance of starting therapy; live vaccines are contraindicated once a patient initiates anti–TNF-α therapy.

PREGNANCY

Fetal immunity is acquired through selective active transportation of maternal IgG and is at its highest near the time of birth, therefore clinicians are advised to schedule treatments away from the third trimester.[53] In a review of the use of biologics during pregnancy and their effect on the developing immune system, the investigators concluded that insufficient evidence exists to warrant the selective use of one biologic agent over another, because of unknown risks.[54] Even though the data collected thus far on TNF-α antagonist therapy during pregnancy is limited, within the existing data set there has not been an increase in obvious malformations.[53] The PIANO study, initiated in November 2009, has followed the pregnancy and children of mothers intentionally treated with infliximab, adalimumab, and certolizumab.[55] No significant differences or trends have been identified regarding the use of anti–TNF-α therapy and pregnancy complications, delivery, birth weight, congenital malformations, and developmental milestones at 9 months of age in comparison with unexposed mothers and their children. Of note, fetal exposure to immunomodulator therapy was associated with slower attainment of developmental milestones. Overall, long-term studies are unavailable and the number of children followed to date is few, making it difficult to draw any firm

Table 3
Common side effects of anti–TNF-α agents[74]

Side Effect	Occurrence in IBD Patients Incidence (%)
Serious infections: fungal, parasitic, viral, tuberculosis	2%–4%[75]
Malignancies: lymphoma, leukemia, and solid cancers	Overall, there is no measurable increase in malignancy risk for IBD patients specifically associated with anti–TNF-α therapies[76] 48 pediatric cases 147 cases of leukemia (all ages)
Hypersensitivity reactions	Not uncommon[77]
Demyelinating conditions and other neurologic disorders: optic neuritis, systemic lupus erythematosus, lupus-like syndrome, sarcoidosis, uveitis, thyroiditis, and interstitial lung disease	37 cases overall for IBD patients treated with either IFX or ADA
Injection or infusion reactions	IFX 6.1% ADA 4% CZ 3%
Hematological reactions	Rare
Liver toxicity (IFX, ADA): hepatitis, elevated liver enzymes, liver failure	5 cases overall (1 of which had CD)
Autoimmunity	Common occurrence but not associated with new onset of autoimmune disease[76]
Immunosuppression	Common, hence use of immunomodulator concomitant therapy
Contraindications:	
Acute infectious diseases: latent tuberculosis and hepatitis B virus infections	
Chronic heart failure	
Vaccinations with live organisms	

Abbreviations: ADA, adalimumab; CZ, certolizumab pegol; IBD, inflammatory bowel disease; IFX, infliximab.

conclusions.[56] Nevertheless, anti–TNF-α agents use during pregnancy has been ruled as "safe" by the US FDA and the European Crohn's and Colitis Organization.[57]

Infliximab treatment in pregnancy provides the largest data repository for this information type. To date, there have been no issues; however, the data pool is relatively small. Moreover, it is still early to assess the long-term effects of fetal infliximab exposure on normal childhood development. Infliximab levels have not been detected in either the breast milk or the sera of breast-fed children, indicating that breastfeeding while receiving infusion therapy is feasible.[53,58,59]

Adalimumab levels in breast milk have been reported in a single case thus far.[60] The patient received adalimumab injections throughout her pregnancy, with the last one occurring 8 weeks before delivery at 38 weeks. The onset of a flare 4 weeks after delivery led to adalimumab therapy resumption at the request of the patient. At this time, enzyme-linked immunosorbent assay tests did not find the drug in either the patient's serum or breast milk. Following injection, serum levels of adalimumab peaked by the third day at 4300 ng/mL then decreased to 2000 ng/mL by day 8.

A corresponding adalimumab profile was also seen in the breast milk, although at one hundredth the level of the serum (43 ng/mL). After day 8, the patient opted to discontinue breastfeeding, although the effect of such a small quantity on the infant's immune system was considered to be negligible in theory.

SUMMARY

The introduction of anti–TNF-α agents for the treatment of CD and UC are proving to be effective and successful therapies for patients who may otherwise have suffered the undesirable side effects of systemic corticosteroids or received surgical intervention. Information gleaned in the last 10 years plus developments in antibody engineering have already yielded the second-generation agents, such as golimumab. However, several obstacles remain to be addressed, such as the identification of potential responders versus nonresponders for treatment. Delays in remission induction may lead to additional complications, deaths, and unnecessary expenses for the biologic. Also, a strategy is required to identify which patients will benefit from the top-down versus the traditional step-up treatment algorithms in this new era of individualized medicine. Uncertainty in this area has led to the overtreatment of 30% of patients.[61]

An often overlooked feature of TNF-α antagonist therapy is the assessment of patient compliance; an important issue as they may balance the price tag of each self-administered injection with little appreciation of the increased risk for antibody development. Infusion therapy conducted by medical professionals implies 100% adherence; however, a retrospective review of the Integrated Health Care Information Service claims database from 2002 to 2006 determined that 34.3% of CD patients were nonadherent in their first year of infliximab therapy.[62] Although substantial improvement in treatment options and outcomes for CD and UC have been realized, fundamental issues personalized medicine and drug adherence need to be addressed despite the advent and successes of anti–TNF-α agents.

ACKNOWLEDGMENTS

The authors would like to thank Kathleen Ismond for her expertise in conducting the literature review and preparation of the article.

REFERENCES

1. Dharmani P, Chadee K. Biologic therapies against inflammatory bowel disease: a dysregulated immune system and the cross talk with gastrointestinal mucosa hold the key. Curr Mol Pharmacol 2008;1(3):195–212.
2. Kozuch PL, Hanauer SB. General principles and pharmacology of biologics in inflammatory bowel disease. Gastroenterol Clin North Am 2006;35:757–73.
3. Horiuchi T, Mitoma H, Harashima SI, et al. Transmembrane TNF-{alpha}: structure, function and interaction with anti-TNF agents. Rheumatology (Oxford) 2010;49(7):1215–8.
4. Kaymakcalan Z, Sakorafas P, Bose S, et al. Comparisons of affinities, avidities, and complement activation of adalimumab, infliximab, and etanercept in binding to soluble and membrane tumor necrosis factor. Clin Immunol 2009;131:308–16.
5. Etchevers MJ, Ordas I, Ricart E. Optimizing the use of tumour necrosis factor inhibitors in Crohn's disease: a practical approach. Drugs 2010;70:109–20.
6. Bosani M, Ardizzone S, Porro GB. Biologic targeting in the treatment of inflammatory bowel diseases. Biologics 2009;3:77–97.

7. EvaluatePharma®. Available at: http://www.evaluatepharma.com. Accessed June 8, 2010.
8. Turner D, Mack D, Leleiko N, et al. Severe pediatric ulcerative colitis: a prospective multicenter study of outcomes and predictors of response. Gastroenterology 2010;138(7):2282–91.
9. Hyams JS, Lerer T, Griffiths A, et al. Outcome following infliximab therapy in children with ulcerative colitis. Am J Gastroenterol 2010;105(6):1430–6.
10. Sorrentino D, Paviotti A, Terrosu G, et al. Low-dose maintenance therapy with infliximab prevents postsurgical recurrence of Crohn's disease. Clin Gastroenterol Hepatol 2010;8(7):591–9.
11. Schoepfer AM, Vavricka SR, Binek J, et al. Efficacy and safety of certolizumab pegol induction therapy in an unselected Crohn's disease population: results of the FACTS survey. Inflamm Bowel Dis 2010;16:933–8.
12. Bourne T, Fossati G, Nesbitt A. A PEGylated Fab' fragment against tumor necrosis factor for the treatment of Crohn disease: exploring a new mechanism of action. BioDrugs 2008;22:331–7.
13. Van Assche G, Vermeire S, Rutgeerts P. Mucosal healing and anti TNFs in IBD. Curr Drug Targets 2010;11:227–33.
14. Han X. Intestinal permeability as a clinical surrogate endpoint in the development of future Crohn's disease therapies. Recent Pat Inflamm Allergy Drug Discov 2010;4:159–76.
15. Arijs I, De HG, Lemaire K, et al. Mucosal gene expression of antimicrobial peptides in inflammatory bowel disease before and after first infliximab treatment. PLoS One 2009;4:e7984.
16. Bolignano D, Della TA, Lacquaniti A, et al. Neutrophil gelatinase-associated lipocalin levels in patients with Crohn disease undergoing treatment with infliximab. J Investig Med 2010;58:569–71.
17. Danalioglu A. The frequency of sister chromatid exchanges in patients with Crohn's disease and the effect of therapy with "anti-tumor necrosis factor" on this frequency. Hepatogastroenterology 2009;56:729–33.
18. Hvas CL, Kelsen J, Agnholt J, et al. Discrete changes in circulating regulatory T cells during infliximab treatment of Crohn's disease. Autoimmunity 2010;43:325–33.
19. Li Z, Arijs I, De Hertogh G, et al. Reciprocal changes of Foxp3 expression in blood and intestinal mucosa in IBD patients responding to infliximab. Inflamm Bowel Dis 2010;16(8):1299–310.
20. Verri WA Jr, Souto FO, Vieira SM, et al. IL-33 induces neutrophil migration in rheumatoid arthritis and is a target of anti-TNF therapy. Ann Rheum Dis 2010;69(9):1697–703.
21. Pastorelli L, Garg RR, Hoang SB, et al. Epithelial-derived IL-33 and its receptor ST2 are dysregulated in ulcerative colitis and in experimental Th1/Th2 driven enteritis. Proc Natl Acad Sci U S A 2010;107:8017–22.
22. Bouchaud G, Mortier E, Flamant M, et al. Interleukin-15 and its soluble receptor mediate the response to infliximab in patients with Crohn's disease. Gastroenterology 2010;138(7):2378–87.
23. Crisafulli C, Galuppo M, Cuzzocrea S. Effects of genetic and pharmacological inhibition of TNF-alpha in the regulation of inflammation in macrophages. Pharmacol Res 2009;60:332–40.
24. Olsen T, Cui G, Goll R, et al. Infliximab therapy decreases the levels of TNF-alpha and IFN-gamma mRNA in colonic mucosa of ulcerative colitis. Scand J Gastroenterol 2009;44:727–35.

25. Jurgens M, Laubender RP, Hartl F, et al. Disease activity, ANCA, and IL23R geno-type status determine early response to infliximab in patients with ulcerative colitis. Am J Gastroenterol 2010;105(8):1811–9.
26. Krebs S, Omer TN, Omer B. Wormwood (*Artemisia absinthium*) suppresses tumour necrosis factor alpha and accelerates healing in patients with Crohn's disease—a controlled clinical trial. Phytomedicine 2010;17:305–9.
27. Aerts NE, Ebo DG, Bridts CH, et al. T cell signal transducer and activator of tran-scription (STAT) 4 and 6 are affected by adalimumab therapy in rheumatoid arthritis. Clin Exp Rheumatol 2010;28:208–14.
28. Klotz U, Teml A, Schwab M. Clinical pharmacokinetics and use of infliximab. Clin Pharmacokinet 2007;46:645–60.
29. Fasanmade AA, Adedokun OJ, Olson A, et al. Serum albumin concentration: a predictive factor of infliximab pharmacokinetics and clinical response in patients with ulcerative colitis. Int J Clin Pharmacol Ther 2010;48:297–308.
30. Fasanmade AA, Adedokun OJ, Ford J, et al. Population pharmacokinetic analysis of infliximab in patients with ulcerative colitis. Eur J Clin Pharmacol 2009;65:1211–28.
31. Abbott Laboratories. Humira®—medication guide. North Chicago (IL): Abbott Laboratory; 2009.
32. Bendtzen K, Ainsworth M, Steenholdt C, et al. Individual medicine in inflammatory bowel disease: monitoring bioavailability, pharmacokinetics and immunogenicity of anti-tumour necrosis factor-alpha antibodies. Scand J Gastroenterol 2009;44:774–81.
33. Kornbluth A, Sachar DB. Ulcerative colitis practice guidelines in adults. American College of Gastroenterology, Practice Parameters Committee. Am J Gastroenterol 2010;105:501–23.
34. Lichtenstein GR, Hanauer SB, Sandborn WJ. Management of Crohn's disease in adults. Am J Gastroenterol 2009;104:465–83.
35. Sadowski DC, Bernstein CN, Bitton A, et al. Canadian Association of Gastroenter-ology Clinical Practice Guidelines: The use of tumour necrosis factor-alpha antag-onist therapy in Crohn's disease. Can J Gastroenterol 2009;23:185–202.
36. Pollono EN, Lopez-Olivo MA, Lopez JA, et al. A systematic review of the effect of TNF-alpha antagonists on lipid profiles in patients with rheumatoid arthritis. Clin Rheumatol 2010;29(9):947–55.
37. Bartelds GM, Wijbrandts CA, Nurmohamed MT, et al. Anti-infliximab and anti-adalimumab antibodies in relation to response to adalimumab in infliximab switchers and anti-tumour necrosis factor naive patients: a cohort study. Ann Rheum Dis 2010;69:817–21.
38. Cassinotti A, Travis S. Incidence and clinical significance of immunogenicity to infliximab in Crohn's disease: a critical systematic review. Inflamm Bowel Dis 2009;15:1264–75.
39. Karmiris K, Paintaud G, Noman M, et al. Influence of trough serum levels and immunogenicity on long-term outcome of adalimumab therapy in Crohn's disease. Gastroenterology 2009;137:1628–40.
40. Schreiber S, Rutgeerts P, Fedorak RN, et al. A randomized, placebo-controlled trial of certolizumab pegol (CDP870) for treatment of Crohn's disease. Gastroen-terology 2005;129:807–18.
41. Lichtenstein GR, Thomsen OO, Schreiber S, et al. Continuous therapy with certo-lizumab pegol maintains remission of patients with Crohn's disease for up to 18 months. Clin Gastroenterol Hepatol 2010;8(7):600–99.
42. Colombel JF, Sandborn WJ, Reinisch W, et al. Infliximab, azathioprine, or combi-nation therapy for Crohn's disease. N Engl J Med 2010;362:1383–95.

43. Feagan BG, McDonald JW, Panaccione R, et al. Methotrexate for the prevention of antibodies to infliximab in patients with Crohn's disease (abstract: S1051). Gastroenterology 2010;138:S167–8.

44. Lichtenstein GR, Diamond RH, Wagner CL, et al. Clinical trial: benefits and risks of immunomodulators and maintenance infliximab for IBD-subgroup analyses across four randomized trials. Aliment Pharmacol Ther 2009;30:210–26.

45. Moss AC, Kim KJ, Fernandez-Becker N, et al. Impact of concomitant immuno-modulator use on long-term outcomes in patients receiving scheduled mainte-nance infliximab. Dig Dis Sci 2010;55:1413–20.

46. Ochenrider MG, Patterson DJ, Aboulafia DM. Hepatosplenic T-cell lymphoma in a young man with Crohn's disease: case report and literature review. Clin Lymphoma Myeloma Leuk 2010;10:144–8.

47. Rosh JR, Lerer T, Markowitz J, et al. Retrospective evaluation of the safety and effect of adalimumab therapy (RESEAT) in pediatric Crohn's disease. Am J Gas-troenterol 2009;104:3042–9.

48. Afif W, Leighton JA, Hanauer SB, et al. Open-label study of adalimumab in patients with ulcerative colitis including those with prior loss of response or intol-erance to infliximab. Inflamm Bowel Dis 2009;15:1302–7.

49. Hanauer SB, Panes J, Colombel JF, et al. Clinical trial: impact of prior infliximab therapy on clinical response to certolizumab pegol maintenance therapy for Crohn's disease. Aliment Pharmacol Ther 2010;32(3):384–93.

50. Sandborn WJ, Abreu MT, D'Haens G, et al. Certolizumab pegol in patients with moderate to severe Crohn's disease and secondary failure to infliximab. Clin Gas-troenterol Hepatol 2010;8(8):688–95.

51. Allez M, Vermeire S, Mozziconacci N, et al. The efficacy and safety of a third anti-TNF monoclonal antibody in Crohn's disease after failure of two other anti-TNF antibodies. Aliment Pharmacol Ther 2010;31:92–101.

52. Wallis RS. Reactivation of latent tuberculosis by TNF blockade: the role of inter-feron gamma. J Investig Dermatol Symp Proc 2007;12:16–21.

53. Gisbert JP. Safety of immunomodulators and biologics for the treatment of inflam-matory bowel disease during pregnancy and breast-feeding. Inflamm Bowel Dis 2010;16:881–95.

54. Kane SV, Acquah LA. Placental transport of immunoglobulins: a clinical review for gastroenterologists who prescribe therapeutic monoclonal antibodies to women during conception and pregnancy. Am J Gastroenterol 2009;104:228–33.

55. Mahadevan U, Martin CF, Sandler RS, et al. One year newborn outcomes among offspring of women with inflammatory bowel disease: The PIANO Registry (abstract: 764). Gastroenterology 2010;138:106.

56. O'Donnell S, O'Morain C. Review article: use of antitumour necrosis factor therapy in inflammatory bowel disease during pregnancy and conception. Aliment Pharmacol Ther 2008;27:885–94.

57. El Mourabet M, El-Hachem S, Harrison JR, et al. Anti-TNF antibody therapy for inflammatory bowel disease during pregnancy: a clinical review. Curr Drug Targets 2010;11:234–41.

58. Stengel JZ, Arnold HL. Is infliximab safe to use while breastfeeding? World J Gas-troenterol 2008;14:3085–7.

59. Kane S, Ford J, Cohen R, et al. Absence of infliximab in infants and breast milk from nursing mothers receiving therapy for Crohn's disease before and after delivery. J Clin Gastroenterol 2009;43:613–6.

60. Ben-Horin S, Yavzori M, Katz L, et al. Adalimumab level in breast milk of a nursing mother. Clin Gastroenterol Hepatol 2010;8:475–6.

61. Lin MV, Blonski W, Lichtenstein GR. What is the optimal therapy for Crohn's disease: step-up or top-down? Expert Rev Gastroenterol Hepatol 2010;4:167–80.
62. Kane SV, Chao J, Mulani PM. Adherence to infliximab maintenance therapy and health care utilization and costs by Crohn's disease patients. Adv Ther 2009;26: 936–46.
63. Regueiro M, Siemanowski B, Kip KE, et al. Infliximab dose intensification in Crohn's disease. Inflamm Bowel Dis 2007;13:1093–9.
64. Sandborn WJ, Schreiber S, Hanauer SB, et al. Reinduction with certolizumab pegol in patients with relapsed Crohn's disease: results from the PRECiSE 4 study. Clin Gastroenterol Hepatol 2010;8(8):696–702.
65. Hanauer SB, Feagan B, Lichtenstein GR, et al. Maintenance infliximab for Crohn's disease: the ACCENT I randomised trial. Lancet 2002;359:1541–9.
66. Sands BE, Blank MA, Diamond RH, et al. Maintenance infliximab does not result in increased abscess development in fistulizing Crohn's disease: results from the ACCENT II study. Aliment Pharmacol Ther 2006;23:1127–36.
67. Hanauer SB, Sandborn WJ, Rutgeerts P, et al. Human anti-tumor necrosis factor monoclonal antibody (adalimumab) in Crohn's disease: the CLASSIC I trial. Gastroenterology 2006;130:323–33.
68. Sandborn WJ, Hanauer SB, Rutgeerts P, et al. Adalimumab for maintenance treatment of Crohn's disease: results of the CLASSIC II trial. Gut 2007;56:1232–9.
69. Colombel JF, Sandborn WJ, Rutgeerts P, et al. Comparison of two adalimumab treatment schedule strategies for moderate-to-severe Crohn's disease: results from the CHARM trial. Am J Gastroenterol 2009;104:1170–9.
70. Sandborn WJ, Feagan BG, Stoinov S, et al. Certolizumab pegol for the treatment of Crohn's disease. N Engl J Med 2007;357:228–38.
71. Schreiber S, Khaliq-Kareemi M, Lawrance IC, et al. Maintenance therapy with certolizumab pegol for Crohn's disease. N Engl J Med 2007;357:239–50.
72. Rutgeerts P, Sandborn WJ, Feagan BG, et al. Infliximab for induction and maintenance therapy for ulcerative colitis. N Engl J Med 2005;353:2462–76.
73. Clare DF, Alexander FC, Mike S, et al. Accelerated infliximab infusions are safe and well tolerated in patients with inflammatory bowel disease. Eur J Gastroenterol Hepatol 2009;21:71–5.
74. Hoentjen F, van Bodegraven AA. Safety of anti-tumor necrosis factor therapy in inflammatory bowel disease. World J Gastroenterol 2009;15:2067–73.
75. Peyrin-Biroulet L. Anti-TNF therapy in inflammatory bowel diseases: a huge review. Minerva Gastroenterol Dietol 2010;56:233–43.
76. Stallmach A, Hagel S, Bruns T. Adverse effects of biologics used for treating IBD. Best Pract Res Clin Gastroenterol 2010;24:167–82.
77. Campi P, Benucci M, Manfredi M, et al. Hypersensitivity reactions to biological agents with special emphasis on tumor necrosis factor-alpha antagonists. Curr Opin Allergy Clin Immunol 2007;7:393–403.

Clinical Pharmacology of 5-ASA Compounds in Inflammatory Bowel Disease

Irene Sonu, MD[a], Ming Valerie Lin, MD[b],
Wojciech Blonski, MD, PhD[c,d], Gary R. Lichtenstein, MD[c,*]

KEYWORDS

- Mesalamine • Sulfasalazine • 5-Aminosalicylic acid
- Ulcerative colitis

The 5-aminosalicylic acid (5-ASA, mesalamine) class of drugs has been recommended as the first line of therapy in patients with mild to moderate ulcerative colitis (UC).[1,2] Mesalamine's mechanism of action is not fully understood, but it has been shown to be successful in the induction and maintenance of clinical remission in patients with UC. Since the discovery of sulfasalazine, there have been several newer preparations of 5-ASA with different modes of delivery on the market, all aimed at minimal systemic absorption and maximal topical application.

Rectal administration of gels, foams, and enemas containing 5-ASA is the most effective way to achieve maximal topical efficacy. Topical mesalamine has been

Potential conflict of interest declaration: Gary R. Lichtenstein, MD. Consultant, Abbott Corporation; Consultant, Alaven; Research, Bristol-Myers Squibb; Consultant, Research, Centocor, Inc; Consultant, Elan; Consultant, Research, Ferring; Consultant, Millenium Pharmaceuticals; Consultant, Research, Proctor and Gamble; Consultant, Research, Prometheus Laboratories, Inc; Consultant, Research, Salix Pharmaceuticals; Consultant, Schering-Plough Corporation; Consultant, Research, Shire Pharmaceuticals; Consultant, Research, UCB; Consultant, Wyeth.

[a] University of Pennsylvania School of Medicine, Suite 100, Stemmler Hall, 3450 Hamilton Walk, Philadelphia, PA 19104, USA
[b] Department of Internal Medicine, Pennsylvania Hospital, University of Pennsylvania Health System, 800 Spruce Street, Philadelphia, PA 19107, USA
[c] Division of Gastroenterology, University of Pennsylvania, 3400 Spruce Street, Philadelphia, PA 19104, USA
[d] Department of Gastroenterology, Medical University, Wroclaw, Poland
* Corresponding author. Gastroenterology Division, Hospital of the University of Pennsylvania, University of Pennsylvania School of Medicine, 3400 Spruce Street, 3rd Floor Ravdin Building, Philadelphia, PA 19104-4283.
E-mail address: grl@uphs.upenn.edu

Gastroenterol Clin N Am 39 (2010) 559–599
doi:10.1016/j.gtc.2010.08.011
0889-8553/10/$ – see front matter © 2010 Elsevier Inc. All rights reserved.

demonstrated to be effective in treating patients with active proctosigmoiditis and left-sided colitis. However, patient tolerability of rectal administration is poor because of difficulty in administration, problems with retention and leakage, and patient discomfort. Thus, despite evidence suggesting a superiority of topical mesalamine to oral aminosalicylates alone in achieving clinical improvement in patients with mild to moderate distal colitis,[3–5] the therapeutic plan is often guided largely by patient preferences with the oral route of administration preferred over rectal therapy. Oral 5-ASA in its unformulated form is rapidly absorbed in the small intestine, leaving a minimal concentration of drug to treat the colon (**Fig. 1**). Various formulations have thus been manufactured to ensure maximal delivery of 5-ASA to the site of inflammation. Sulfasalazine, olsalazine, and balsalazide are azo-bonded prodrugs, in which 5-ASA (the active moiety) is linked by an azo bond to the carrier moiety (**Fig. 2**). The bond is cleaved by colonic bacterial azoreductase, resulting in release of the 2 constituent moieties. Other oral formulations such as Asacol, which is coated with a gastroresistant and a pH-sensitive acrylic-based resin (Eudragit-S), delay release of the drug until it reaches the terminal ileum, where the pH is consistently 7 or higher. Similarly, Apriso also consists of a delayed-release mechanism and offers once-daily dosing[6] with a capsule containing granules composed of mesalamine in a polymer matrix with an enteric (outer) coating, Eudragit-L.[6] The outer coating dissolves in the terminal ileum (pH ≥6), while the polymer matrix core facilitates slow, sustained release throughout the colon (**Fig. 3**).[7] Pentasa, formulated as ethylcellulose-coated controlled-release capsules, is released throughout the gastrointestinal tract. Lialda contains a "Multi Matrix System Technology" (MMX) with lipophilic and hydrophilic matrices to provide delayed release of mesalamine. Lialda contains Eudragit-S, which enables mesalamine release at pH 7 or higher in the terminal ileum, and its release continues throughout the colon.[8] Despite the variety of delivery mechanisms employed, the

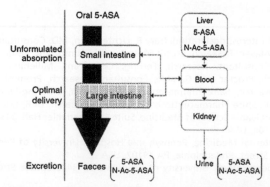

Fig. 1. Proposed metabolic pathway of 5-ASA after oral administration. The shaded area (large intestine) indicates the site of topical action. Unformulated 5-ASA is absorbed rapidly from the small intestine, and many current formulations are designed to delay release of 5-ASA until the terminal ileum or proximal colon. 5-ASA, 5-aminosalicylic acid; N-AC-5-ASA, N-acetyl-5-ASA. (*Reprinted from* Lichtenstein GR, Kamm MA. Review article: 5-aminosalicylate formulations for the treatment of ulcerative colitis—methods of comparing release rates and delivery of 5-aminosalicylate to the colonic mucosa. Aliment Pharmacol Ther 2008;28(6):663–73; copyright 2008, Wiley-Blackwell; with permission.)

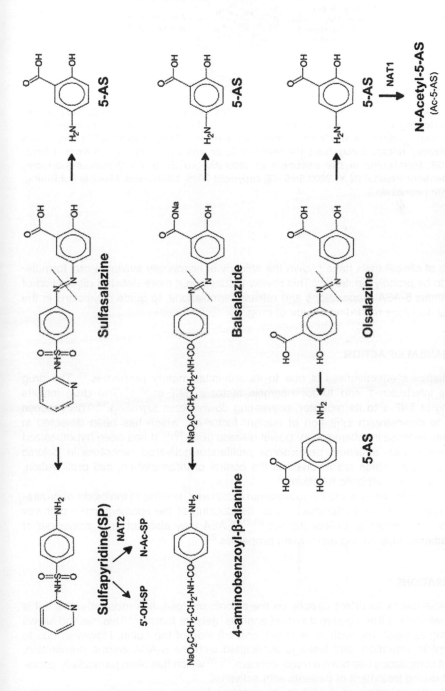

Fig. 2. Structure of different prodrugs of 5-AS and part of their metabolism. (*Reprinted from* Klotz U, Schwab M. Topical delivery of therapeutic agents in the treatment of inflammatory bowel disease. Adv Drug Deliv Rev 2005;57:267–79; copyright 2005, Elsevier; with permission.)

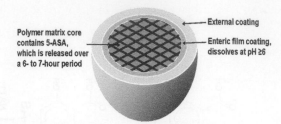

Polymer matrix core
contains 5-ASA,
which is released over
a 6- to 7-hour period

External coating

Enteric film coating,
dissolves at pH ≥6

Fig. 3. The formulation of mesalamine granules. The external coating protects the granules from dissolving in the stomach. On encountering a pH of at least 6 in the terminal ileum, the enteric coating dissolves and initiates mesalamine release. The polymer matrix core allows for extended release throughout the terminal ileum and colon. (*Reprinted from* Lichtenstein GR. Mesalamine in the treatment of ulcerative colitis: novel therapeutic options. Gastroenterol Hepatol (N Y) 2009;5:65–73; copyright 2009, Millennium Medical Publishing, Inc; with permission.)

results of clinical trials have shown the efficacy of historically available oral formulations to be broadly similar.[9,10] This review focuses on a more detailed discussion of the various 5-ASA preparations and release formulations, to guide physicians in the clinical decisions regarding choice of drug.

MECHANISM OF ACTION

Mesalamine's effectiveness is due to its anti-inflammatory properties.[11] The drug blocks interleukin-1 and tumor necrosis factor-α (TNF-α).[12–14] The drug inhibits binding of TNF-α to its receptor, preventing downstream signaling.[15] This process leads to downstream inhibition of nuclear factor-κB, which has been detected in inflamed mucosa in inflammatory bowel disease (IBD).[16,17] It has been hypothesized that 5-ASA also activates peroxisome proliferator-activated receptors in colonic epithelial cells, which are involved in the control of inflammation, cell proliferation, apoptosis, and metabolic function.[18]

The drug also inhibits the cyclooxygenase pathway, leading to inhibition of prostaglandin E_2 in inflamed intestine.[19] Also, its blocking of the lipooxygenase pathway inhibits the production of leukotrienes.[20,21] 5-ASA may also act as a scavenger of free radicals, thus having antioxidant properties.[22]

PREPARATIONS

As 5-ASA exerts its effect directly on the colonic mucosa, it is most effective if it is administered via the rectal route using enemas, gels, or foams.[23] This method allows the drug to reach the rectum, sigmoid, and left side of the colon. However, due to discomfort, retention, and leakage associated with the 5-ASA enema preparation, patient compliance has been a major concern,[24–26] which has been particularly appreciated during treatment of patients with active UC.

Oral administration of 5-ASA in its simplest form is not effective because the majority of the drug is absorbed by the small bowel, resulting in insufficient concentration of drug by the time it reaches the large intestine.[18] In addition, acetylation in the gut epithelium and liver inactivates the drug. Sulfasalazine was the first aminosalicy-late to be used for the treatment of patients with IBD; however, it was associated with many adverse effects and frequent allergic reactions. The majority were attribut-able to its carrier moiety, sulfapyridine.[27] To address this problem, new oral formula-tions have been developed that allow enough drug to reach the distal bowel in therapeutic concentrations. Mesalamine, olsalazine, and balsalazide are the other 3 available oral preparations of 5-ASA. A summary of various 5-ASA formulations is presented in **Table 1**.

The mucosal concentration of 5-ASA is inversely correlated with severity of inflam-mation in patients with UC.[28–30] Patients with none or mild endoscopic and micro-scopic colonic inflammation had significantly higher mucosal concentrations of 5-ASA when compared with those having moderate and severe macroscopic ($P = .03$) and microscopic ($P<.01$) activity of UC.[28] On the other hand, levels of soluble

Table 1
5-ASA formulations and release sites

Name Formulation	Release Site	Dosage Per Tablet
Sulfasalazine/ Azulfidine	5-ASA linked to sulfapyridine by an azo bond	500 mg
Asacol/delayed release mesalamine	Enclosed in enteric "film" (Eudragit-S) releasing at pH ≥7 in the terminal ileum and colon	400 mg (Asacol)
		800 mg (Asacol HD)
Salofalk, Claversal	Enclosed Eudragit-L releasing at pH ≥6 in the jejunum, ileum, and colon	250 mg (Salofalk) 500 mg (Salofalk and Claversal)
Pentasa	Microspheres within a moisture-sensitive, ethylcellulose, semipermeable membrane releasing mesalamine in the duodenum, jejunum, ileum, and colon	250 mg and 500 mg capsules
Apriso	The outer coating (Eudragit-L) dissolves in the jejunum, ileum, and colon (pH ≥6), while a polymer matrix core facilitates slow, sustained release throughout the colon	375 mg
Olsalazine/Dipentum	Two molecules of 5-ASA linked by an azo bond between their amino groups cleaved by azoreductase	250 mg
Balsalazide disodium/ Colazal	5-ASA linked by an azo bond to 4-amino-benzoyl-β-alanine cleaved by azoreductase	750 mg
Lialda, Mezavant	Has lipophilic and hydrophilic matrices to provide delayed release of mesalamine. Has Eudragit-S, which enables mesalamine release at pH ≥7 in the terminal ileum and continues throughout the colon	1200 mg
Salofalk Granustix, Pentasa sachets	Micropellet formulations	500 mg sachets

interleukin-2 receptor, which is a proinflammatory cytokine, were significantly lower in patients with high mucosal concentrations of 5-ASA when compared with those with low mucosal concentrations.[28] A study of 18 patients with UC and high risk of relapse has demonstrated that increased 5-ASA doses lead to an improved clinical course of UC.[30] It has been suggested that mucosal concentrations of 5-ASA depend not only on the dose of the drug but also on other factors.[31] A phase 2 study of MMX mesalamine observed higher 5-ASA mucosal concentrations in the sigmoid colon and rectum in patients with UC after treatment at a once-daily dose of 4.8 g when compared with one daily dose of 1.2 or 2.4 g.[32] On the other hand, a biopsy study has demonstrated that patients with UC treated with balsalazide at the daily dose of 6.75 g (equivalent to pH dependent mesalamine at the daily dose of 2.4 g) had a 96% higher mean mucosal concentrations of 5-ASA in the distal colon than in those receiving pH-dependent mesalamine at the daily dose of 3.74 g.[33] Therefore, mucosal concentrations of 5-ASA may depend on its formulation and be independent of dose-plasma concentration relationships.[23] Studies[34–37] have demonstrated interindividual variability in 5-ASA mucosal concentrations, which may be caused by local pH conditions, transit rates, and activities of enzymes and transporters involved in metabolism of 5-ASA within colonic mucosa.[23] It has been suggested that the mucosal concentration of 5-ASA might be inversely related to the risk of relapse in patients receiving maintenance treatment.[23]

Sulfasalazine

Sulfasalazine/Azulfidine (Pharmacia & Upjohn Co, New York) consists of 5-ASA linked to sulfapyridine by an azo bond (see **Fig. 2**).[18] The bond is cleaved by colonic bacterial azoreductase. In 1977, Azad Khan and colleagues[38] published data of a nonplacebo controlled trial to discern if sulfasalazine's efficacy is a result of the parent molecule or its metabolites, sulfapyridine and 5-ASA. The study consisted of a blind nonplacebo controlled trial in patients with UC given retention enemas of sulfasalazine, sulfapyridine, or 5-ASA daily for 2 weeks. The primary end point was histologic improvement, which was observed in 30% of patients receiving sulfasalazine or 5-ASA, but only 5% of those receiving sulfapyridine. Thus, the study concluded that the active moiety was the 5-ASA metabolite of sulfasalazine.[38] In addition, the sulfapyridine moiety is absorbed systemically, leading to adverse effects, whereas the 5-ASA moiety is less well absorbed from the distal small intestine and thus reaches high concentrations (1–100 mmol/L) in the lumen of the colon and rectum.[28]

Mesalamine

Mesalamine (termed mesalazine in Europe) is otherwise known as 5-ASA.

Formulations

There are various formulations of mesalamine enclosed within an enteric coat or "film" such as Eudragit-S (used in Asacol and Lialda) or Eudragit-L (used in Apriso) (Röhm GmbH & Co KG, Pharma Polymers, Darmstadt, Germany).[39] The enteric coating (Eudragit-L) is broken down in the jejunum, terminal ileum, or cecum when a change in pH (at ≥ 6) causes it to disintegrate and release the active drug. Similarly, the enteric coating (Eudragit-S) is broken down in the terminal ileum, or cecum when a change in pH (at ≥ 7) causes it to disintegrate and release the active drug. Asacol (Procter & Gamble Pharmaceuticals, Cincinnati, OH, USA), Salofalk (Axcan Pharma, Mont St Hilaire, Quebec, Canada and Falk Pharma, Freiburg, Germany), Claversal (Merckle GMbH, Ulm, Germany), Mesasal (GlaxoSmithKline, Mississauga, ON, Canada), Ipocol

(Sandoz Pharmaceuticals, Bordon, Hampshire, UK), and Mesren (Ivax Pharmaceuticals Limited, Runcorn, Cheshire, UK), use the enteric coated approach.[39]

Pentasa (Shire Pharmaceuticals Inc, Wayne, PA, USA, licensed from Ferring A/S, Copenhagen, Denmark) is another mesalamine-containing drug, but instead of having an enteric coat it is composed of microspheres containing 5-ASA enclosed within a moisture-sensitive, ethylcellulose, semipermeable membrane, allowing for pH-independent release of the drug.[39] Drug release begins in the duodenum (unlike the other drugs mentioned, which release further down the bowel).[39]

Apriso (Salix Pharmaceuticals Inc, Morrisville, NC, USA) is composed of gelatin capsules that dissolve, releasing granules of the drug into the stomach.[6] The delayed-release coating (Eudragit-L) on the granules dissolves at a pH of 6 or higher. The granules contain an extended-release polymer matrix core that swells and gradually distributes mesalamine throughout the colon. Apriso is the newest of the 5-ASAs to be approved by the Food and Drug Administration (FDA), with the main benefit of it being administered once a day.[6,40] This medication is currently FDA approved for maintenance of remission for patients with ulcerative colitis. Two randomized, double-blind, placebo-controlled, multicenter trials were conducted on patients in remission from mild to moderate UC where Apriso was given at 1.5 g/d and compared with placebo.[41] The primary end point was remaining relapse free at 6 months (defined using Sutherland Disease Activity Index [DAI] of rectal bleeding subscale score of ≥ 1 and mucosal appearance score ≥ 2). Of the 562 patients enrolled, 70% ($P = .001$) were relapse-free at month 6 compared with 56% in the placebo arm.[41] The recommended dose is 4 0.375-g capsules once daily (a total of 1.5 g daily). Adverse effects include renal impairment, headache, diarrhea, upper abdominal pain, nausea, nasopharyngitis, influenza, influenza-like illness, and sinusitis. Hepatic failure was very rarely noted to occur in patients with preexisting liver disease.[41]

Olsalazine/Dipentum (Alaven Pharmaceuticals, Marietta, GA) consists of 2 molecules of 5-ASA linked by an azo bond between their amino groups. The azo bond is split by bacterial azoreductase in the distal small bowel and colon, releasing the active moiety (see **Fig. 2**).[18]

Benzalazine, balsalazide/Colazide (Astra Zeneca), and balsalazide disodium/Colazal (Salix Pharmaceuticals) is comprised of 5-ASA linked by an azo bond to 4-amino-benzoy-β-alanine which, similar to Olsalazine, is cleaved by bacterial azoreductase in the distal bowel, thus releasing the active 5-ASA. The 4-amino-benzoy-β-alanine is inert and poorly absorbed, causing few side effects (see **Fig. 2**).[18]

The MMX technology (previously known as SPD476, now marketed as Lialda in the United States and Mezavant in Canada; Shire Pharmaceuticals Inc, Wayne, PA) is a high-strength formulation of 5-ASA (1.2 g per tablet).[42] This system uses lipophilic and hydrophilic matrices, all enclosed within a gastroresistant, pH-dependent coating (Eudragit-S), allowing drug release at pH 7 or higher in the terminal ileum.[43] After the coating disintegrates, an interaction between the hydrophilic matrix and intestinal fluids occurs leading to swelling of the drug and formation of a viscous gel mass allowing for slow diffusion and release of active drug down the colon.[43] The hydrophilic matrix also adheres to the colonic mucosa.[44,45] Several randomized placebo-controlled studies have investigated the efficacy and safety of the MMX formulation in comparison with placebo.[42,43,46-48] In 2007, Kamm and colleagues[43] published a double-blind, multicenter study comparing MMX mesalamine to placebo for treatment of active UC (with an Asacol internal reference arm). Patients with active mild to moderate UC (n = 343) who received 2.4 g/d or 4.8 g/d of MMX once daily, Asacol 2.4 g/d divided into 3 doses, or placebo for 8 weeks. The study reported 40.5% ($P = .01$) of the 2.4 g/d MMX and 41.2% ($P = .007$) of the 4.8 g/d MMX achieved clinical and endoscopic remission at week 8, compared with 22.1% in the placebo group.[43] In addition, Sandborn and colleagues[46] pooled data from 2 phase 3, randomized placebo-controlled trials assessing the efficacy of MMX for inducing remission of mild to moderately active UC performed by Kamm and colleagues[43] and Lichtenstein and colleagues.[49] A total of 517 patients were randomized to receive 8 weeks of therapy with either MMX 2.4 g/d (every day or divided twice daily (n = 172), MMX 4.8 g/d (every day) (n = 174) or placebo (n = 171).[43,49] The proportion of patients in remission (defined as UC DAI ≤1) at week 8 was 2-fold higher in the MMX treated arm regardless of dose (37.2% for lower dose and 35.1% for higher dose) when compared with placebo (17.5%, $P<.001$).[43,49] Likewise, patients treated with MMX had 2-fold higher rates of complete mucosal healing than placebo recipients at week 8 (32% vs 16%, P value-not reported).[43,49] The percentages in remission were significantly greater ($P<.05$) in the MMX group compared with placebo when stratified for disease extent, disease severity, and gender as well as among patients not previously receiving low-dose ASA.[43,49] MMX at 4.8 g/d was also more successful than placebo in patients transferring from prior low-dose oral 5-ASA, but not on 2.5 g/d MMX. The study concluded that MMX mesalamine was efficacious for active UC regardless of disease extent, severity, gender, and previous low-dose 5-ASA therapy.[48] Adverse effects of MMX included abnormal liver function tests, angina pectoris, pulmonary edema, cerebral infarction, abdominal pain, diarrhea, flatulence, nausea, nasopharyngitis, and headache. The safety profile of MMX is similar to that of other oral nonsulfa-5-ASA therapies.[43,50] The clinical studies demonstrate that MMX mesalamine (at either 2.4 g/d or 4.8 g/d dose) is effective for inducing clinical and endoscopic remission in patients with active mild to moderate UC.[51] For patients who do not respond to initial 8 weeks of therapy benefit from an additional 8 weeks of therapy.[52] Extended therapy beyond 8 weeks may prevent escalation to steroids or biologics. MMX mesalamine is successful in maintaining remission for at least 12 months.[51] Given MMX mesalamine's simplified dosing regimen and ability to induce and maintain clinical and endoscopic remission in patients with mild to moderate UC, this formulation is commonly recommended to patients with active UC. Lower pill burden aids compliance and, hopefully, better clinical outcomes. Prospective, community-based studies will evaluate adherence to MMX mesalamine. Trials comparing the various 5-ASA formulations are needed to further evaluate the efficacy of these different medications.[51]

Salofalk Granustix sachets (Falk Pharma) and Pentasa sachets (Ferring Pharmaceuticals) are micropellet formulations of 5-ASA that allow for less frequent dosing and an easy-to-swallow drug.[40,53] The Salofalk granustix sachets release 5-ASA in the ileocecal region, which is similar to the Salofalk tablets; however, there is a prolonged release of 5-ASA from the sachet compared with the tablet.[40] The Pentasa sachets contain mesalamine and also have a prolonged release; the drug is released in the terminal ileum and ascending colon.[53]

Dosing of mesalamine

Dose response studies for mild to moderate active UC reported additional benefit of 2.4 g/d compared with 1.6 g/d,[54] and another study showed added benefit of 4.8 g/d dosing compared with 1.6 g/d.[55] Two meta-analyses recommended dosing 3 g/d or greater for mild to moderate active UC.[36,56] The regimen commonly used by clinicians is to administer a 2.4 g/d dose for mild to moderate active UC, with an increase to a maximum of 4.8 g/d if patients are not responsive to the lower dose. The Assessing the Safety & Clinical Efficacy of New Dose of 5-ASA (ASCEND) trials involved 2 randomized, double-blind placebo-controlled trials comparing 4.8 g and 2.4 g/d dosing of mesalamine.[57,58] The ASCEND I trial involved 301 patients with mild to moderately active UC with a primary end point of overall improvement (complete remission or clinical response to therapy) at week 6 of treatment in the format of a noninferiority trial. The results revealed significant improvement on the higher dose compared with the lower dose for those with moderately active UC (57% in 2.4 g/d, 72.4% in 4.8 g/d; P = .0384).[57] The ASCEND II trial involved moderately active UC only (286 patients), and patients were randomized to the 2.4 g/d dose or 4.8 g/d daily dose of mesalamine; the primary end point was the same as that of the ASCEND I trial.[58] Results yielded a significant treatment success in those on the 4.8 g/d dose (72%, 89/124 patients) compared with those on the 2.4 g/d dose (59%, 77/130 patients, P = .036). Adverse events were similar in both groups. The studies suggested that the higher dose is more effective at providing acute response and remission in patients with moderately active UC, while the lower dose is sufficient in patients with mildly active UC.[57,58]

The notion that a higher dose (4.8 g of mesalamine) is superior to 2.4 g of mesalamine is not true in all populations studied. The primary end point of the ASCEND II and III studies was overall improvement at 6 weeks, which was determined by the Physician's Global Assessment (PGA), which encompassed the clinical assessments of rectal bleeding, stool frequency, and sigmoidoscopy findings.

In ASCEND III, only patients with moderately active UC were studied. Overall, 70% of patients (n = 273/389) achieved overall improvement with Asacol HD at 4.8 g/d compared with 66% of patients (n = 251/383) who took Asacol 400 mg tablets at 2.4 g/d.[59] (In ASCEND II, 72% of patients [n = 89/124] achieved overall improvement with Asacol HD at 4.8 g/d at 6 weeks, as compared with 59% of patients [n = 77/130] who took Asacol 400 mg tablets at 2.4 g/d [P = .036]).[58] Thus, when compared with each other, 2.4 g of mesalamine in the formulation of delayed-release mesalamine has similar efficacy as compared with 4.8 g of mesalamine for active treatment of ulcerative colitis. In a post hoc analysis there is, however, a suggestion that certain subsets of patients may benefit from high dose (4.8 g of mesalamine). In particular, in the ASCEND III trial there is a therapeutic advantage for the 4.8 g/d dose compared with the 2.4 g daily dose observed among patients previously treated with corticosteroids, oral mesalamines, rectal therapies, or multiple UC medications.[59]

The convention that dosing 5-ASA compounds multiple times a day was challenged initially by studies of Kamm colleagues[43] and Lichtenstein colleagues[49] using MMX mesalamine in assessing efficacy of induction of response and remission. Similarly, a once daily formulation was found to be effective for maintenance of remission by using Apriso for maintenance of remission in 2 6-month maintenance studies.[41]

The same findings were reproduced in a study evaluating delayed release mesalamine by Sandborn and colleagues.[60] This multicenter, randomized, investigator-blinded, 12-month, active-control trial involved 1023 patients and compared once daily (QD) dosing to twice daily (BID) dosing of delayed-release mesalamine (Asacol) 1.6 to 2.4 g/d in patients with UC and who were currently in clinical remission (for at least 3 months).[60] The primary end point was maintenance of clinical remission at 6 months.[60] At month 6, 90.5% (428/483) of patients on the QD dose and 91.8% (435/474) on the BID dose maintained remission (95% confidence interval [CI] for BID-QD, −2.3, 4.9, respectively).[60] The study was designed to be a noninferiority design trial.[60] At month 12, 85.4% (379/444) or patients on the QD dose and 85.4% (380/445) of the BID dose maintained clinical remission (95% CI for BID-QD, −4.6, 4.7 respectively).[60] Withdrawals due to adverse events were similar in both groups. The study concluded that once-daily dosing of Asacol at doses of 1.6 to 2.4 g/d was effective for the maintenance of clinical remission in patients with UC.[60]

Foam versus liquid enema

Rectal administration of 5-ASA has been advocated as the treatment of choice in proctitis, proctosigmoiditis, and left-sided UC[61,62] because local concentrations and active drug at the affected site are sufficiently high for therapeutic activity, and in addition, systemic absorption is considerably lower. Other advantages include a generally quicker response time and less frequent dosing schedule. Different meta-analyses of controlled trials have also indicated a superiority of topical mesalamine over oral 5-ASA alone in achieving clinical improvement in patients with mild to moderate distal colitis.[3-5] However, in practice, rectal application often serves as an alternative or add-on therapy to oral 5-ASA.

Mesalamine rectal suppositories have been shown effective in the treatment of proctitis and maintenance of remission; however, their use is limited because they do not provide sufficient spread of the active ingredient beyond the distal colon. The spread of mesalamine liquid enema formulation is generally good, and has been shown to be effective in inducing and maintaining remission in distal colitis.[63-66] However, patient acceptance may be compromised by difficulties with self-administration, retention, discomfort, or the necessity for prolonged bed rest. Rectal mesalamine foam was developed to optimize drug delivery and improve patient acceptance. The rectal foam has a higher viscosity than the liquid enema, which favors retention, enhances mucosal adhesion, and provides wider mucosal spread.[67]

An internal pharmaceutical company report assessed the extent of dispersion of the rectal foam in a gamma scintigraphic study in healthy volunteers. It was found that immediately after dosing, the foam had spread through the rectum and sigmoid colon, reaching the upper descending colon after 12 hours.[68]

Pokrotnieks and colleagues[69] in a multicenter, randomized, double-blind parallel-group study showed that mesalamine foam was well tolerated and more effective than placebo in patients with distal UC. In this study, 111 patients with mild to moderately active proctitis, proctosigmoiditis, or left-sided UC received mesalamine foam or placebo enema for 6 weeks.[70] Clinical remission was more frequent in the mesalamine than the placebo group (65% vs 40%; $P = .0082$).[69] The frequency of endoscopic remission was also higher in the mesalamine group (57%) than in the placebo group (37%).[69] In comparing the efficacy of mesalamine foam with mesalamine liquid enema, Cortot and colleagues[70] conducted a multicenter investigator-blinded clinical trial and randomized 375 patients with mild to moderate UC to rectal foam or liquid enema for 4 weeks. Eligible patients were 18 years and older with newly diagnosed or relapsing active mild to moderate left-sided UC, with a disease extension of at least 5 cm from the anal margin and not above the splenic flexure.[70] Remission rates at week 4 in mesalamine foam versus mesalamine liquid enema were 68.3% versus 73.6% in the per protocol (PP) population (lower limit of 97.5% CI −15.1%) and 66.7% versus 70.5% in the intention-to-treat (ITT) population (97.5% CI −13.4%).[70] Remission rates at week 2 were 48.1% versus 50.6% in ITT (97.5% CI −12.8%) and 49.1% versus 52.1% in PP (97.5% CI −13.8%) in foam versus liquid enema, respectively.[70] Both treatments were well tolerated with minimal adverse events. Although the noninferiority of mesalamine foam could not be strictly demonstrated at week 4 in the PP analysis, it was achieved in the ITT population and at week 2 in both populations.[70] Mesalamine foam represents a clinically efficient and well tolerated therapeutic alternative to mesalamine liquid enema in patients with mild to moderately active proctitis and proctosigmoiditis. It may be especially appropriate in cases of poor tolerance of enemas because of acute rectal inflammation.

EFFICACY OF 5-ASA AGENTS

The oral formulations of 5-ASA have several disadvantages. First, several formulations of these drugs require frequent dosing of 2 to 4 times daily, resulting in a high pill burden on the patient and impacting patient compliance and disease control.[71–73] Also, it has been suggested that therapeutic doses of the drugs may not reach the left colon; with measured concentrations being the highest in the right side of the colon.[74,75] Several double-blind randomized clinical trials have evaluated the efficacy and safety of various oral 5-ASA formulations in inducing[76–93] (**Table 2**) and maintaining (**Table 3**) remission of UC.[34,94–105]

Several studies have compared the efficacy of sulfasalazine and the other 5-ASA formulations, and meta-analyses have been published analyzing past studies. Rahimi and colleagues[106] compared mesalamine and balsalazide in the induction and maintenance of remission in patients with UC in a meta-analysis (**Tables 4** and **5**). The study involved 6 randomized placebo-controlled trials, including 653 patients. Pooling of 3 trials for symptomatic remission resulted in a significant relative risk (RR) of 1.23 (95% CI 1.03–1.47, $P = .02$), and for complete remission the RR was 1.3 (95% CI 1.002–1.68, $P = .048$). Pooling of 2 trials for outcome of relapse revealed a nonsignificant RR of 0.77 (95% CI 0.56–1.07, $P = .12$). For adverse events, 5 studies were pooled revealing a nonsignificant RR of 0.87 (95% CI 0.75–1.001, $P = .53$). All 6 studies were pooled for withdrawals due to adverse events, yielding a nonsignificant RR of 0.69 (95% CI 0.37–1.29, $P = .24$). This meta-analysis concluded that balsalazide is more effective than mesalamine in the induction of remission, but there is no difference between the 2 drugs for the prevention of relapse. Adverse events and withdrawals due to severe adverse events were similar for both drugs.[106]

Nikfar and colleagues[107] published a meta-analysis in 2009 comparing the efficacy of sulfasalazine compared with 5-ASA compounds (mesalamine, olsalazine, and balsalazide) for the induction and maintenance of remission in patients with mild to moderate UC. The outcomes of sulfasalazine versus 5-ASA formulations are presented in **Tables 6–8**.[107] Data from 1966 to 2008 and 20 randomized, placebo-controlled trials were collected. Comparison of sulfasalazine with mesalamine yielded a nonsignificant RR of 1.04 (95% confidence interval of 0.89–1.21, $P = .63$) for overall improvement, a nonsignificant RR of 0.98 (95% CI 0.78–1.23, $P = .85$) for relapse, a nonsignificant RR of 0.76 (95% CI 0.54–1.07, $P = .11$) for any adverse events, and a nonsignificant RR of 0.78 (95% CI 0.46–1.3, $P = .33$) for withdrawals due to adverse events.[107] Comparison of sulfasalazine with olsalazine yielded a nonsignificant RR of 1.14 (95% CI 0.91–1.43, $P = .25$) for overall improvement, a nonsignificant RR of 0.93 (95% CI 0.77–1.12, $P = .42$) for relapse, a nonsignificant RR of 1.21 (95% CI 0.9–1.61, $P = .20$) for any adverse events, and a nonsignificant RR of 1.53 (95% CI 0.93–2.52, $P = .09$) for withdrawals due to adverse events.[107] Thus, the meta-analysis concluded that sulfasalazine was not more efficacious or more tolerable than mesalamine or olsalazine. Adverse events were significantly lower for balsalazide compared with sulfasalazine. Due to the cost-effectiveness of sulfasalazine compared with the 5-ASA compounds, the study recommended using sulfasalazine as a first-choice treatment for UC, and to use the 5-ASA compounds if the patient does not tolerate sulfasalazine.[107] It is important, however, to recognize that balsalazide is currently also available in generic form.

Sutherland and MacDonald[9,10] published 2 Cochrane database reviews assessing the efficacy, dose-responsiveness, and safety of the newer release formulations of 5-ASA compared with placebo or sulfasalazine in the induction and maintenance of remission for UC. For induction of remission the meta-analysis reported that 5-ASA

Table 2
Randomized double-blind controlled trials comparing therapy with various oral 5-ASA formulations in inducing remission of UC

Reference	Treatment Arm	Daily Dose	No. of Patients	Study Duration	Primary End Point	Results	Adverse Events	Withdrawals	Comments
Fleig et al, 1988[76]	Sulfasalazine	3.0 g	21	6 wk	Improvement in mean stool frequency (A) and consistency (B) macroscopic (C) and microscopic (D) appearance of colonic mucosa measured at wk 0 and 6	A: 6.9 ± 3.4 vs 3.0 ± 1.9 (P<.05); B: significant improvement; C: improvement 8 pts, no change: 8 pts, worsening: 0 pts; D: improvement: 8 pts, no change: 7 pts, worsening: 2 pts	Nausea (3 pts) Pruritus (1 pt) Generalized exanthema (1 pt)	Side effects (generalized exanthema) (1 pt)	No statistical difference in efficacy between sulfasalazine and benzalazine. Changes in macroscopic and microscopic appearance of colonic mucosa
	Benzalazine	2.16 g	22			A: 6.8 ± 2.1 vs 4.0 ± 2.7 (P<.05); B: significant improvement; C: improvement 11 pts no change: 5 pts, worsening: 0 pts; D: improvement: 8 pts, no change: 7 pts, worsening: 0 pts	3 pts: nausea and vomiting	Rapid worsening of disease (3 pts) Lost to follow-up (2 pts)	
Riley et al, 1988[77]	Sulfasalazine	2 g	19	4 wk	Improvement in stool frequency, rectal bleeding, macroscopic and microscopic grade of colonic mucosa measured at wk 0 and wk 4	Significant improvement of macroscopic score above 5 cm at wk 4 (P<.05)	Itchy rash (2pts) Headache (6 pts) GI symptoms (anorexia, nausea, vomiting, dyspepsia) (4 pts)	Itchy rash (2 pts)	Improvement in rectal bleeding and macroscopic grade of colonic mucosa at wk 4 was significantly greater in pts treated with high-dose mesalamine than sulfasalazine (P<.05)
	Mesalamine	0.8 g	20			Significant improvement of rectal bleeding (P<.005), macroscopic (P<.01), and microscopic (P<.005) scores at wk 4	Itchy rash (2pts) Headache (4 pts) GI symptoms (anorexia, nausea, vomiting, dyspepsia) (4 pts)		

Study	Drug	Dose	N	Duration	Outcome	Results	Adverse events		Comments
	Mesalamine	2.4 g	21			Significant improvement of stool frequency, (P<.01), rectal bleeding (P<.01), and macroscopic score (P<.005) at wk 4	Headache (5pts) GI symptoms (anorexia, nausea, vomiting, dyspepsia) (7 pts)	Up to 2-fold increase in plasma creatinine (2pts)	
Rachmilewitz 1989[78]	Coated mesalamine	1.5 g	115	8 wk	Clinical and endoscopic remission: clinical and endoscopic activity score ≤4	Clinical remission: wk 4: 50/70 pts (71%) wk 8: 37/50 pts (74%) Endoscopic remission: wk 3 : 20/41 pts (49%)	16/115 pts (14%) Total number of adverse events: 29	7/115 pts (6%)	164 patients were included in the efficacy analysis (87 received coated mesalamine and 77 received sulfasalazine)
	Sulfasalazine	3.g	105			Clinical remission: wk 4: 38/58 pts (66%) (F = .338, vs coated mesalamine) wk 8: 35/43 pts (81%) (P = .835, vs coated mesalamine) Endoscopic remission: wk 8 : 18/38 pts (47%) (P = .272 vs coated mesalamine)	25/105 pts (24%) Total number of adverse events: 47	8/105 pts (8%)	

(continued on next page)

Table 2
(continued)

Reference	Treatment Arm	Daily Dose	No. of Patients	Study Duration	Primary End Point	Results	Adverse Events	Withdrawals	Comments
Rao et al, 1989[79]	Olsalazine	2 g	20	4 wk	Overall improvement defined as a positive change in at least 2 following criteria: -clinical activity index by Truelove and Witts -percentage of bloody stools -sigmoidoscopic appearance of colon -histologic appearance of colonic mucosa	Overall improvement at wk 4 vs wk 0, 15/18 pts (83%) ($P<.01$) Proportion of unformed stools (78% at wk 0 vs 55% at wk 4, $P<.001$) Bloody stools (61% at wk 0 vs 22% at wk 4, $P<.001$) Improvement in sigmoidoscopic score at wk 4 vs wk 0: 83% ($P<.01$) Improvement in histologic score at wk 4 vs wk 0:44% ($P<.01$)	Headache and nasal stuffiness (1 pt) Diarrhea (1 pt)	2	No difference in the overall response between treatment arms significantly greater decrease in proportion of unformed stools at wk 4 in patients treated with sulfasalazine vs olsalazine ($P<.05$) No difference in tolerance between treatment arms
	Sulfasalazine	3 g	17			Overall improvement at wk 4 vs wk 0, 9/13 pts (69%) ($P<.01$) Proportion of unformed stools (72% at wk 0 vs 28% at wk 4, $P<.001$) Bloody stools (67% at wk 0 vs 37% at wk 4, $P<.001$) Improvement in sigmoidoscopic score at wk 4 vs wk 0: 84% ($P<.01$) Improvement in histologic score at wk 4 vs wk 0: 46% ($P<.01$)	Dyspepsia and nausea (2 pts) Exacerbation of bloody diarrhea (1 pt) Myalgia, headache and dizziness (1 pt)	4	

Study	Drug	Dose	Duration	Outcome measure	Result	Result	Result	Result
Munakata et al, 1995[80]	Mesalamine	1.5 g	52	4 wk	Improvement in clinical symptoms and endoscopic findings	Marked and moderate clinical improvement: 30/48 pts (63%)	6/52 pts (11.5%)	Not reported	No difference in clinical and endoscopic improvement between treatment arms General usefulness based on the improvement and safety: mesalamine 65.3% vs. sulfasalazine 45.6% ($P = .042$)
	Sulfasalazine	3.0 g	57			Marked and moderate clinical improvement: 32/52 pts (62%)	16/57 pts (28.1%)	Not reported	—
Kruis et al, 1998[81]	Olsalazine	3 g	88	12 wk	Endoscopic remission: score 0 or 1 on 5-point scale —score 0: normal mucosa with visible vascular pattern, no granularity or friability —score 1: inactive colitis, pink mucosa, no visible blood vessels, faintly granular but no friability	52.2%	41/88 pts (46%)	11/88 pts (13%)	
	Mesalamine	3 g	80			48.8% ($P = .67$, vs olsalazine)	29/80 pts (36%)	9/80 pts (11%)	
Green et al, 1998[82]	Balsalazide	6.75 g	50	12 wk	Complete remission at wk 4, 8, and 12: symptomatic remission with no use of relief medication in the previous 4 days and grade 0 or 1 on sigmoidoscopy [grade 0: normal, vascular pattern clearly visible grade 1: erythema with loss of vascular pattern]	wk 4: 38%* wk 8: 54%** wk 12: 62%***	24/50 pts (48%)*	15/50 pts (30%)* Treatment failure 6/50pts (12%)** AEs 1/50 pts (2%)	—
	Mesalamine	2.4 g	49			wk 4: 12%* wk 8: 22%** wk 12: 37%*** *$P<.01$ **$P<.01$ ***$P<.05$	35/49 pts (71%)* *$P = .024$	23/49 pts (47%)* Treatment failure 16/49 pts (33%)** AEs 1/49 pts (2%) *$P = .068$ **$P = .015$	

(continued on next page)

Table 2
(continued)

Reference	Treatment Arm	Daily Dose	No. of Patients	Study Duration	Primary End Point	Results	Adverse Events	Withdrawals	Comments
Green et al, 2002[83]	Balsalazide	6.75 g	28	12 wk	Remission rates at the end of study or withdrawal/ remission: return to stool frequency (with or without pain) to that before relapse without the presence of blood and confirmed by biopsy	Completed study in remission: 21/28 pts (75%)*	Serious: 2/28 pts (7%) Minor: 27/28 pts (96%)	AEs 2/28 pts (7%)* Treatment failure: 1/28 pts (4%)** Lost to follow-up: 0/28 (0%)***	
	Sulfasalazine	3 g	29			Completed study in remission: 17/29 pts (69%)* *P = .19	Serious: 0/29 pts (0%) Minor: 27/29 pts (93%)	AEs 9/29 pts (31%)* Treatment failure: 1/29 pts (3%)** Lost to follow-up: 1/29 (3%)*** *P = .041 **P >.2 ***P >.2	
Forbes et al, 2005[84]	Asacol-mesalamine in Eudragit-S coating	2.4 g	42	8 wk	Efficacy based on modified St Mark's Colitis Activity Score, macroscopic and microscopic appearance of rectum and physician's global assessment (PGA). Clinical remission defined from PGA	Decrease in St Mark's Colitis Activity Score: −2.3* Clinical remission wk 8: 28.6%** Improvement in sigmoidoscopy score: 54.8%*** Improvement in histologic score: 31%****	31/42 pts (73.8%)	11/42 pts (26.1%)	
	Ipocol-mesalamine in Eudragit-S coating	2.4 g	46			Decrease in St Mark's Colitis Activity Score: −1.5* Clinical remission wk 8: 26.1%** Improvement in sigmoidoscopy score: 50.0%*** Improvement in histologic score: 0.4%**** *P = ns **P = ns ***P = ns ****P = ns	34/46 pts (73.9%)	9/46 pts (19.6%)	
Pruitt et al, 2002[85]	Balsalazide	6.75 g	84	8 wk	Symptomatic remission: patient functional assessment ratings of normal or mild and absence of rectal bleeding at wk 8 or early completion of	38/73 pts (52%) 39/84 pts (46%)	45/84 pts (54%)	AEs: 3/84 pts (4%)	73 pts in efficacy evaluable population 84 pts in intention to treat population
	Mesalamine	2.4 g	89			38/77 pts (49%) 38/89 pts (44%)	57/89 pts (64%)	AEs: 6/89 pts (7%)	77 pts in efficacy evaluable population 89 pts in intention to treat

Levine at al. 2002[86]	Balsalazide	6.75 g	53	8 wk	Improvement in rectal bleeding and in at least one other sign or symptom at wk 8	Improvement in rectal bleeding: 65%*, ● Improvement in stool frequency: 53%** Improvement in sigmoidoscopic score: 79%***, ●● Improvement in PGA: 74%****, ●●● Improvement in overall symptom assessment: 65% ●●●● Improvement in patient functional assessment: 71% ●●●●●	23/53 pts (43%)	16/53 pts (30%)	49 pts in efficacy evaluable population 53 pts in intention to treat population
	Balsalazide	2.25 g	50			Improvement in rectal bleeding : 32%* Improvement in stool frequency: 29%** Improvement in sigmoidoscopic score: 53%**** Improvement in PGA: 51%****, ●●● $*P = .006$ $**P = .006$ $***P = .015$ $****P = .030$	27/50 pts (54%)	17/50 pts (34%)	49 pts in efficacy evaluable population 50 pts in intention to treat population
	Mesalamine	2.4 g	51			Improvement in rectal bleeding: 53% ● Improvement in sigmoidoscopic score: 51% ●● Improvement in PGA: 62% ●●● Improvement in overall symptom assessment 58% ●●●● Improvement in patient functional assessment: 61% ●●●●● $●P = ns$ $●●P = ns$ $●●●P = ns$ $●●●●P = ns$ $●●●●●P = ns$	26/51 pts (51%)	15/51 pts (29%)	49 pts in efficacy evaluable population 51 pts in intention to treat population

(continued on next page)

Table 2
(continued)

Reference	Treatment Arm	Daily Dose	No. of Patients	Study Duration	Primary End Point	Results	Adverse Events	Withdrawals	Comments
Mansfield et al, 2002[87]	Balsalazide	6.75 g	26	8 wk	Remission defined as a stool frequency of ≤2/d without blood and with normal colonic mucosa or minimal erythema on sigmoidoscopy at wk 8	13/26 pts (50%)	17/26 pts (65%)*	AEs 1/26 pts (4%)* Treatment ineffective 2/26 pts (7.5%) Protocol violation 2/26 pts (7.5%)	
	Sulfasalazine	3 g	24			9/24 pts (38%)	21/24 pts (88%)* *P = .10	AEs 9/24 pts (38%)* Treatment ineffective 3/24 pts (12%) Protocol violation 1/24 pts (4%) *P = .004	
Raedler et al, 2004[88]	Mesalamine micropellets	3 g	181	8 wk	Clinical remission: Clinical Activity Index according to Rachmilewitz ≤2 at wk 8	67%* (intention to treat population) 64.4%** (according to protocol population)	56/181 pts (30.9%)*	Not reported	179 pts in intention to treat population 160 pts in according to protocol population 181 pts in safety population
	Mesalamine tablets	3 g	181			62.9%* (intention to treat population) 64.2%** (according to protocol population) *OR = 1.199 (95% CI 0.758–1.897) **OR = 1.008 (95% CI 0.623–1.632)	43/181 pts (23.8%)* P = .43	not reported	178 pts in intention to treat population 162 pts in according to protocol population 181 pts in safety population

Study	Drug	Dose	Duration	Endpoint	Results		Adverse events/withdrawals	Comments
Tursi et al, 2004[89]	Balsalazide + VSL # 3	2.25 g + 3 g VSL #3	30	8 wk	Symptomatic remission: patient functional assessment of normal bowel movements and absence of rectal bleeding	24/30 pts (80%)* (95% CI: 59–91)	Not reported	Protocol violation 1/30 pts (3%) Protocol ineffectiveness 1/30 pts (3%)
	Balsalazide	4.5 g	30			21/30 pts (70%)* (95% CI: 43–81)	Not reported	Protocol violation 1/30 pts (3%) Protocol ineffectiveness 3/30 pts (10%)
	Mesalamine	2.4 g	30			16/30 pts (53.3%)* (95% CI: 42–62) $P<.02$	Not reported	Protocol violation 2/30 pts (6%) Protocol ineffectiveness 4/30 pts (13%) AEs 2/30 pts (6%)
Jiang and Cui, 2004[90]	Olsalazine	1 g	21	8 wk	Complete remission: decrease in clinical symptoms with relative normal appearance of colonic mucosa	Complete remission: 16/21 pts (76%)*	Not reported	Not reported	—
	Sulfasalazine	1 g	21			Complete remission: 13/21 pts (48%)* *$P<.05$	Not reported	Not reported	
Marakhouski et al, 2005[91]	Mesalamine pellets	1.5 g – 3.0 g	115	8 wk	Clinical remission: clinical activity index ≤4	At 3 wk: 54/114 pts (47%)* At 8 wk: 76/114 pts (67%)**	36/114 pts (32%)	1/114 pts (0.9%)(AE)	114 pts in intention to treat and safety analysis *daily dose 1.5 g **includes pts with dose escalation to 3 g/d in nonresponders to initial dose of 1.5 g/d (n = 44) and pts treated with daily dose of 1.5 g (n = 70)
	Mesalamine tablets	1.5 g – 3.0 g	118			At 3 wk: 48/115 pts (42%)* At 8 wk: 78/115 pts (68%)**	42/118 pts (36%)	4/118 pts (3.4%) (AE)	115 pts in intention to treat analysis 118 pts in safety analysis *daily dose 1.5 g **includes pts with dose escalation to 3 g/d in nonresponders to initial dose of 1.5 g/d (n = 52) and pts treated with daily dose of 1.5 g (n = 63)

(continued on next page)

Table 2
(continued)

Reference	Treatment Arm	Daily Dose	No. of Patients	Study Duration	Primary End Point	Results	Adverse Events	Withdrawals	Comments
Gibson et al, 2006[92]	Eudragit-L coated mesalamine	3 g	131	8 wk	Clinical remission; clinical activity index ≤4	69%	74/131 pts (57%)	16/131 pts (12%)	—
	Ethylcellulose-coated mesalamine	3 g	127			69%	66/127 pts (52%)	14/127 pts (11%)	
Ito et al, 2010[93]	pH-dependent release mesalamine	2.4 g	66	8 wk	Decrease in UC activity index	Mean decrease: 1.5 (95% CI 0.7, 2.3) ●	56/66 pts (84.8%)	Not reported	
	pH-dependent release mesalamine	3.6 g	64			Mean decrease 2.9 (95% CI 2.3, 3.5)*	53/64 pts (82.8%)	Not reported	
	Time-dependent release mesalamine	2.25 g	63			1.3 (95% CI 0.6, 2.1)*, ● *P = .003 ●difference 0.2 (95% CI −0.8, 1.2)	55/65 pts (84.6%)	Not reported	

Abbreviations: AE, adverse event; CI, confidence interval; GI, gastrointestinal; ns, not significant; OR, odds ratio; pt(s), patient(s).
Data from Fleig WE, Laudage G, Sommer H, et al. Prospective, randomized, double-blind comparison of benzalazine and sulfasalazine in the treatment of active ulcerative colitis. Digestion 1988;40:173–80.

was superior to placebo with regard to the endoscopic, global, or clinical measures of improvement or complete remission as defined by the authors of each study. For the failure to induce global/clinical improvement or remission, the pooled Peto odds ratio was 0.40 (95% CI, 0.30–0.53) and a dose-response trend for 5-ASA was also observed. When 5-ASA was compared with sulfasalazine, the pooled Peto odds ratio was 0.83 (95% CI 0.60–1.13) for the failure to induce global/clinical improvement or remission, and 0.66 (95% CI 0.42–1.04) for the failure to induce endoscopic improvement. Sulfasalazine was shown to be not as well tolerated as 5-ASA. In conclusion, the newer 5-ASA preparations were superior to placebo and tended toward therapeutic benefit over sulfasalazine. However, taking cost into consideration, sulfasalazine may be the preferred option if tolerated by the patient.[10] It should be emphasized, however, that since the publication of these meta-analyses balsalazide has been released in generic formulations and at lower cost.

For the maintenance of remission of UC, the Peto odds ratio for the failure to maintain clinical or endoscopic remission (withdrawals and relapses) for 5-ASA versus placebo was 0.47 (95% CI, 0.36–0.62) with a number-needed-to-treat (NNT) value of 6.[9] These values were also calculated for the trials in which sulfasalazine and 5-ASA were compared, revealing an odds ratio of 1.29 (95% CI, 1.05–1.57), with a negative NNT value (−19), suggesting a higher degree of therapeutic effectiveness for sulfasalazine. Sulfasalazine and 5-ASA had similar adverse event profiles, with odds ratios of 1.16 (95% CI 0.62–2.16), and 1.31 (95% CI 0.86–1.99), respectively.[9] The investigators noted that trials comparing 5-ASA and sulfasalazine may have been biased in favor of sulfasalazine, because most of the trials enrolled patients who were known to be tolerant to sulfasalazine and this may have minimized sulfasalazine-related adverse events. The meta-analysis concluded that newer 5-ASA preparations were superior to placebo for maintenance therapy. However, the newer preparations had a statistically significant therapeutic inferiority relative to sulfasalazine.[9]

Recent studies have suggested that combination therapy with both rectal and oral 5-ASA is more effective than oral administration alone in patients with extensive mild or moderate active UC.[108] Safdi and colleagues[109] were one of the first groups to demonstrate the superior efficacy of combining oral (Asacol) and rectal mesalamine therapy in producing earlier and more complete relief of rectal bleeding in patients with mild to moderate distal UC compared with using either agent alone. Subsequently, several investigators observed a significantly higher concentration of 5-ASA in the distal colonic mucosa in patients receiving both oral and enema therapy, supporting their positive therapeutic effect.[30,75]

Marteau and colleagues[108] conducted a randomized, double-blind placebo-controlled trial investigating the efficacy of adding mesalamine enema to oral mesalamine in patients with extensive mild to moderate active UC. The trial consisted of 127 patients with UC who were randomized to Pentasa or placebo enema in addition to oral Pentasa 2 g twice daily. Remission was achieved in 64% (95% CI 50%, 76%) of the mesalamine group versus 43% (95% CI 28%, 58%) of the placebo group at 8 weeks (P = .03). Improvement was seen as early as 4 weeks with 89% (95% CI 78%, 96%) of the mesalamine group versus 62% (95% CI 46%, 75%) of the placebo group (P = .0008), and in 86% (95% CI 75%, 94%) of the mesalamine group versus 68% (95% CI 53%, 81%) of the placebo group at 8 weeks (P = .026). In particular, time to cessation of rectal bleeding was significantly shorter for patients treated with the mesalamine enema who had any bleeding (P = .0025) or frank bleeding at baseline (P = .0031). The acceptability of combination therapy was similar in both groups, 84% and 85% in enema and placebo groups, respectively. During the course

Table 3
Randomized double blind controlled trials comparing therapy with various oral 5-ASA formulations in maintaining remission of UC

References	Treatment Arms	No. of Patients in Each Arm	Dosage	Study Duration	Primary End Point	Results	Efficacy	Adverse Events	Withdrawals	Description of Side Effects
McIntyre et al, 1988[94]	Balsalazide	41	1 g/d	6 mo	To compare balsalazide and sulfasalazine for efficacy and tolerance in the long-term maintenance of remission in patients with UC. A relapse was defined as the recurrence of previous symptoms.	51% remission	No statistical significance in the maintenance in remissions between the 2 groups (P<.1), thus concluded that coated 5-ASA is a safe, effective therapy for maintaining UC in remission	2	0	
	Sulfasalazine	38	1 g/d			63% remission		10	2	Rash and abdominal pain
Rutgeerts et al, 1989[95]	5-ASA	131	0.75 g/d	12 mo	To compare 5-ASA with sulfasalazine in maintaining UC remission. Remission was assessed by symptoms and colonoscopy at investigator's discretion	28% relapsed	No statistical significance in the cumulative rate of relapse between the 2 groups. Thus concluded that balsalazide was not significantly different from sulfasalazine in maintaining remission in patients with UC	24	9	Diarrhea, nausea, other GI symptoms, skin hypersensitivity, CNS and cardiovascular
	Sulfasalazine	142	1.5-2.0 g/d			23% relapsed		20	7	

| Mulder et al, 1988[34] | 5-ASA | 41 | 1.5 g/d | 12 mo | To compare the efficacy and safety of 5-ASA with sulfasalazine for maintenance of remission in UC. Patients were assessed clinically, endoscopically (recto/sigmoidoscopy) and histologically. Remission was considered when data obtained at each visit were assessed as "normal" or "in remission." Relapse is when patients were prescribed for additional treatment or abnormality in haf of the assessment groups (clinical, endoscopic, histology) | 54% remission | No statistical difference between the remission rate between the 2 groups (P>.70), thus concluded that 5-ASA is equally effective as sulfasalazine in maintenance of remission of UC | 0 | 0 | |
| | Sulfasalazine | 34 | 3 g/d | | | 46% remission | | 4 | 4 | Erythroderma, anxiety, backache, laboratory abnormality |

(continued on next page)

Table 3
(continued)

References	Treatment Arms	No. of Patients in Each Arm	Dosage	Study Duration	Primary End Point	Results	Efficacy	Adverse Events	Withdrawals	Description of Side Effects
Rijk et al, 1992[96]	Sulfasalazine	23	4 g/d	48 weeks	To assess the relapse-preventing properties and the safety of sulfasalazine and olsalazine in patients with UC in remission. A sigmoidoscopy with biopsies was performed to determine whether the colitis was in remission at the inclusion and the 48-wk visit	30.4% relapse	No statistical significance in the relapse rate between the 2 groups (P = .15), thus concluded that sulfasalazine and olsalazine are equally effective in maintaining remission of UC with a similar incidence of adverse effects	7	3	Upper abdominal complaints, rash
	Olsalazine	23	2 g/d			26.1% relapse		9	3	Loose stools
Kiilerich et al, 1992[97]	Olsalazine	114	0.5 g twice daily	12 mo	The relapse preventing effect of olsalazine compared with sulfasalazine over 1 year in patient with UC in remission. Remission was defined by: (1) no visible blood in the stools for more than 3 days within the last week, and/or (2) less than 3 stools per day for at least 4 days within the last week, and (3) sigmoidoscopy grade 1–2 at admission (no spontaneous bleeding without or with distinct vessels in the mucosa)	46.9% relapse rate	Cumulative relapse rate similar in both groups (P = .54), thus concluded that olsalazine 500 mg twice daily is equally effective and has the same incidence of adverse reactions as sulfasalazine 1 g twice daily in the maintenance therapy for ulcerative colitis	9	9	Diarrhea, abdominal pain, constipation, urticaria, nausea, dyspepsia
	Sulfasalazine	112	1 g twice daily			42.4% relapse rate		6	6	Diarrhea, abdominal pain, constipation, urticaria, nausea, dyspepsia

Study	Drug	N	Dose	Duration	Aim/Definition	Failure/Relapse rate	Conclusion			Side effects
Nilsson et al, 1995[98]	Olsalazine	161	1 g/d	18 mo	To compare the relapse-preventing effect of olsalazine and sulfasalazine in patients with UC. Relapse was defined as macroscopic changes in the rectum of grade 3 or 4	54.7% failure rate	No statistical significance in the remission curve ($P = .19$), thus concluded that relapse-preventing effect of olsalazine and sulfasalazine did not differ	39	12	Diarrhea, abdominal pain/cramps, vomiting, eczema, rheumatic symptoms (polyarthritis fever and sacroiliitis), impotence
	Sulfasalazine	161	2 g/d			47.2% failure rate		26	8	Diarrhea, eczema, rheumatic symptoms (polyarthritis fever and sacroiliitis), drowsiness, dizziness, vertigo, loss of taste, lack of concentration, psychological discomfort, impotence
Ardizzone et al, 1995[99]	5-ASA	44	0.5 g twice daily	12 mo	The prevention of relapse in patients with quiescent UC. Relapse of the disease was defined as appearance of bloody diarrhea with endoscopic signs of inflammation requiring systemic steroids	20.5% (6 mo) and 38.4% (12 mo) relapse rate	No statistically significant differences in the relapse rate between the 2 groups after 6 and 12 months ($P = .32$ and $P = .18$), thus concluded that 5-ASA is as effective as sulfasalazine in maintaining remission of UC	5	5	Urticaria and arthralgia
	Sulfasalazine	44	1.0 g twice daily			27.5% (6 mo) and 51% (12 mo) relapse rate		3	3	Severe diarrhea

(continued on next page)

Table 3
(continued)

References	Treatment Arms	No. of Patients in Each Arm	Dosage	Study Duration	Primary End Point	Results	Efficacy	Adverse Events	Withdrawals	Description of Side Effects
Riley et al, 1998[100]	5-ASA	48	0.8 g/d, 1.2 g/d, 1.6 g/d	48 weeks	The long-term efficacy and toxicity of delayed-release mesalamine and enteric coated sulfasalazine in the maintenance of UC remission. Clinical assessment including sigmoidoscopy and biopsy, and symptomatic deterioration (6 variables used to assess the severity-stool frequency, rectal bleeding, hemoglobin concentration, ESR and sigmoidoscopy and histologic grade)	37.5% relapse	No statistically significant differences in the relapse rate or mean time to relapse between the 2 groups and a better tolerability in the mesalamine group ($P>.90$), thus concluded that delayed-release 5-ASA is as effective as sulfasalazine in maintaining remission of UC	20	0	Headache and upper GI upset
	Sulfasalazine	44	2 g/d, 3 g/d, 4 g/d			38.6% relapse		26	1	Headache and upper GI upset

Study	Group	N	Dose	Duration	Description	Result	Conclusion			Adverse events
Green et al, 1998[101]	Balsalazide	49	3 g/d	12 mo	The efficacy and safety of balsalazide (Colazide) compared with mesalamine (Asacol) in maintaining UC remission. A symptomatic relapse was defined as the recurrence of moderate or severe symptoms on the patients' overall evaluation	58% remission	Equal proportion of patients in each treatment group remained in remission ($P = .4275$) and similar proportion of adverse events ($P = .8317$), thus concluded that balsalazide 3 g daily is at least as effective, and equally well tolerated and accepted by patients as a long-term maintenance treatment of UC, as delayed-release mesalamine 1.2 g daily	30	2	Headaches, GI symptoms, respiratory infections, abnormal laboratory test, fracture, hernia
	5-ASA	46	1.2 g/d			58% remission		30	0	Headaches, GI symptoms, respiratory infections, abnormal laboratory test, suspected UTI, UC complications, cardiac arrest
Kruis et al, 2001[102]	Balsalazide (low dose)	49	1.5 g twice daily	26 weeks	To compare the relapse preventing effect and safety profile of the 2 doses of balsalazide and mesalamine. Efficacy assessments were clinical activity index (CAI) and endoscopic score according to Rachmilewitz, and a histologic score	43.8% clinical remission	The difference in clinical remission was statistically significant ($P = .006$), thus concluded that high-dose balsalazide was superior in maintaining remission in pts with UC. All 3 treatments were safe and well tolerated	3	3	Headache, hypertension, malaise, dizziness, abdominal pain, pruritus and rashes
	Balsalazide (high dose)	40	3.0 g twice daily			77.5% clinical remission		2	2	Pancreatitis, gingivitis, alopecia, nail disorder
	5-ASA	44	0.5 g 3 times daily			56.8% clinical remission		4	4	Palpitation, hypotension, tenesmus, nausea, impotence, diarrhea, alopecia

(continued on next page)

Table 3
(continued)

References	Treatment Arms	No. of Patients in Each Arm	Dosage	Study Duration	Primary End Point	Results	Efficacy	Adverse Events	Withdrawals	Description of Side Effects
Mahmud et al, 2002[103]	5-ASA	20	1.2 g/d	9 mo	To compare/evaluate the renal function (by the measurement of GFR, microalbuminuria and urinary GST) in patients with UC receiving either mesalazine or olsalazine	GFR, microalbuminuria and urinary GST activity were not statistically different between the 2 groups	No statistically significant difference in GFR and urinary GST activity from the baseline in the 2 treatment groups (P = ns). The adjusted baseline microalbumin levels were significantly lower in the mesalamine groups (P = .024), thus concluded that treatment with mesalamine or olsalazine for 9 months had no significant impact on GFR	2	2	Abdominal pain, abdominal distension, dyspepsia, nausea
	Olsalazine	20	1.0 g/d					2	2	Backache, generalized body aches and pains, insomnia, hypotension
Kohn et al, 2009 (abstract)[104]	5-ASA	221	2.4 g/d	12 mo	To evaluate the efficacy and safety of the 2 groups. Clinical remission was defined as a score of ≤1 on the UC DAI for at least 1 month and endoscopic remission was defined as no endoscopic evidence of active disease	51.4% clinical remission; 41.9% clinical and endoscopic remission	Statistically significant difference between the clinical remission rate (P = .026), but not the clinical and endoscopic remission rate (P = .13), thus concluded that 5-ASA MMX is efficacious as a long-term maintenance therapy in pts with mild to moderate UC (it has a significantly higher number of patients in remission, with a comparable safety profile)	n/a	n/a	
	5-ASA	221	2.4 g/d			36.4% clinical remission; 31.8% clinical and endoscopic remission		n/a	n/a	

Prantera et al, 2009[105]	5-ASA	162	2.4 g/d	12 mo	To assess the proportion of patients in clinical, and clinical and endoscopic remission at the end of the study period. Clinical remission was defined as a combined score of ≤1 on the UC DAI scale and endoscopic remission was defined as clinical remission, with a normal mucosal appearance on endoscopic examination	68% clinical remission; 60.9% clinical and endoscopic remission	No statistical significance between both groups in clinical or clinical and endoscopic remission ($P = .69$), thus concluded that 5-ASA MMX is similarly effective with a comparable safety profile to delayed-released 5-ASA for the maintenance treatment of UC	92	3	Melena
	5-ASA	169	2.4 g/d			65.9% clinical remission, 61.7% clinical and endoscopic remission		99	3	Laboratory abnormality and epistaxis
Ito et al, 2010[93]	5-ASA	65	2.4 g/d	48 weeks	Percent of patients without bloody stools: Each patient would record the condition of their bloody stools, stool frequency and drug compliance in their diary	76.9% without bloody stool	No significant difference in the time to bloody stools ($P = .27$), thus concluded that the pH- and time-dependent release of mesalamine formulations were similarly safe and effective	62	1	Nasopharyngitis, diarrhea, abnormal laboratory values
	5-ASA	66	2.25 g/d			69.2% without bloody stool		62	3	Nasopharyngitis, diarrhea, abnormal laboratory values

Abbreviations: CNS, central nervous system; DAI, Disease Activity Index; ESR, erythrocyte sedimentation rate; GFR, glomerular filtration rate; GST, glutathione-S-transferase; MMX, Multi Matrix System; n/a, not available; UTI, urinary tract infection.

Table 4
Outcome of remission

| Study | Symptomatic Remission | | Complete Remission | |
	Balsalazide	Mesalamine	Balsalazide	Mesalamine
Tursi et al	21/26	16/22	—	—
Levin et al	—	—	21/98	9/49
Pruitt et al	38/73	38/77	34/73	32/77
Green et al	44/50	28/49	31/50	18/49

Data from Rahimi R, Nikfar S, Rezaie A, et al. Comparison of mesalamine and balsalazide in induction and maintenance of remission in patients with ulcerative colitis: a meta-analysis. Dig Dis Sci 2009;54:714.

of the 8-week study period, 24 of 71 patients (34%) in the mesalamine enema group and 28 of 56 patients (50%) in the placebo enema group had at least one adverse event after the start of treatment. The majority of adverse events were of mild or moderate intensity. The most common adverse events considered drug related were diarrhea (in 4% of patients), headache (4%), and vomiting (3%) in the mesalamine enema group. In the placebo enema group, the most common drug-related adverse event was abdominal pain (4%). Three patients (4%) in the mesalamine enema group and one patient (2%) in the placebo enema group had a serious adverse event, all of the gastrointestinal system (aggravation of ulcerative colitis, painful defecation, vomiting, abdominal pain, and/or bloody diarrhea) and all considered unrelated to the study drug. There were no deaths during the course of the study.

Safdi and colleagues[109] also investigated the efficacy of combination versus monotherapy, comparing mesalamine rectal suspension enema (Rowasa; nightly dosing) or oral mesalamine (Asacol, dose: 2.4 mg/d) alone versus in combination. The double-blind study was conducted on 60 patients with mild to moderate distal UC (at least 5 cm above the anal verge and not more than 50 cm, with total DAI score between 4 and 10). Patients' total DAI were evaluated at weeks 3 and 6 and their abbreviated

Table 5
Outcome of relapse

| Study | Relapse | |
	Balsalazide	Mesalamine
Kruis et al	36/88	19/34
Green et al	16/49	18/46

Data from Rahimi R, Nikfar S, Rezaie A, et al. Comparison of mesalamine and balsalazide in induction and maintenance of remission in patients with ulcerative colitis: a meta-analysis. Dig Dis Sci 2009;54:714.

Table 6			
Outcomes investigated for sulfasalazine versus mesalamine			
Outcome	Study	Sulfasalazine	Mesalamine
Overall improvement	Munkata et al	40/57	37/52
	Rachmilewitz	35/43	37/50
	Riley et al	10/19	16/20
	Androlei et al	3/6	4/6
Relapse	Ardizzone et al	18/35	15/39
	Eliakim et al	8/20	6/18
	Rutgeerts	29/126	30/107
	Mulder et al	17/31	19/41
	Riley et al	17/44	18/48
	Androlei et al	1/6	3/7
Adverse events	Munkata et al	16/57	6/52
	Eliakim et al	3/20	3/18
	Rutgeerts	20/167	24/167
	Rachmilewitz	25/105	16/115
	Androlei et al	1/6	1/7
Withdrawals because of adverse events	Ardizzone et al	1/44	2/44
	Munakata et al	7/57	3/52
	Eliakim et al	0/22	0/20
	Rutgeerts	7/142	9/131
	Rachmilewitz	8/36	7/38
	Mulder et al	2/34	0/41
	Riley et al	2/19	0/20
	Riley et al	1/44	0/48

Data from Nikfar S, Rahimi R, Rezaie A, et al. A meta-analysis of the efficacy of sulfasalazine in comparison with 5-aminosalicylates in the induction of improvement and maintenance of remission in patients with ulcerative colitis. Dig Dis Sci 2008;54:1157–70.

DAI evaluated at weeks 1 and 2, and patients recorded the amount of blood in stools, urgency, straining at stools, and abdominal pain daily.[109] At week 6 combination therapy produced a greater improvement in DAI (−5.2) than monotherapy with Asacol (−3.9) or Rowasa (−4.4), with similar results at week 3. In addition, patients on combination therapy reported absence of bloody stool sooner than patients on monotherapy.[109] Overall, the results from this as well as the study by Marteau and colleagues[108] demonstrated that the combination strategy was more effective and safe, and it is not unreasonable to consider this approach in patients with mild to moderate left sided or extensive UC.[109]

Ito and colleagues[93] performed a multicenter, double-blind randomized study comparing the efficacy and safety of the pH-dependent release formulation of mesalamine (Asacol at doses 2.4 g or 3.6 g) with the time-dependent release formulation of mesalamine (Pentasa at 2.25 g) as well as with placebo. The study involved 229 patients with mild to moderate UC, and the primary end point was the decrease in the UC DAI over the course of 8 weeks. Results indicated a superiority of Asacol at a dose of 3.6 g over Pentasa at 2.25 g ($P = .003$) in the induction of remission for mild to moderate UC. In addition, Asacol was preferable to Pentasa for patients with proctitis.[93]

Table 7
Outcomes investigated for sulfasalazine versus olsalazine

Outcome	Study	Sulfasalazine	Olsalazine
Overall improvement	Jiang and Cui	14/21	20/21
	Rao et al	9/13	15/18
	Willoughby et al	17/25	12/21
Relapse	Kruis et al	7/31	16/78
	Nilsson et al	72/161	63/161
	Rijk et al	7/23	6/23
	Kiilerich et al	47/112	42/114
	Ireland et al	10/82	16/82
Adverse events	Kruis et al	5/40	16/111
	Nilsson et al	26/161	39/161
	Rijk et al	8/23	9/23
	Rao et al	4/17	2/20
	Ireland et al	20/82	21/82
Withdrawals because of adverse events	Kruis et al	1/40	5/111
	Nilsson et al	8/161	12/161
	Rijk et al	3/23	3/23
	Ireland et al	9/82	16/82
	Willoughby et al	2/30	2/26

Data from Nikfar S, Rahimi R, Rezaie A, et al. A meta-analysis of the efficacy of sulfasalazine in comparison with 5-aminosalicylates in the induction of improvement and maintenance of remission in patients with ulcerative colitis. Dig Dis Sci 2008;54:1157–70.

ADVERSE EFFECTS

The most common side effects include nausea, vomiting, dyspepsia, malaise, and headaches. Up to one-third of patients cannot tolerant this class of drugs.[18] Less common adverse effects include blood dyscrasias, male infertility, and rashes.

To compare the short-term adverse effects among the 5-ASA agents (mesalamine, olsalazine, balsalazide), Loftus and colleagues[110] performed a meta-analysis of 46

Table 8
Outcomes investigated for sulfasalazine versus balsalazide

Outcome	Study	Sulfasalazine	Balsalazide
Overall improvement	Manfield et al	9/24	13/26
	Green et al	17/29	21/28
Relapse	Mcintyre et al	8/30	17/41
Withdrawals because of adverse events	Manfield et al	9/24	1/26
	Green et al	9/29	2/28
	Mcintyre et al	2/38	0/41

Data from Nikfar S, Rahimi R, Rezaie A, et al. A meta-analysis of the efficacy of sulfasalazine in comparison with 5-aminosalicylates in the induction of improvement and maintenance of remission in patients with ulcerative colitis. Dig Dis Sci 2008;54:1157–70.

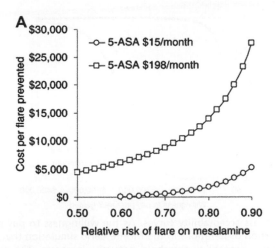

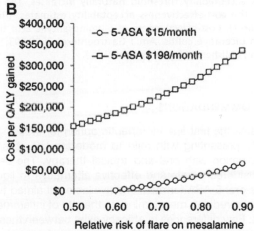

Fig. 4. Two-way sensitivity analyses examining the impact of the relative risk of flare on maintenance 5-ASA and the cost of 5-ASA on the cost/flare prevented (*A*), and the cost/ QALY (quality-adjusted life year) gained (*B*). A 5-ASA cost of $198 per month represents the base case, and $15 per month represents the cost of sulfasalazine. At $15 per month (the cost of sulfasalazine) and a relative risk of flare less than 0.60, maintenance 5-ASA became cost-saving. (*Reprinted from* Yen EF, Kane SV, Ladabaum U. Cost-effectiveness of 5-aminosalicylic acid therapy for maintenance of remission in ulcerative colitis. Am J Gastroenterol 2008;103(12):3094–105; copyright 2008, Macmillan Publishers Ltd; with permission.)

randomized trials for mild to moderate active UC. The study concluded that all 3 5-ASA formulations produce similar adverse effects in the short term. Patients on mesalamine experience fewer adverse events or withdrawals due to serious side effects than those on sulfasalazine. Similar results were found comparing balsalazide with sulfasalazine. Lastly, patients on olsalazine did not significantly experience more adverse effects or withdrawals than patients on sulfasalazine.[110]

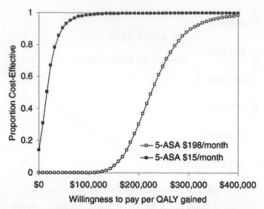

Fig. 5. Cost-effectiveness acceptability curves. As the willingness to pay per QALY gained increases, the proportion of iterations in the Monte Carlo simulation that falls at or below the cost-effectiveness acceptability threshold naturally increases. The cost of 5-ASA has a dramatic effect on the cost-effectiveness acceptability estimates. (*Reprinted from* Yen EF, Kane SV, Ladabaum U. Cost-effectiveness of 5-aminosalicylic acid therapy for maintenance of remission in ulcerative colitis. Am J Gastroenterol 2008;103(12):3094–105; copyright 2008, Macmillan Publishers Ltd; with permission.)

SUMMARY AND RECOMMENDATIONS

5-ASA therapy remains the first-line therapeutic option for inducing and maintaining remission in patients presenting with mild to moderate UC. It is more efficacious when used in combination with oral and topical therapy. The use of mesalamine foam should be considered a safe and effective alternative to liquid enema. There are currently various oral 5-ASA formulations available, all aimed to ensure maximal delivery of the active ingredient, mesalamine, to the site of inflammation with minimal systemic absorption. Few differences in efficacy exist between these different preparations. The initial treatment choice should be based on patient preference, tolerability, and the patient's ability to comply with the prescribed regimen. The cost of 5-ASA plays an important role in the management of the patient. Recent decision analysis has shown that maintenance therapy with sulfasalazine is cost-effective, provided that this agent would yield similar efficacy and safety profiles to the newer 5-ASA compounds (**Figs. 4** and **5**).[111]

REFERENCES

1. Baron JH, Connell AM, Lennard-Jones JE, et al. Sulphasalazine and salicylazo-sulphadimidine in ulcerative colitis. Lancet 1962;1:1094–6.
2. Misiewicz J, Lennard-Jones J, Conell A, et al. Controlled trial of sulphasalazine in maintenance therapy for ulcerative colitis. Lancet 1965;i:185–8.
3. Cohen RD, Woseth DM, Thisted RA, et al. A meta-analysis and overview of the literature on treatment options for left-sided ulcerative colitis and ulcerative proctitis. Am J Gastroenterol 2000;95:1263–76.
4. Regueiro M, Loftus EV Jr, Steinhart AH, et al. Clinical guidelines for the medical management of left-sided ulcerative colitis and ulcerative proctitis: summary statement. Inflamm Bowel Dis 2006;12:972–8.

5. Regueiro M, Loftus EV Jr, Steinhart AH, et al. Medical management of left-sided ulcerative colitis and ulcerative proctitis: critical evaluation of therapeutic trials. Inflamm Bowel Dis 2006;12:979–94.
6. Safdi A, Pieniaszek H, Grigston A, et al. Mulitiple-dose pharmacokinetics of granulated mesalamine, a unique formulation providing delayed and extended release of 5-ASA. Am J Gastroenterol 2008;103(S1):S439–40.
7. Lichtenstein G. Mesalamine in the treatment of ulcerative colitis: novel therapeutic options. Gastroenterol Hepatol (N Y) 2009;5:65–73.
8. Wilding IR, Behrens C, Tardif SJ, et al. Combined scintigraphic and pharmacokinetic investigation of enteric-coated mesalazine micropellets in healthy subjects. Aliment Pharmacol Ther 2003;17:1153–62.
9. Sutherland L, Macdonald JK. Oral 5-aminosalicylic acid for maintenance of remission in ulcerative colitis. Cochrane Database Syst Rev 2006;2:CD000544.
10. Sutherland L, Macdonald JK. Oral 5-aminosalicylic acid for induction of remission in ulcerative colitis. Cochrane Database Syst Rev 2006;2:CD000543.
11. Qureshi AI, Cohen RD. Mesalamine delivery systems: do they really make much difference? Adv Drug Deliv Rev 2005;57:281–302.
12. Cominelli F, Nast CC, Duchini A, et al. Recombinant interleukin-1 receptor antagonist blocks the proinflammatory activity of endogenous interleukin-1 in rabbit immune colitis. Gastroenterology 1992;103:65–71.
13. Rachmilewitz D, Karmeli F, Schwartz LW, et al. Effect of aminophenols (5-ASA and 4-ASA) on colonic interleukin-1 generation. Gut 1992;33:929–32.
14. Mahida YR, Lamming CF, Gallagher A, et al. 5 Aminosalicylic acid is a potent inhibitor of interleukin 1 beta production in organ culture of colonic biopsy specimens from patients with inflammatory bowel disease. Gut 1991;32:50–4.
15. Shanahan F, Niederlehner A, Carramanzana N, et al. Sulfasalazine inhibits the binding of TNF alpha to its receptor. Immunopharmacology 1990;20:217–24.
16. Barnes PJ, Karin M. Nuclear factor-kappaB: a pivotal transcription factor in chronic inflammatory diseases. N Engl J Med 1997;336:1066–71.
17. Rogler G, Brand K, Vogl D, et al. Nuclear factor kappaB is activated in macrophages and epithelial cells of inflamed intestinal mucosa. Gastroenterology 1998;115:357–69.
18. Desreumaux P, Ghosh S. Review article: mode of action and delivery of 5-aminosalicylic acid - new evidence. Aliment Pharmacol Ther 2006;24(Suppl 1):2–9.
19. Sharon P, Ligumsky M, Rachmilewitz D, et al. Role of prostaglandins in ulcerative colitis. Enhanced production during active disease and inhibition by sulfasalazine. Gastroenterology 1978;75:638–40.
20. Stenson WF, Lobos E. Sulfasalazine inhibits the synthesis of chemotactic lipids by neutrophils. J Clin Invest 1982;69:494–7.
21. Stenson WF. Role of eicosanoids as mediators of inflammation in inflammatory bowel disease. Scand J Gastroenterol 1990;172:13–8.
22. Ahnfelt-Ronne I, Nielsen OH, Christensen A, et al. Clinical evidence supporting the radical scavenger mechanism of 5-aminosalicylic acid. Gastroenterology 1990;98:1162–9.
23. Lichtenstein GR, Kamm MA. Review article: 5-aminosalicylate formulations for the treatment of ulcerative colitis—methods of comparing release rates and delivery of 5-aminosalicylate to the colonic mucosa. Aliment Pharmacol Ther 2008;28:663–73.
24. Cohen RD. Review article: evolutionary advances in the delivery of aminosalicylates for the treatment of ulcerative colitis. Aliment Pharmacol Ther 2006;24:465–74.

25. Eliakim R, Tulassay Z, Kupcinskas L, et al. Clinical trial: randomized-controlled clinical study comparing the efficacy and safety of a low-volume vs. a high-volume mesalazine foam in active distal ulcerative colitis. Aliment Pharmacol Ther 2007;26:1237–49.

26. Segars LW, Gales BJ. Mesalamine and olsalazine: 5-aminosalicylic acid agents for the treatment of inflammatory bowel disease. Clin Pharm 1992; 11:514–28.

27. Nielsen OH. Sulfasalazine intolerance. A retrospective survey of the reasons for discontinuing treatment with sulfasalazine in patients with chronic inflammatory bowel disease. Scand J Gastroenterol 1982;17:389–93.

28. Frieri G, Giacomelli R, Pimpo M, et al. Mucosal 5-aminosalicylic acid concentration inversely correlates with severity of colonic inflammation in patients with ulcerative colitis. Gut 2000;47:410–4.

29. Frieri G, Pimpo M, Galletti B, et al. Long-term oral plus topical mesalazine in frequently relapsing ulcerative colitis. Dig Liver Dis 2005;37:92–6.

30. Naganuma M, Iwao Y, Ogata H, et al. Measurement of colonic mucosal concentrations of 5-aminosalicylic acid is useful for estimating its therapeutic efficacy in distal ulcerative colitis: comparison of orally administered mesalamine and sulfasalazine. Inflamm Bowel Dis 2001;7:221–5.

31. Hussain FN, Ajjan RA, Riley SA. Dose loading with delayed-release mesalazine: a study of tissue drug concentrations and standard pharmacokinetic parameters. Br J Clin Pharmacol 2000;49:323–30.

32. D'Haens G, Hommes D, Engels L, et al. Once daily MMX mesalazine for the treatment of mild-to-moderate ulcerative colitis: a phase II, dose-ranging study. Aliment Pharmacol Ther 2006;24:1087–97.

33. Kornbluth A, Cuffari C, George J, et al. A prospective, blinded assessment of distal colonic mucosal concentrations of 5-ASA and NAC-5ASA in UC patients treated with either balsalazide (Colazal) Or a pH-dependent mesalamine (Asacol). Gastroenterology 2006;130:A209.

34. Mulder CJ, Tytgat GN, Weterman IT, et al. Double-blind comparison of slow-release 5-aminosalicylate and sulfasalazine in remission maintenance in ulcerative colitis. Gastroenterology 1988;95:1449–53.

35. Kruis W, Judmaier G, Kayasseh L, et al. Double-blind dose-finding study of olsalazine versus sulphasalazine as maintenance therapy for ulcerative colitis. Eur J Gastroenterol Hepatol 1995;7:391–6.

36. Sutherland LR, May GR, Shaffer EA. Sulfasalazine revisited: a meta-analysis of 5-aminosalicylic acid in the treatment of ulcerative colitis. Ann Intern Med 1993; 118:540–9.

37. Travis SP, Tysk C, de Silva HJ, et al. Optimum dose of olsalazine for maintaining remission in ulcerative colitis. Gut 1994;35:1282–6.

38. Azad Khan AK, Piris J, Truelove SC. An experiment to determine the active therapeutic moiety of sulphasalazine. Lancet 1977;2:892–5.

39. Sandborn WJ. Oral 5-ASA therapy in ulcerative colitis: what are the implications of the new formulations? J Clin Gastroenterol 2008;42:338–44.

40. Brunner M, Greinwald R, Kletter K, et al. Gastrointestinal transit and release of 5-aminosalicylic acid from [153]Sm-labelled mesalazine pellets vs. tablets in male healthy volunteers. Aliment Pharmacol Ther 2003;17:1163–9.

41. APRISO [prescribing information]. Morrisville, NC: Salix Pharmaceuticals Inc; 2008.

42. Prantera C, Viscido A, Biancone L, et al. A new oral delivery system for 5-ASA: preliminary clinical findings for MMx. Inflamm Bowel Dis 2005;11:421–7.

43. Kamm MA, Sandborn WJ, Gassull M, et al. Once-daily, high-concentration MMX mesalamine in active ulcerative colitis. Gastroenterology 2007;132:66–75, quiz 432–3.

44. Mohammadi-Samani S, Bahri-Najafi R, Yousefi G. Formulation and in vitro evaluation of prednisolone buccoadhesive tablets. Farmaco 2005;60:339–44.

45. Ali J, Khar RK, Ahuja A. Formulation and characterisation of a buccoadhesive erodible tablet for the treatment of oral lesions. Pharmazie 1998;53:329–34.

46. Sandborn WJ, Kamm MA, Lichtenstein GR, et al. MMX Multi Matrix System mesalazine for the induction of remission in patients with mild-to-moderate ulcerative colitis: a combined analysis of two randomized, double-blind, placebo-controlled trials. Aliment Pharmacol Ther 2007;26:205–15.

47. Kamm MA, Lichtenstein GR, Sandborn WJ, et al. Randomised trial of once- or twice-daily MMX mesalazine for maintenance of remission in ulcerative colitis. Gut 2008;57:893–902.

48. Lichtenstein GR, Kamm MA, Sandborn WJ, et al. MMX mesalazine for the induction of remission of mild-to-moderately active ulcerative colitis: efficacy and tolerability in specific patient subpopulations. Aliment Pharmacol Ther 2008; 27:1094–102.

49. Lichtenstein GR, Kamm MA, Boddu P, et al. Effect of once- or twice-daily MMX mesalamine (SPD476) for the induction of remission of mild to moderately active ulcerative colitis. Clin Gastroenterol Hepatol 2007;5:95–102.

50. Sutherland L, Roth D, Beck P, et al. Oral 5-aminosalicylic acid for maintenance of remission in ulcerative colitis. Cochrane Database Syst Rev 2002;4.CD000544.

51. Schreiber S, Kamm MA, Lichtenstein GR. Mesalamine with MMX technology for the treatment of ulcerative colitis. Expert Rev Gastroenterol Hepatol 2008;2: 299–314.

52. Kamm MA, Lichtenstein GR, Sandborn WJ, et al. Effect of extended MMX mesalamine therapy for acute, mild-to-moderate ulcerative colitis. Inflamm Bowel Dis 2009;15:1–8.

53. Wilding IR, Kenyon CJ, Hooper G. Gastrointestinal spread of oral prolonged-release mesalazine microgranules (Pentasa) dosed as either tablets or sachet. Aliment Pharmacol Ther 2000;14:163–9.

54. Sninsky CA, Cort DH, Shanahan F, et al. Oral mesalamine (Asacol) for mildly to moderately active ulcerative colitis. A multicenter study. Ann Intern Med 1991; 115:350–5.

55. Schroeder KW, Tremaine WJ, Ilstrup DM. Coated oral 5-aminosalicylic acid therapy for mildly to moderately active ulcerative colitis. A randomized study. N Engl J Med 1987;317:1625–9.

56. Sutherland L, Roth D, Beck P. Alternatives to sulfasalazine: a meta-analysis of 5-ASA in the treatment of ulcerative colitis. Inflamm Bowel Dis 1997;3(2): 65–78.

57. Hanauer SB, Sandborn WJ, Dallaire C, et al. Delayed-release oral mesalamine 4.8 g/d (800 mg tablets) compared to 2.4 g/d (400 mg tablets) for the treatment of mildly to moderately active ulcerative colitis: the ASCEND I trial. Can J Gastroenterol 2007;21:827–34.

58. Hanauer SB, Sandborn WJ, Kornbluth A, et al. Delayed-release oral mesalamine at 4.8 g/d (800 mg tablet) for the treatment of moderately active ulcerative colitis: the ASCEND II trial. Am J Gastroenterol 2005;100:2478–85.

59. Sandborn WJ, Regula J, Feagan BG, et al. Delayed-release oral mesalamine 4.8 g/d (800-mg tablet) is effective for patients with moderately active ulcerative colitis. Gastroenterology 2009;137:1934–43, e1–3.

60. Sandborn WJ, Korzenik J, Lashner B, et al. Once-daily dosing of delayed-release oral mesalamine (400-mg tablet) is as effective as twice-daily dosing for maintenance of remission of ulcerative colitis. Gastroenterology 2010;138: 1286–96 96, e1–3.

61. Ardizzone S, Bianchi Porro G. A practical guide to the management of distal ulcerative colitis. Drugs 1998;55:519–42.

62. Azad Khan AK, Howes DT, Piris J, et al. Optimum dose of sulphasalazine for maintenance treatment in ulcerative colitis. Gut 1980;21:232–40.

63. Campieri M, De Franchis R, Bianchi Porro G, et al. Mesalazine (5-aminosalicylic acid) suppositories in the treatment of ulcerative proctitis or distal proctosigmoiditis. A randomized controlled trial. Scand J Gastroenterol 1990;25:663–8.

64. D'Arienzo A, Panarese A, D'Armiento FP, et al. 5-Aminosalicylic acid suppositories in the maintenance of remission in idiopathic proctitis or proctosigmoiditis: a double-blind placebo-controlled clinical trial. Am J Gastroenterol 1990;85: 1079–82.

65. Sutherland LR, Martin F, Greer S, et al. 5-Aminosalicylic acid enema in the treatment of distal ulcerative colitis, proctosigmoiditis, and proctitis. Gastroenterology 1987;92:1894–8.

66. Marshall JK, Irvine EJ. Rectal aminosalicylate therapy for distal ulcerative colitis: a meta-analysis. Aliment Pharmacol Ther 1995;9:293–300.

67. Campieri M, Corbelli C, Gionchetti P, et al. Spread and distribution of 5-ASA colonic foam and 5-ASA enema in patients with ulcerative colitis. Dig Dis Sci 1992;37:1890–7.

68. Ferring Pharmaceuticals, Mesalazine foam: internal data. In: Clinical study report PPL 469. Ferring Pharmaceuticals; 2002.

69. Pokrotnieks J, Marlicz K, Paradowski L, et al. Efficacy and tolerability of mesalazine foam enema (Salofalk foam) for distal ulcerative colitis: a double-blind, randomized, placebo-controlled study. Aliment Pharmacol Ther 2000;14:1191–8.

70. Cortot A, Maetz D, Degoutte E, et al. Mesalamine foam enema versus mesalamine liquid enema in active left-sided ulcerative colitis. Am J Gastroenterol 2008;103:3106–14.

71. Kane SV. Systematic review: adherence issues in the treatment of ulcerative colitis. Aliment Pharmacol Ther 2006;23:577–85.

72. Kane SV, Brixner D, Rubin DT, et al. The challenge of compliance and persistence: focus on ulcerative colitis. J Manag Care Pharm 2008;14:s2–12, quiz s3–5.

73. Kane SV, Cohen RD, Aikens JE, et al. Prevalence of nonadherence with maintenance mesalamine in quiescent ulcerative colitis. Am J Gastroenterol 2001;96: 2929–33.

74. De Vos M, Verdievel H, Schoonjans R, et al. Concentrations of 5-ASA and Ac-5-ASA in human ileocolonic biopsy homogenates after oral 5-ASA preparations. Gut 1992;33:1338–42.

75. Frieri G, Pimpo MT, Palumbo GC, et al. Rectal and colonic mesalazine concentration in ulcerative colitis: oral vs. oral plus topical treatment. Aliment Pharmacol Ther 1999;13:1413–7.

76. Fleig WE, Laudage G, Sommer H, et al. Prospective, randomized, double-blind comparison of benzalazine and sulfasalazine in the treatment of active ulcerative colitis. Digestion 1988;40:173–80.

77. Riley SA, Mani V, Goodman MJ, et al. Comparison of delayed release 5 aminosalicylic acid (mesalazine) and sulphasalazine in the treatment of mild to moderate ulcerative colitis relapse. Gut 1988;29:669–74.

78. Rachmilewitz D. Coated mesalazine (5-aminosalicylic acid) versus sulphasala-zine in the treatment of active ulcerative colitis: a randomised trial. BMJ 1989; 298:82–6.

79. Rao SS, Dundas SA, Holdsworth CD, et al. Olsalazine or sulphasalazine in first attacks of ulcerative colitis? A double blind study. Gut 1989;30:675–9.

80. Munakata A, Yoshida Y, Muto T, et al. Double-blind comparative study of sulfa-salazine and controlled-release mesalazine tablets in the treatment of active ulcerative colitis. J Gastroenterol 1995;30(Suppl 8):108–11.

81. Kruis W, Brandes JW, Schreiber S, et al. Olsalazine versus mesalazine in the treatment of mild to moderate ulcerative colitis. Aliment Pharmacol Ther 1998; 12:707–15.

82. Green JR, Lobo AJ, Holdsworth CD, et al. Balsalazide is more effective and better tolerated than mesalamine in the treatment of acute ulcerative colitis. The Abacus Investigator Group. Gastroenterology 1998;114:15–22.

83. Green JR, Mansfield JC, Gibson JA, et al. A double-blind comparison of balsa-lazide, 6.75 g daily, and sulfasalazine, 3 g daily, in patients with newly diagnosed or relapsed active ulcerative colitis. Aliment Pharmacol Ther 2002;16:61–8.

84. Forbes A, Al-Damluji A, Ashworth S, et al. Multicentre randomized-controlled clinical trial of Ipocol, a new enteric-coated form of mesalazine, in comparison with Asacol in the treatment of ulcerative colitis. Aliment Pharmacol Ther 2005;21:1099–104.

85. Pruitt R, Hanson J, Safdi M, et al. Balsalazide is superior to mesalamine in the time to improvement of signs and symptoms of acute mild-to-moderate ulcera-tive colitis. Am J Gastroenterol 2002;97:3078–86.

86. Levine DS, Riff DS, Pruitt R, et al. A randomized, double blind, dose-response comparison of balsalazide (6.75 g), balsalazide (2.25 g), and mesalamine (2.4 g) in the treatment of active, mild-to-moderate ulcerative colitis. Am J Gas-troenterol 2002;97:1398–407.

87. Mansfield JC, Glaffer MH, Cann PA, et al. A double-blind comparison of balsa-lazide, 6.75 g, and sulfasalazine, 3 g, as sole therapy in the management of ulcerative colitis. Aliment Pharmacol Ther 2002;16:69–77.

88. Raedler A, Behrens C, Bias P. Mesalazine (5-aminosalicylic acid) micropellets show similar efficacy and tolerability to mesalazine tablets in patients with ulcer-ative colitis—results from a randomized-controlled trial. Aliment Pharmacol Ther 2004;20:1353–63.

89. Tursi A, Brandimarte G, Giorgetti GM, et al. Low-dose balsalazide plus a high-potency probiotic preparation is more effective than balsalazide alone or mesalazine in the treatment of acute mild-to-moderate ulcerative colitis. Med Sci Monit 2004;10:PI126–31.

90. Jiang XL, Cui HF. Different therapy for different types of ulcerative colitis in China. World J Gastroenterol 2004;10:1513–20.

91. Marakhouski Y, Fixa B, Holoman J, et al. A double-blind dose-escalating trial comparing novel mesalazine pellets with mesalazine tablets in active ulcerative colitis. Aliment Pharmacol Ther 2005;21:133–40.

92. Gibson PR, Fixa B, Pekarkova B, et al. Comparison of the efficacy and safety of Eudragit-L-coated mesalazine tablets with ethylcellulose-coated mesalazine tablets in patients with mild to moderately active ulcerative colitis. Aliment Phar-macol Ther 2006;23:1017–26.

93. Ito H, Iida M, Matsumoto T, et al. Direct comparison of two different mesalamine formulations for the induction of remission in patients with ulcerative colitis: a double-blind, randomized study. Inflamm Bowel Dis 2010;16(9):1567–74.

· 94. McIntyre PB, Rodrigues CA, Lennard-Jones JE, et al. Balsalazide in the mainte-nance treatment of patients with ulcerative colitis, a double-blind comparison with sulphasalazine. Aliment Pharmacol Ther 1988;2:237–43.

95. Rutgeerts P. Comparative efficacy of coated, oral 5-aminosalicylic acid (Claver-sal) and sulphasalazine for maintaining remission of ulcerative colitis. Interna-tional Study Group. Aliment Pharmacol Ther 1989;3:183–91.

96. Rijk MC, van Lier HJ, van Tongeren JH. Relapse-preventing effect and safety of sulfasalazine and olsalazine in patients with ulcerative colitis in remission: a prospective, double-blind, randomized multicenter study. The Ulcerative Colitis Multicenter Study Group. Am J Gastroenterol 1992;87:438–42.

97. Kiilerich S, Ladefoged K, Rannem T, et al. Prophylactic effects of olsalazine v sulphasalazine during 12 months maintenance treatment of ulcerative colitis. The Danish Olsalazine Study Group. Gut 1992;33:252–5.

98. Nilsson A, Danielsson A, Lofberg R, et al. Olsalazine versus sulphasalazine for relapse prevention in ulcerative colitis: a multicenter study. Am J Gastroenterol 1995;90:381–7.

99. Ardizzone S, Petrillo M, Molteni P, et al. Coated oral 5-aminosalicylic acid (Claver-sal) is equivalent to sulfasalazine for remission maintenance in ulcerative colitis. A double-blind study. J Clin Gastroenterol 1995;21:287–9.

100. Riley SA, Mani V, Goodman MJ, et al. Comparison of delayed-release 5-amino-salicylic acid (mesalazine) and sulfasalazine as maintenance treatment for patients with ulcerative colitis. Gastroenterology 1988;94:1383–9.

101. Green JR, Gibson JA, Kerr GD, et al. Maintenance of remission of ulcerative colitis: a comparison between balsalazide 3 g daily and mesalazine 1.2 g daily over 12 months. ABACUS Investigator group. Aliment Pharmacol Ther 1998;12:1207–16.

102. Kruis W, Schreiber S, Theuer D, et al. Low dose balsalazide (1.5 g twice daily) and mesalazine (0.5 g three times daily) maintained remission of ulcerative colitis but high dose balsalazide (3.0 g twice daily) was superior in preventing relapses. Gut 2001;49:783–9.

103. Mahmud N, O'Toole D, O'Hare N, et al. Evaluation of renal function following treatment with 5-aminosalicylic acid derivatives in patients with ulcerative colitis. Aliment Pharmacol Ther 2002;16:207–15.

104. Kohn A, Prantera C, Caprilli R, et al. Maintenance treatment of ulcerative colitis with 5-aminosalicylic acid (5-ASA): Results from the Italian population of a one year, randomized, multinational study comparing MMx® with Asacol®. Gastro-enterology 2009;136(Suppl 1):A65.

105. Prantera C, Kohn A, Campieri M, et al. Clinical trial: ulcerative colitis mainte-nance treatment with 5-ASA: a 1-year, randomized multicentre study comparing MMX with Asacol. Aliment Pharmacol Ther 2009;30:908–18.

106. Rahimi R, Nikfar S, Rezaie A, et al. Comparison of mesalazine and balsalazide in induction and maintenance of remission in patients with ulcerative colitis: a meta-analysis. Dig Dis Sci 2009;54:712–21.

107. Nikfar S, Rahimi R, Rezaie A, et al. A meta-analysis of the efficacy of sulfasala-zine in comparison with 5-aminosalicylates in the induction of improvement and maintenance of remission in patients with ulcerative colitis. Dig Dis Sci 2009;54:1157–70.

108. Marteau P, Probert CS, Lindgren S, et al. Combined oral and enema treatment with Pentasa (mesalazine) is superior to oral therapy alone in patients with extensive mild/moderate active ulcerative colitis: a randomised, double blind, placebo controlled study. Gut 2005;54:960–5.

109. Safdi M, DeMicco M, Sninsky C, et al. A double-blind comparison of oral versus rectal mesalamine versus combination therapy in the treatment of distal ulcerative colitis. Am J Gastroenterol 1997;92:1867–71.
110. Loftus EV Jr, Kane SV, Bjorkman D. Systematic review: short-term adverse effects of 5-aminosalicylic acid agents in the treatment of ulcerative colitis. Aliment Pharmacol Ther 2004;19:179–89.
111. Yen EF, Kane SV, Ladabaum U. Cost-effectiveness of 5-aminosalicylic acid therapy for maintenance of remission in ulcerative colitis. Am J Gastroenterol 2008;103:3094–105.

Targeted Therapeutic Agents for Colorectal Cancer

Cheng E. Chee, MD[a], Frank A. Sinicrope, MD[a,b,*]

KEYWORDS

- Colorectal cancer • Targeted therapy • VEGF • EGFR

Colorectal cancer (CRC) is the third most incident cancer and cause of cancer-related deaths in the United States. In 2009, the number of new cases of CRC in the United States was estimated at 146,970 with 49,920 deaths expected from this malignancy.[1] The incidence and mortality rate of CRC have continued to decline largely owing to improved screening efforts that lead to early detection and removal of precancerous polyps and improvements in anticancer treatment. Despite current therapies, approximately 40% to 50% of patients with CRC who undergo potentially curative surgery ultimately relapse and die of metastatic disease.[2] In addition, approximately 20% of patients with CRC present with metastases (stage IV disease) at diagnosis, for which palliative systemic therapy is the primary treatment modality.[3] Although the medical management of CRC has steadily improved, the focus of this review is on the use of molecular targeted agents for the treatment of CRC. The objective of targeted anticancer therapeutics is to disrupt specific steps in the molecular pathway of tumorigenesis, with the goal of tumor regression while producing minimal systemic toxicity.

SYSTEMIC CHEMOTHERAPY FOR ADVANCED CRC

The backbone of systemic chemotherapy for metastatic CRC consists of 5-fluorouracil (5-FU) and folinic acid (FA, also known as leucovorin), a regimen used for many years that achieves response rates of approximately 20% and a median survival of 11 months compared with 5 months with best supportive care (BSC).[4] The platinum analogue oxaliplatin and irinotecan (CPT-11), a topoisomerase 1 inhibitor, were later added to the 5-FU/FA backbone, and it was observed that the combination

Funding support: None.

The authors have nothing to disclose.

[a] Division of Oncology, Mayo Clinic, 200 First Street SW, Rochester, MN 55905, USA

[b] Division of Gastroenterology & Hepatology, Mayo Clinic, Rochester, MN, USA

* Corresponding author. Divisions of Oncology, Gastroenterology & Hepatology, Mayo Clinic, 200 First Street SW, Rochester, MN 55905.

E-mail address: sinicrope.frank@mayo.edu

doi:10.1016/j.gtc.2010.08.017

chemotherapy produced higher response rates (35%–53%) and prolonged progression-free survival (PFS) (5–8 months) and overall survival (14–18 months).[5–8] The standard combination chemotherapy in the first-line setting includes 5-FU/FA and oxaliplatin (FOLFOX) or 5-FU/FA and irinotecan (FOLFIRI). FOLFOX and FOLFIRI have shown equivalent clinical activity but have different safety profiles, with peripheral sensory neuropathy occurring with oxaliplatin and gastrointestinal toxicity being more frequent with irinotecan.[9,10] Substitution of 5-FU/FA with the oral fluoropyrimidine capecitabine (Xeloda) has been tested in combination with oxaliplatin (XELOX) or with irinotecan (XELIRI), and the capecitabine-based combinations have shown similar efficacy to their equivalent 5-FU–based combinations.[11–13] Capecitabine is an oral agent that is metabolized to 5-FU in vivo and has been shown to be at least as effective as intravenous 5-FU.[14–16] The side-effect profile of capecitabine differs from bolus 5-FU in that a lower incidence of myelosuppression, mucositis, and diarrhea is observed, but the incidence of hand-foot syndrome was higher in the capecitabine treatment arms.[14,16]

TARGETED THERAPY IN CRC

The 2 signaling pathways important in the growth and metastatic potential of human CRCs include the vascular endothelial growth factor (VEGF) and epidermal growth factor receptor (EGFR) pathways. Molecular targeted agents against VEGF and EGFR have been developed, and in clinical trials, they have shown to enhance the efficacy of cytotoxic chemotherapy in patients with advanced CRC . Based on these data, anti-VEGF (bevacizumab, Avastin) and anti-EGFR (cetuximab, Erbitux; panitumumab, Vectibix) monoclonal antibodies were approved by the US Food and Drug Administration (FDA) for the treatment of advanced CRC.

Angiogenesis Inhibitors

Angiogenesis results in the formation of new blood vessels, and in tumors, this process promotes tumor growth and metastasis. The VEGF family, composed of VEGFs and VEGF receptors (VEGFRs), regulates the process of angiogenesis, and various strategies have evolved to inhibit this signaling pathway.[17] Bevacizumab is a humanized monoclonal antibody that binds to VEGF-A, thereby preventing the binding of this growth factor to its associated VEGFRs.[17,18] Besides inhibiting angiogenesis, it has been postulated that anti-VEGF therapy can transiently normalize tumor vasculature and improve drug and oxygen delivery to tumor cells, making them more chemosensitive and radiosensitive.[19] The potential role for bevacizumab in the treatment of CRC was initially shown in a phase 2 trial that compared 2 doses of bevacizumab in combination with 5-FU/FA with 5-FU/FA alone in patients with metastatic CRC. This study showed that the bevacizumab combinations produced improved response rates and extended median time to disease progression and median survival rates and favored the lower bevacizumab dose of 5 mg/kg.[20] This study led to the pivotal randomized phase 3 trial that gained the approval of bevacizumab in the United States in 2004 as the first-line agent in the treatment of metastatic CRC **(Table 1)**.[21] When compared with the irinotecan and 5-FU/FA combination (coined IFL), the addition of bevacizumab to IFL showed improved median survival (20.3 vs 15.6 months, hazard ratio [HR] 0.66, $P<.001$), response rates (44.8% vs 34.8%, $P = .004$), and median duration of response (10.4 vs 7.1 months, HR 0.62, $P = .001$).[21] Grade 3 hypertension was more common in the bevacizumab group but was easily treated with antihypertensives.[21] Bevacizumab has also shown

Table 1
Targeted therapy in metastatic colorectal cancer

Study	No. of Patients	Study Type	Response Rate	Median TTP	Median PFS	Median OS	References
First-line Therapy							
5-FU/FA	36	Phase 2	17%	5.2 mo	—	13.8 mo	20
5-FU/FA and Bevacizumab[a]	35		40% (P = .029)	9.0 mo (P = .005)	—	21.5 mo	
IFL	411	Phase 3	34.8%	—	6.2 mo	15.6 mo	21
IFL/Bevacizumab	402		44.8% (P = .004)	—	10.6 mo (P<.001)	20.3 mo (P<.001)	
FOLFOX-4 or XELOX	701	Phase 3	49%	—	8.0 mo	19.9 mo	23
FOLFOX-4 or XELOX with Bevacizumab	699		47% (P = .31)	—	9.4 mo (P = .002)	21.3 mo (P = .08)	
Second-line Therapy							
FOLFOX-4	291	Phase 3	8.6%	—	4.7 mo	10.8 mo	26
FOLFOX-4/Bevacizumab	286		22.7% (P<.0001)	—	7.3 mo (P<.0001)	12.9 mo (P = .001)	
Cetuximab	111	Phase 2	10.8%	1.5	—	6.9 mo	41
Cetuximab/Irinotecan	218		22.9% (P = .007)	4.1 mo (P<.001)	—	8.6 mo	
BSC	285	Phase 2	0%	—	—	4.6 mo	45
Cetuximab/BSC	287		8% (P<.001)	—	—	6.1 mo (P = .005)	
BSC	232	Phase 3	0%	—	1.8 mo	—	48
Panitumumab/BSC	231		10% (P<.0001)	—	2.0 mo (P<.0001)	—	
Cetuximab/Bevacizumab	40	Phase 2	20%	4.9 mo	—	11.4 mo	64
Cetuximab/Bevacizumab/Irinotecan	43		37%	7.3 mo	—	14.5 mo	

Abbreviations: BSC, best supportive care; IFL, irinotecan, bolus 5-fluorouracil and folinic acid; OS, overall survival; TTP, time to progression; PFS, progression free survival.
[a] Using bevacizumab at 5 mg/kg.

improved clinical efficacy with a comparable safety profile, when combined with the current standard oxaliplatin- and irinotecan-based regimens for advanced CRC.[21-23]

Bevacizumab is at present approved by the FDA for use in the first and second-line treatment of metastatic CRC. At present, in the United States, first-line therapy for patients with advanced CRC is combination chemotherapy of FOLFOX, XELOX or FOLFIRI, all given in combination with bevacizumab. The role of bevacizumab beyond the first progression was analyzed in the Bevacizumab Regimens: Investigation of Treatment Effects (BRiTE) study, which showed an improved overall survival with continued VEGF inhibition with bevacizumab beyond the initial progression of disease.[24] This study supports the hypothesis that continued suppression of the VEGF pathway may be important to maximize the clinical benefit of bevacizumab in metastatic CRC.[24] Further data supporting this hypothesis include observations of a rebound increase in VEGF concentration in human tumors and rapid tumor growth in mouse xenograft models after stopping the administration of a VEGF inhibitor.[25] Bevacizumab was approved as a second-line agent in metastatic CRC treatment after the Eastern Cooperative Oncology Group (ECOG) 3200 trial demonstrated that the combination of FOLFOX with bevacizumab significantly improved PFS (7.3 vs 4.7 months) and median survival (12.9 vs 10.8 months) compared with FOLFOX alone.[26] The role of bevacizumab in addition to chemotherapy to increase the resectability of liver metastasis has been explored by several small studies.[27,28] One study showed that the use of bevacizumab with chemotherapy in a preoperative setting can achieve a high objective tumor response rate of 73% and the treatment was also safe, whereby the incidence of wound and bleeding complications and liver dysfunction was not increased.[28] Confirmation of the ability of bevacizumab to enable more patients to undergo resection of hepatic metastases requires larger studies.

The most common side effects from bevacizumab are hypertension, which is seen in 11% to 24% of cases, and the potential for bleeding, gastrointestinal perforations (1.5%–2% of patients), arterial thrombotic events (approximately 4%–5%), and proteinuria.[29,30] In clinical practice, bevacizumab can be given to patients with advanced CRC with intact primary tumors, and in circumstances in which surgery is planned, the drug administration is generally stopped 4 weeks before surgery so as not to increase bleeding or interfere with wound healing.[31] At present, there are no predictive biomarkers available to predict which patient cohorts may benefit most from bevacizumab therapy. Expression of VEGF protein in human CRC tissues has not correlated with the clinical outcome of bevacizumab therapy.[32]

A variety of novel molecules, which target the VEGF signaling pathway, are currently under investigation. Vatalanib and axitinib are tyrosine kinase inhibitors that block VEGFR-1, VEGFR-2, and VEGFR-3. Vatalanib was studied in the first and second-line setting in the Colorectal Oral Novel Therapy for the Inhibition of Angiogenesis and Retarding of Metastases (CONFIRM) 1 and 2 trials, respectively, and no significant benefit was observed in the treatment of metastatic CRC when vatalanib was combined with FOLFOX.[33,34] Targeted agents, which are currently being tested in the first-line setting for metastatic CRC, include a phase 1 or 2 trial of axitinib and bevacizumab, a phase 3 trial of cediranib (tyrosine kinase inhibitor to VEGFR-1, VEGFR-2, VEGFR-3, and c-kit) with FOLFOX,[35] a phase 2 trial of aflibercept (VEGF Trap) and FOLFOX,[35] and a phase 3 trial of sunitinib (oral multitarget tyrosine kinase inhibitor) with FOLFIRI.[35] In the second-line setting, ongoing clinical trials include a phase 3 trial of aflibercept and FOLFIRI,[35] a phase 3 trial of brivanib (dual kinase inhibitor of VEGFR-2 and fibroblast growth factor) with cetuximab,[35] a phase 2 trial of axitinib with FOLFOX or FOLFIRI,[35] and a phase 1b study of AMG 706 (tyrosine kinase inhibitor to VEGF, platelet-derived growth factor, and c-kit) with panitumumab in addition to FOLFOX or FOLFIRI.[36]

EGFR Inhibitors

EGFR expression in tumor cell membranes is detected in approximately two-thirds of human CRC and is an adverse prognostic marker in this malignancy.[37] Cetuximab is a chimeric IgG1 monoclonal antibody against EGFR.[38,39] By binding to the extracellular domain of the human EGFR, cetuximab competitively inhibits the binding of epidermal growth factor (EGF) and other ligands to EGFR, blocking receptor phosphorylation and activation of receptor-associated kinases, thereby inhibiting downstream signal transduction and resulting in the inhibition of cell proliferation, induction of apoptosis, and reduction in angiogenesis.[38–40] EGFR is upregulated in 60% to 80% of CRC cases.[41,42] Initial in vivo studies on human colon cancer cells xenografted into nude mice indicated that cetuximab enhanced antitumor activity when combined with irinotecan.[43] Subsequent clinical trials validated these findings. In a phase 2 clinical trial, single-agent cetuximab was used to treat patients with advanced and treatment-refractory CRC with prior exposure to irinotecan either alone or in a combination regimen. Partial response was achieved in 10.5% of 57 evaluable patients, and the median survival time was 6.4 months.[44] The activity of cetuximab in combination with irinotecan in refractory metastatic CRC was confirmed in the Bowel Oncology with Cetuximab Antibody (BOND) trial that showed a significantly higher response rate and median time to progression (TTP) in the combination arm compared with cetuximab alone (22.9% versus 10.8%, $P = .007$ and 4.1 versus 1.5 months, $P<.001$, respectively) (see **Table 1**).[41] In contrast to bevacizumab, cetuximab shows activity as monotherapy with an approximate 10% response rate in patients with advanced CRC.[26,41] Cetuximab monotherapy was shown to be superior to BSC in patients who had been either previously treated with a fluoropyrimidine-, irinotecan-, and oxaliplatin-based regimen or had contraindications to treatment with these drugs.[45] In this study, cetuximab improved overall survival (HR 0.77; 95% confidence interval [CI], 0.64–0.92; $P = .005$) with a median survival of 6.1 months in the cetuximab group compared with 4.6 months in the BSC group and it also preserved quality-of-life measures.[45] The administration of anti-EGFR monoclonal antibodies can cause an acneiform rash in more than 80% of patients, with the incidence of grade 3 or 4 skin rash in less than 10% of patients.[25] Other side effects include hypomagnesemia, diarrhea, and hypersensitivity reactions, particularly with the chimeric antibody cetuximab.[30] Cetuximab is FDA approved as a single agent in metastatic CRC treatment after the failure of both irinotecan- and oxaliplatin-based regimens or in patients who are intolerant to irinotecan-based regimens. Cetuximab is also approved in combination with irinotecan in patients with metastatic CRC who are refractory to irinotecan-based chemotherapy.

Panitumumab is a high-affinity fully human IgG2 monoclonal antibody that also targets EGFR.[46] In a phase 2 trial of heavily pretreated patients with metastatic CRC, single-agent panitumumab had a median PFS of 14 weeks and median overall survival of 9 months.[47] The overall response rate of 9% was similar to single-agent cetuximab. Skin toxicities occurred in 95% of patients but were rarely severe, and there was a very low incidence of hypersensitivity reactions (1 of 148 patients) when compared with cetuximab.[47] This led to a pivotal phase 3 trial that led to the approval of panitumumab as a single-agent salvage therapy for patients with metastatic CRC in the United States (see **Table 1**).[48] In this study, patients previously exposed to fluoropyrimidine-, irinotecan-, or oxaliplatin-based treatment were randomized to panitumumab and BSC versus BSC alone. Results demonstrated that panitumumab, in a third-line setting, was superior to BSC alone with a response rate of 10% and PFS of 8 weeks versus 7.3 weeks (HR 0.54; 95% CI, 0.44–0.66; $P<.0001$). Overall survival was not significantly different because 76% of the patients crossed over from the BSC arm to the panitumumab arm.[48] Panitumumab monotherapy was approved in patients with metastatic CRC with progression on or after fluoropyrimidine-, oxaliplatin-, and irinotecan-containing chemotherapy.

Predictive Biomarkers for Anti-EGFR Therapy

The use of biomarkers to predict the clinical outcomes of EGFR-targeted therapy in metastatic CRC has been highlighted recently. Several trials with cetuximab and panitumumab have noted an intriguing correlation between rash intensity and survival outcomes, whereby the higher the grade of skin rash, the better the clinical outcome.[41,44,48] This finding suggests that the intensity of the skin rash induced by anti-EGFR antibodies can serve as a predictive marker of therapeutic efficacy.

The most important recent development is the finding that the mutational status of KRAS oncogene is a predictive biomarker for the efficacy of anti-EGFR therapies.[49–53] KRAS encodes for the RAS protein, which functions as a GTPase that is involved in signal transduction events, and loss of RAS is associated with hyperproliferation.[54,55] Mutation in the codons 12 and 13 of KRAS gene is present in approximately 40% of human CRCs and is an early event in tumorigenesis such that the frequency of mutation is not affected by the tumor stage.[55] When KRAS status was determined on archived tissue from completed anti-EGFR clinical trials in CRC, improved clinical outcomes were observed in patients with wild-type KRAS tumors but not in those with mutant KRAS tumors.[49,51,56,57] When cetuximab was compared with BSC, overall survival was nearly doubled in tumors with wild-type KRAS compared with CRCs with mutated KRAS (9.5 vs 4.8 months; HR 0.55; 95% CI, 0.41–0.74; $P<.001$).[51] Importantly, patients whose tumors had mutated KRAS showed no significant difference in outcomes between cetuximab therapy and BSC.[51] Similar observations have been noted with panitumumab. Using archived tissue from a phase 3 trial comparing panitumumab monotherapy with BSC, patients with wild-type KRAS tumors who were treated with panitumumab had a response rate of 17% and a median PFS of 12.3 weeks versus 7.3 weeks in patients with wild-type KRAS tumors who were in the BSC group (HR 0.45; 95% CI, 0.34–0.59; $P<.0001$).[49] In the patients with mutated KRAS tumors, the response rate was 0% and PFS was identical, that is, 7.4 weeks versus 7.3 weeks (HR 0.99; 95% CI, 0.73–1.36) in the panitumumab versus BSC study arms.[49]

The RAS/RAF/MAPK signaling pathway occurs downstream from EGFR pathway. Once RAS is activated, it recruits the oncogene RAF that phosphorylates MAP2K-1 and MAP2K-2, thus initiating MAPK signaling that ultimately leads to expression of proteins involved in cell proliferation, differentiation, and survival.[58–60] More recently, mutations in the BRAF oncogene have been shown to be another potential predictive marker for response to anti-EGFR therapy. Mutations in BRAF oncogene are detected in approximately 10% of sporadic CRCs.[61,62] Tumors with mutations in the BRAF gene do not respond to EGFR inhibitors, and patients with mutant BRAF tumors have been shown to have significantly shorter PFS and overall survival rates compared with patients whose tumors carry wild-type BRAF.[61,62] Although mutations in BRAF and loss of PTEN expression seem to be associated with resistance to EGFR-targeted monoclonal-antibody treatment, these markers require validation before they can be used in clinical practice.[63] At present, all patients with a new diagnosis of metastatic CRC should be tested for KRAS mutation in the tumor sample, and the use of cetuximab or panitumumab should be restricted to patients with CRCs containing wild-type KRAS.

Based on the results outlined earlier, the idea of combining the agents targeting both VEGF and EGFR pathways has been tested. The use of combined targeted therapy in refractory CRC was an attractive concept, with the potential to eliminate the use of conventional cytotoxic drugs. This concept was first highlighted in the BOND-2 study, in which the combination of bevacizumab and cetuximab was used as a salvage therapy in heavily pretreated patients with metastatic CRC.[64] This study showed a modest response rate of 20% for combined targeted therapy with a 4.9-month median TTP when compared with an approximate 10% response rate and 1.5-month median TTP reported in previous studies.[41,44] Two prospective randomized phase 3 trials, Capecitabine, Irinotecan, and Oxaliplatin in advanced colorectal cancer (CAIRO)-2 and Panitumumab Advanced Colorectal Cancer Evaluation (PACCE), were subsequently performed in an attempt to validate these findings but showed inferior outcomes and increased toxicities with the combination of anti-VEGF and anti-EGFR treatment and chemotherapy.[65,66] Based on these results, anti-VEGF and anti-EGFR antibodies should not be used concurrently in patients with CRC in clinical practice outside a clinical trial. Other strategies under investigation include combining an anti-EGFR antibody with a small molecule such as a tyrosine kinase inhibitor against EGFR, such as erlotinib (Tarceva). In preclinical studies, this combination has shown synergistic effects compared with either drug alone, and phase 2 trials are currently ongoing to evaluate this strategy.[67–69]

ADJUVANT THERAPY

Patients with stage II and III (lymph node-positive) CRC, resected with curative intent, are candidates for adjuvant systemic chemotherapy. As 5-FU/FA was the standard treatment of advanced CRC, this regimen was later evaluated in the adjuvant setting and found to be effective, with 2 studies demonstrating an improvement in 3-year overall survival by 5%, when 5-FU/FA was compared with observation only.[70–73] In the late 1990s, when FOLFOX showed superiority over 5-FU/FA alone in the metastatic setting, the use of FOLFOX in the adjuvant setting was then evaluated in the Multicenter International Study of Oxaliplatin/5-fluorouracil/Leucovorin in the Adjuvant Treatment of Colon Cancer (MOSAIC) trial.[74] This was a European multi-institution trial that compared infusional 5-FU/FA with and without the addition of oxaliplatin in stage II and III disease.[74] The overall 5-year disease-free survival (DFS) was 73.3% versus 67.4%, with and without oxaliplatin, respectively, for stage II and III disease combined. For stage III disease, 6-year overall survival rates were 78.5% and 76% in the FOLFOX and 5-FU/FA groups, respectively (HR 0.84; 95% CI, 0.71–1.00; $P = .046$), with no significant difference in the stage II group.[75] Peripheral neuropathy, a known side effect of oxaliplatin, was well tolerated and generally reversible. The MOSAIC data were later confirmed by the National Surgical Adjuvant Breast and Bowel Project (NSABP) C-07 trial revealing a 6% benefit in 4-year DFS for the oxaliplatin-containing regimen in stage II and III disease.[76] A similar 20% reduction in recurrence was seen in both the stages. Based on these data, the US FDA approved the use of oxaliplatin in adjuvant therapy, and FOLFOX has now become the new standard of care for stage III disease. Besides stage III disease, considerations for adjuvant therapy should be made in the treatment of high-risk stage II disease. However, in rectal cancer, preoperative or neoadjuvant chemoradiation is a standard approach in the United States because of the potential advantages of increased radiosensitivity in the unoperated pelvis and enhanced sphincter preservation.[77]

Despite its enhanced efficacy with advanced CRC, bevacizumab has not been shown to be active in an adjuvant setting. The NSABP C-08 trial reported that the addition of bevacizumab to modified FOLFOX-6 in patients with stage II and III CRC did not significantly prolong DFS, although a transient benefit was seen during the 1-year interval when bevacizumab was used.[78] Furthermore, grade 3+ toxicities such as hypertension, wound complications, pain, and proteinuria may not substantiate its use and tolerability in the long term in this patient population.[29] Although it is possible that a longer duration of bevacizumab therapy may be required to obtain potential benefit, it must be emphasized that this drug, given in combination with a standard adjuvant regimen, was ineffective in the adjuvant setting. The results of the AVANT study, another adjuvant trial using bevacizumab and chemotherapy in patients with high-risk stage II and III CRC, will be reported soon. The North Central Cancer Treatment Group conducted a phase 3 intergroup trial (N0147) assessing the potential benefit of adding the anti-EGFR antibody cetuximab to a modified FOLFOX-6 regimen as adjuvant therapy in patients with completely resected stage III colon cancer.[79] The recently reported results of this study showed that the addition of cetuximab to modified FOLFOX-6 was of no benefit for patients with resected stage III wild-type *KRAS* CRC.[80]

SUMMARY

The development of molecular targeted therapies has greatly affected the current treatment of patients with advanced CRC. Agents targeting the VEGF or EGFR pathways have been shown to increase the efficacy of cytotoxic chemotherapy resulting in the extension of survival and have led to newer regimens that are now the standard of care for the treatment of metastatic CRC. Although associated with some adverse effects, these agents are considerably better tolerated than conventional cytotoxic agents. Regrettably, attempts to move targeted therapies to earlier stage disease have yet to show any clinical benefit. Another important advance is the identification of predictive biomarkers for anti-EGFR therapies. Specifically, clinical benefit of anti-EGFR antibody therapy is restricted to CRCs with wild-type *KRAS* oncogene, and *KRAS* testing should now be performed in tumor samples of all patients with metastatic CRC. These data, as well as emerging data for other predictive biomarkers, can enable individualized treatment decisions and more personalized therapeutic approaches. The continued development of molecular targeted therapies holds much promise for further improvement in patient outcomes and in quality of life for patients with CRC.

REFERENCES

1. Jemal A, Siegel R, Ward E, et al. Cancer statistics, 2009. CA Cancer J Clin 2009; 59(4):225–49.
2. Obrand DI, Gordon PH. Incidence and patterns of recurrence following curative resection for colorectal carcinoma. Dis Colon Rectum 1997;40(1):15–24.
3. Wagner AD, Arnold D, Grothey AA, et al. Anti-angiogenic therapies for metastatic colorectal cancer. Cochrane Database Syst Rev 2009;3:CD005392.
4. Scheithauer W, Rosen H, Kornek GV, et al. Randomised comparison of combination chemotherapy plus supportive care with supportive care alone in patients with metastatic colorectal cancer. BMJ 1993;306(6880):752–5.
5. de Gramont A, Figer A, Seymour M, et al. Leucovorin and fluorouracil with or without oxaliplatin as first-line treatment in advanced colorectal cancer. J Clin Oncol 2000;18(16):2938–47.
6. Douillard JY, Cunningham D, Roth AD, et al. Irinotecan combined with fluorouracil compared with fluorouracil alone as first-line treatment for metastatic colorectal cancer: a multicentre randomised trial. Lancet 2000;355(9209):1041–7.
7. Giacchetti S, Perpoint B, Zidani R, et al. Phase III multicenter randomized trial of oxaliplatin added to chronomodulated fluorouracil-leucovorin as first-line treatment of metastatic colorectal cancer. J Clin Oncol 2000;18(1):136–47.

8. Saltz LB, Cox JV, Blanke C, et al. Irinotecan plus fluorouracil and leucovorin for metastatic colorectal cancer. Irinotecan study group. N Engl J Med 2000; 343(13):905–14.

9. Tournigand C, Andre T, Achille E, et al. FOLFIRI followed by FOLFOX6 or the reverse sequence in advanced colorectal cancer: a randomized GERCOR study. J Clin Oncol 2004;22(2):229–37.

10. Colucci G, Gebbia V, Paoletti G, et al. Phase III randomized trial of FOLFIRI versus FOLFOX4 in the treatment of advanced colorectal cancer: a multicenter study of the gruppo oncologico dell'italia meridionale. J Clin Oncol 2005; 23(22):4866–75.

11. Cassidy J, Clarke S, Diaz-Rubio E, et al. Randomized phase III study of capecitabine plus oxaliplatin compared with fluorouracil/folinic acid plus oxaliplatin as first-line therapy for metastatic colorectal cancer. J Clin Oncol 2008;26(12):2006–12.

12. Porschen R, Arkenau HT, Kubicka S, et al. Phase III study of capecitabine plus oxaliplatin compared with fluorouracil and leucovorin plus oxaliplatin in metastatic colorectal cancer: a final report of the AIO Colorectal Study Group. J Clin Oncol 2007;25(27):4217–23.

13. Skof E, Rebersek M, Hlebanja Z, et al. Capecitabine plus Irinotecan (XELIRI regimen) compared to 5-FU/LV plus Irinotecan (FOLFIRI regimen) as neoadjuvant treatment for patients with unresectable liver-only metastases of metastatic colorectal cancer: a randomised prospective phase II trial. BMC Cancer 2009;9:120.

14. Van Cutsem E, Twelves C, Cassidy J, et al. Oral capecitabine compared with intravenous fluorouracil plus leucovorin in patients with metastatic colorectal cancer: results of a large phase III study. J Clin Oncol 2001;19(21):4097–106.

15. Van Cutsem E, Hoff PM, Harper P, et al. Oral capecitabine vs intravenous 5-fluorouracil and leucovorin: integrated efficacy data and novel analyses from two large, randomised, phase III trials. Br J Cancer 2004;90(6):1190–7.

16. Hoff PM, Ansari R, Batist G, et al. Comparison of oral capecitabine versus intravenous fluorouracil plus leucovorin as first-line treatment in 605 patients with metastatic colorectal cancer: results of a randomized phase III study. J Clin Oncol 2001;19(8):2282–92.

17. Kim KJ, Li B, Winer J, et al. Inhibition of vascular endothelial growth factor-induced angiogenesis suppresses tumour growth in vivo. Nature 1993;362(6423):841–4.

18. Gordon MS, Margolin K, Talpaz M, et al. Phase I safety and pharmacokinetic study of recombinant human anti-vascular endothelial growth factor in patients with advanced cancer. J Clin Oncol 2001;19(3):843–50.

19. Jain RK. Normalization of tumor vasculature: an emerging concept in antiangiogenic therapy. Science 2005;307(5706):58–62.

20. Kabbinavar F, Hurwitz HI, Fehrenbacher L, et al. Phase II, randomized trial comparing bevacizumab plus fluorouracil (FU)/leucovorin (LV) with FU/LV alone in patients with metastatic colorectal cancer. J Clin Oncol 2003;21(1):60–5.

21. Hurwitz H, Fehrenbacher L, Novotny W, et al. Bevacizumab plus irinotecan, fluorouracil, and leucovorin for metastatic colorectal cancer. N Engl J Med 2004; 350(23):2335–42.

22. Hochster HS, Hart LL, Ramanathan RK, et al. Safety and efficacy of oxaliplatin and fluoropyrimidine regimens with or without bevacizumab as first-line treatment of metastatic colorectal cancer: results of the TREE Study. J Clin Oncol 2008; 26(21):3523–9.

23. Saltz LB, Clarke S, Diaz-Rubio E, et al. Bevacizumab in combination with oxaliplatin-based chemotherapy as first-line therapy in metastatic colorectal cancer: a randomized phase III study. J Clin Oncol 2008;26(12):2013–9.

24. Grothey A, Sugrue MM, Purdie DM, et al. Bevacizumab beyond first progression is associated with prolonged overall survival in metastatic colorectal cancer: results from a large observational cohort study (BRiTE). J Clin Oncol 2008; 26(33):5326–34.

25. Van Cutsem E. First-line treatment: approaches with cytotoxic and biologic agents. In: Chu E, editor. New treatment strategies for metastatic colorectal cancer. New York: CMPMedica; 2008. p. 21–46.

26. Giantonio BJ, Catalano PJ, Meropol NJ, et al. Bevacizumab in combination with oxaliplatin, fluorouracil, and leucovorin (FOLFOX4) for previously treated metastatic colorectal cancer: results from the eastern cooperative oncology group study E3200. J Clin Oncol 2007;25(12):1539–44.

27. Emmanouilides C, Sfakiotaki G, Androulakis N, et al. Front-line bevacizumab in combination with oxaliplatin, leucovorin and 5-fluorouracil (FOLFOX) in patients with metastatic colorectal cancer: a multicenter phase II study. BMC Cancer 2007;7:91.

28. Gruenberger B, Tamandl D, Schueller J, et al. Bevacizumab, capecitabine, and oxaliplatin as neoadjuvant therapy for patients with potentially curable metastatic colorectal cancer. J Clin Oncol 2008;26(11):1830–5.

29. Allegra CJ, Yothers G, O'Connell MJ, et al. Initial safety report of NSABP C-08: a randomized phase III study of modified FOLFOX6 with or without bevacizumab for the adjuvant treatment of patients with stage II or III colon cancer. J Clin Oncol 2009;27(20):3385–90.

30. Grothey A. Recognizing and managing toxicities of molecular targeted therapies for colorectal cancer. Oncology (Williston Park) 2006;20(14 Suppl 10):21–8.

31. Kesmodel SB, Ellis LM, Lin E, et al. Preoperative bevacizumab does not significantly increase postoperative complication rates in patients undergoing hepatic surgery for colorectal cancer liver metastases. J Clin Oncol 2008;26(32):5254–60.

32. Jubb AM, Hurwitz HI, Bai W, et al. Impact of vascular endothelial growth factor-A expression, thrombospondin-2 expression, and microvessel density on the treatment effect of bevacizumab in metastatic colorectal cancer. J Clin Oncol 2006; 24(2):217–27.

33. Hecht JR, Trarbach T, Jaeger E, et al. A randomized, double-blind, placebo-controlled, phase III study in patients (Pts) with metastatic adenocarcinoma of the colon or rectum receiving first-line chemotherapy with oxaliplatin/5-fluorouracil/leucovorin and PTK787/ZK 222584 or placebo (CONFIRM-1). J Clin Oncol 2005;23(16S):LBA3.

34. Kohne K, Bajetta E, Lin E, et al. Final results of CONFIRM 2: A multinational, randomized, double-blind, phase III study in 2nd line patients (pts) with metastatic colorectal cancer (mCRC) receiving FOLFOX4 and PTK787/ZK 222584 (PTK/ZK) or placebo. J Clin Oncol. 2007;25(18S):4033.

35. US National Institute of Health. Available at: www.clinicaltrials.gov. Accessed March 11, 2010.

36. Schwartzberg LS, Hurwitz H, Stephenson J, et al. Safety and pharmacokinetics (PK) of AMG 706 with panitumumab plus FOLFIRI or FOLFOX for the treatment of patients (pts) with metastatic colorectal cancer (mCRC). J Clin Oncol 2007; 25(18S):4081.

37. Rego RL, Foster NR, Smyrk TC, et al. Prognostic effect of activated EGFR expression in human colon carcinomas: comparison with EGFR status. Br J Cancer 2010;102(1):165–72.

38. Baselga J. The EGFR as a target for anticancer therapy–focus on cetuximab. Eur J Cancer 2001;37(Suppl 4):S16–22.

39. Goldstein NI, Prewett M, Zuklys K, et al. Biological efficacy of a chimeric antibody to the epidermal growth factor receptor in a human tumor xenograft model. Clin Cancer Res 1995;1(11):1311–8.
40. Graham J, Muhsin M, Kirkpatrick P. Cetuximab. Nat Rev Drug Discov 2004;3(7): 549–50.
41. Cunningham D, Humblet Y, Siena S, et al. Cetuximab monotherapy and cetuximab plus irinotecan in irinotecan-refractory metastatic colorectal cancer. N Engl J Med 2004;351(4):337–45.
42. Messa C, Russo F, Caruso MG, et al. TGF-alpha, and EGF-R in human colorectal adenocarcinoma. Acta Oncol 1998;37(3):285–9.
43. Prewett MC, Hooper AT, Bassi R, et al. Enhanced antitumor activity of anti-epidermal growth factor receptor monoclonal antibody IMC-C225 in combination with irinotecan (CPT-11) against human colorectal tumor xenografts. Clin Cancer Res 2002;8(5):994–1003.
44. Saltz LB, Meropol NJ, Loehrer PJ Sr, et al. Phase II trial of cetuximab in patients with refractory colorectal cancer that expresses the epidermal growth factor receptor. J Clin Oncol 2004;22(7):1201–8.
45. Jonker DJ, O'Callaghan CJ, Karapetis CS, et al. Cetuximab for the treatment of colorectal cancer. N Engl J Med 2007;357(20):2040–8.
46. Yang XD, Jia XC, Corvalan JR, et al. Development of ABX-EGF, a fully human anti-EGF receptor monoclonal antibody, for cancer therapy. Crit Rev Oncol Hematol 2001;38(1):17–23.
47. Hecht JR, Patnaik A, Berlin J, et al. Panitumumab monotherapy in patients with previously treated metastatic colorectal cancer. Cancer 2007;110(5):980–8.
48. Van Cutsem E, Peeters M, Siena S, et al. Open-label phase III trial of panitumumab plus best supportive care compared with best supportive care alone in patients with chemotherapy-refractory metastatic colorectal cancer. J Clin Oncol 2007;25(13):1658–64.
49. Amado RG, Wolf M, Peeters M, et al. Wild-type KRAS is required for panitumumab efficacy in patients with metastatic colorectal cancer. J Clin Oncol 2008; 26(10):1626–34.
50. Lievre A, Bachet JB, Le Corre D, et al. KRAS mutation status is predictive of response to cetuximab therapy in colorectal cancer. Cancer Res 2006;66(8):3992–5.
51. Karapetis CS, Khambata-Ford S, Jonker DJ, et al. K-ras mutations and benefit from cetuximab in advanced colorectal cancer. N Engl J Med 2008;359(17): 1757–65.
52. Di Fiore F, Van Cutsem E, Laurent-Puig P, et al. Role of KRAS mutation in predicting response, progression-free survival, and overall survival in irinotecan-refractory patients treated with cetuximab plus irinotecan for a metastatic colorectal cancer: Analysis of 281 individual data from published series. J Clin Oncol. 2008;26(Suppl 20):4035.
53. Lievre A, Bachet JB, Boige V, et al. KRAS mutations as an independent prognostic factor in patients with advanced colorectal cancer treated with cetuximab. J Clin Oncol 2008;26(3):374–9.
54. Bos JL. Ras oncogenes in human cancer: a review. Cancer Res 1989;49(17): 4682–9.
55. Fearon ER, Vogelstein B. A genetic model for colorectal tumorigenesis. Cell 1990; 61(5):759–67.
56. Bokemeyer C, Bondarenko I, Hartmann JT, et al. KRAS status and efficacy of first-line treatment of patients with metastatic colorectal cancer (mCRC) with FOLFOX with or without cetuximab: the OPUS experience. J Clin Oncol 2008;26(15S):4000.

57. Van Cutsem E, Lang I, D'haens G, et al. KRAS status and efficacy in the first-line treatment of patients with metastatic colorectal cancer (mCRC) treated with FOL-FIRI with or without cetuximab: the CRYSTAL experience. J Clin Oncol 2008; 26(15S):2.

58. Yarden Y, Sliwkowski MX. Untangling the ErbB signalling network. Nat Rev Mol Cell Biol 2001;2(2):127–37.

59. Scaltriti M, Baselga J. The epidermal growth factor receptor pathway: a model for targeted therapy. Clin Cancer Res 2006;12(18):5268–72.

60. McCubrey JA, Steelman LS, Abrams SL, et al. Roles of the RAF/MEK/ERK and PI3K/PTEN/AKT pathways in malignant transformation and drug resistance. Adv Enzyme Regul 2006;46:249–79.

61. Di Nicolantonio F, Martini M, Molinari F, et al. Wild-type BRAF is required for response to panitumumab or cetuximab in metastatic colorectal cancer. J Clin Oncol 2008;26(35):5705–12.

62. Tol J, Nagtegaal ID, Punt CJ. BRAF mutation in metastatic colorectal cancer. N Engl J Med 2009;361(1):98–9.

63. Siena S, Sartore-Bianchi A, Di Nicolantonio F, et al. Biomarkers predicting clinical outcome of epidermal growth factor receptor-targeted therapy in metastatic colorectal cancer. J Natl Cancer Inst 2009;101(19):1308–24.

64. Saltz LB, Lenz HJ, Kindler HL, et al. Randomized phase II trial of cetuximab, bevacizumab, and irinotecan compared with cetuximab and bevacizumab alone in irinotecan-refractory colorectal cancer: the BOND-2 study. J Clin Oncol 2007; 25(29):4557–61.

65. Tol J, Koopman M, Cats A, et al. Chemotherapy, bevacizumab, and cetuximab in metastatic colorectal cancer. N Engl J Med 2009;360(6):563–72.

66. Hecht JR, Mitchell E, Chidiac T, et al. A randomized phase IIIB trial of chemotherapy, bevacizumab, and panitumumab compared with chemotherapy and bevacizumab alone for metastatic colorectal cancer. J Clin Oncol 2009;27(5):672–80.

67. Bos M, Mendelsohn J, Kim YM, et al. PD153035, a tyrosine kinase inhibitor, prevents epidermal growth factor receptor activation and inhibits growth of cancer cells in a receptor number-dependent manner. Clin Cancer Res 1997; 3(11):2099–106.

68. Matar P, Rojo F, Cassia R, et al. Combined epidermal growth factor receptor targeting with the tyrosine kinase inhibitor gefitinib (ZD1839) and the monoclonal antibody cetuximab (IMC-C225): superiority over single-agent receptor targeting. Clin Cancer Res 2004;10(19):6487–501.

69. Huang S, Armstrong EA, Benavente S, et al. Dual-agent molecular targeting of the epidermal growth factor receptor (EGFR): combining anti-EGFR antibody with tyrosine kinase inhibitor. Cancer Res 2004;64(15):5355–62.

70. Wolmark N, Rockette H, Fisher B, et al. The benefit of leucovorin-modulated fluorouracil as postoperative adjuvant therapy for primary colon cancer: results from National Surgical Adjuvant Breast and Bowel Project protocol C-03. J Clin Oncol 1993;11(10):1879–87.

71. Efficacy of adjuvant fluorouracil and folinic acid in colon cancer. International Multicentre Pooled Analysis of Colon Cancer Trials (IMPACT) investigators. Lancet 1995;345(8955):939–44.

72. O'Connell MJ, Mailliard JA, Kahn MJ, et al. Controlled trial of fluorouracil and low-dose leucovorin given for 6 months as postoperative adjuvant therapy for colon cancer. J Clin Oncol 1997;15(1):246–50.

73. Zaniboni A, Labianca R, Marsoni S, et al. GIVIO-SITAC 01: a randomized trial of adjuvant 5-fluorouracil and folinic acid administered to patients with colon

carcinoma–long term results and evaluation of the indicators of health-related quality of life. Gruppo Italiano Valutazione Interventi in Oncologia. Studio Italiano Terapia Adiuvante Colon. Cancer 1998;82(11):2135–44.

74. Andre T, Boni C, Mounedji-Boudiaf L, et al. Oxaliplatin, fluorouracil, and leucovorin as adjuvant treatment for colon cancer. N Engl J Med 2004;350(23):2343–51.

75. Andre T, Boni C, Navarro M, et al. Improved overall survival with oxaliplatin, fluorouracil, and leucovorin as adjuvant treatment in stage II or III colon cancer in the MOSAIC trial. J Clin Oncol 2009;27(19):3109–16.

76. Kuebler JP, Wieand HS, O'Connell MJ, et al. Oxaliplatin combined with weekly bolus fluorouracil and leucovorin as surgical adjuvant chemotherapy for stage II and III colon cancer: results from NSABP C-07. J Clin Oncol 2007;25(16): 2198–204.

77. Sauer R, Becker H, Hohenberger W, et al. Preoperative versus postoperative chemoradiotherapy for rectal cancer. N Engl J Med 2004;351(17):1731–40.

78. Wolmark N, Yothers G, O'Connell MJ, et al. A phase III trial comparing mFOLFOX6 to mFOLFOX6 plus bevacizumab in stage II or III carcinoma of the colon: results of NSABP protocol C-08. J Clin Oncol 2009;27(18S):LBA4.

79. Alberts SR, Sinicrope FA, Grothey A. N0147: a randomized phase III trial of oxaliplatin plus 5-fluorouracil/leucovorin with or without cetuximab after curative resection of stage III colon cancer. Clin Colorectal Cancer 2005;5(3):211–3.

80. Alberts SR, Sargent DJ, Smyrk TC, et al. Adjuvant mFOLFOX6 with or without cetuxiumab (Cmab) in KRAS wild-type (WT) patients (pts) with resected stage III colon cancer (CC): results from NCCTG Intergroup Phase III Trial N0147. J Clin Oncol 2010;28(Suppl 18):CRA3507.

New Pharmacologic Therapies for Gastroenteropancreatic Neuroendocrine Tumors

Ben Lawrence, MBChB, MSc[a,b], Bjorn I. Gustafsson, MD, PhD[c,d],
Mark Kidd, PhD[b], Irvin Modlin, MD, PhD, DSc, FRCS (Eng & Ed)[b,*]

KEYWORDS

- Antineoplastic • Biotherapy • Carcinoid • Chemotherapy
- Neuroendocrine tumor

Gastroenteropancreatic neuroendocrine tumors (GEP-NETs) are more common than previously thought and second only to colorectal cancers as the most prevalent gastrointestinal cancers.[1,2] Systemic therapy for GEP-NETs is indicated to control symptoms of bioactive peptide and amine hypersecretion and to reduce tumor proliferation in the setting of unresectable or recurrent disease.[3] Although the treatment of individual tumors is often complex and requires multidisciplinary expertise,[4] there are stable themes that guide the choice of systemic treatment of GEP-NETs. These themes are well described in recent consensus statements such as the European Neuroendocrine Tumor Society (ENETS), the UK and Ireland Neuroendocrine Tumor Network, the National Comprehensive Cancer Network, and the European Society of Medical Oncology.[5,6,7,8] Broadly speaking, all systemic treatment is palliative: somatostatin (SST) analogues effectively reduce symptoms of neuroendocrine hypersecretion (eg, carcinoid syndrome), systemic treatment does not markedly change the natural history of well-differentiated tumors, cytotoxic chemotherapy is indicated for poorly differentiated neuroendocrine carcinomas, and systemic therapy should be 1 part of a multimodal intervention that considers surgery, local therapies, and peptide receptor radiolabeled therapy. This article describes recent developments in systemic

The authors have nothing to disclose.

[a] Department of Medical Oncology, Auckland City Hospital, Private Bag 92024, Auckland, New Zealand
[b] Gastrointestinal Pathobiology Research Group, Yale University School of Medicine, PO Box 208602, New Haven, Connecticut, USA
[c] Department of Cancer Research and Molecular Medicine, Norwegian University of Science and Technology, University Hospital, Prinsesse Kristinas Gate 1, 7006 Trondheim, Norway
[d] Department of Gastroenterology, St Olavs University Hospital, Prinsesse Kristinas Gate 1, 7006 Trondheim, Norway
* Corresponding author.
E-mail address: imodlin@yale.edu

Gastroenterol Clin N Am 39 (2010) 615–628
doi:10.1016/j.gtc.2010.08.013
0889-8553/10/$ – see front matter © 2010 Elsevier Inc. All rights reserved.

pharmacotherapy, particularly in the more controversial indolent tumors, with a focus on novel treatments that target specific proteins in cellular proliferation pathways. The lack of globally accepted definitions of what precisely represents a particular grade or stage of tumor has hampered both delineation of treatment strategy and assessment of efficacy and outcome with different treatment regimens.[4]

CLASSIFICATION

The terms used to describe neuroendocrine tumors (NETs) are bewildering in their diversity. NET nomenclature has been difficult, because Obendorfer named the tumor as "karzinoide" or cancer-like before later observing that these tumors were truly malignant. A simplistic classification based on embryologic origin, which classified carcinoids as of fore-, mid-, or hindgut origin, emerged in the 1960s and is still used in some areas.[9] In the current decade, 2 new classifications have emerged, although neither has gained universal acceptance. The World Health Organization (WHO) classification describes tumors by their degree of differentiation and site of origin,[10] and the more recent ENETS classification includes TNM-type staging, augmented by the Ki-67 index of proliferation.[11] However, controversy remains on whether Ki-67 or the precise number (of positive cells) that represents a clinically or therapeutically relevant cipher should be assessed.[12] The changing classification and the natural reluctance of most clinicians to abandon terms associated with a known therapeutic approach have resulted in a variety of names remaining in the pathologist and clinician lexicon. For example, the term neuroendocrine tumor is often used to describe the entire family of tumors, but is now a histologic stage in the WHO classification, in which it describes the well-differentiated and more indolent end of the GEP-NET spectrum. Similarly, the term carcinoid is used interchangeably by clinicians to describe all NETs, only NETs with indolent biologic behavior, or only NETs originating in the small bowel. However, in the WHO classification, carcinoid is now synonymous with NET, and either term describes grade 1 tumors (**Table 1**). However, it is generally agreed that the term carcinoid should be phased out because it denotes an archaic concept that is no longer compatible with the modern biologic understanding of neuroendocrine malignancy.

In this article, the authors group GEP-NETs along the lines of the WHO definition, but they have made slight adjustments to approximate the inclusion criteria of pharmacotherapeutic trials and to separate GEP-NETs by the appropriate therapeutic approaches. This should not imply that the authors believe that this grouping has any inherent value for future classification but simply that it provides a more easily comprehensible system by which the logic of therapeutic strategies can be appreciated. Therefore, the authors combine the WHO grade 1 and 2 tumors and divide them by the site of tumor origin as either well-differentiated carcinoids (ie, of

---

Table 1
WHO Classification of neuroendocrine tumors

WHO Classification	WHO Synonym	Biologic Behavior
Well-differentiated neuroendocrine tumor	Carcinoid	Uncertain malignant potential
Well-differentiated neuroendocrine carcinoma	Malignant carcinoid	Low-grade malignancy
Poorly differentiated neuroendocrine carcinoma		High-grade malignancy

enterochromaffin cell origin) or well-differentiated pancreatic NETs (**Fig. 1**). The group of poorly differentiated tumors (including WHO grade 3) irrespective of the site of origin is discussed separately.

IMPEDIMENTS TO THE DEVELOPMENT OF NEW PHARMACOLOGIC THERAPY FOR GEP-NETS

Although some consensus has emerged on the choice of systemic treatment, the trial literature used to make these decisions is problematic. The incidence of each subtype of GEP-NET is low, and there is broad variability in the biologic behavior within each subtype. The lack of a widely accepted classification and staging system hinders recruitment of homogenous trial participants. Single centers lack sufficient cases of GEP-NET subtypes for adequate recruitment. As a result, most studies are retrospective, include heterogeneous tumor types, often lack standardized entry criteria, reflect single-center experience, and are underpowered.[3] Most trials are uncontrolled, and the few controlled trials do not compare the intervention with best supportive care. Furthermore, most studies are funded by pharmaceutical companies with the unavoidable implications inherent therein. Finally, the more indolent GEP-NETs are difficult to assess using traditional measures of efficacy in trial design. The traditional gold standard for therapeutic efficacy in a nonrandomized trial is the objective response rate, but this measure has uncertain utility when the tumor is slow growing and the action of the therapeutic agent is cytostatic. Nonetheless, this compromised dataset has been used to draw the conclusions that follow, based on the somewhat flawed assertion of "it's the best we have."

WELL-DIFFERENTIATED (LOW-GRADE) CARCINOID TUMORS

Only a few carcinoid tumors are completely resectable,[13] meaning that most carcinoid tumors would benefit from systemic antiproliferative therapy if an effective option existed. Disease symptoms related to the secretion of bioactive peptides and amines were a dominant event in the past, when a far greater percentage of advanced NETs were undetected. Now, only approximately 10% to 20% of carcinoid tumors produce the flushing, diarrhea, bronchospasm, and cardiac fibrosis (previously referred to as the carcinoid syndrome). This group benefits from agents that control hypersecretion, namely, the SST analogue class of drugs,[3] or more specific agents that actually interfere with serotonin secretion.[14]

	INTESTINE	PANCREAS
WELL DIFFERENTIATED	CARCINOID SST Analog/ VEGF inhibitor?	WD PET mTOR inhibitor/ Multi TKI/Alkylator
POORLY DIFFERENTIATED	PD NET/PET Platinum drugs and Etoposide	

Fig. 1. A summary of systemic treatment options for Gastroenteropancreatic neuroendocrine tumors (GEP-NETs based on tumor site and degree of differentiation. All therapies for well differentiated GEP-NETs require further investigation. mTOR, mammalian target of rapamycin; PD, poorly differentiated; PET, pancreatic endocrine tumor; SST, somatostatin; TKI, tyrosine kinase inhibitor; VEGF, vascular endothelial growth factor; WD, well differentiated.

SST Analogues

SST analogues such as octreotide and lanreotide effectively control symptoms of carcinoid syndrome in most cases in which the underlying tumor has a low proliferative index, although in some patients the effect tends to wane over time. This effect reflects either an increase in tumor growth or tachyphylaxis and can be temporarily overcome by incremental dose increases of the SST analogue or the addition of interferon. Long acting octreotide (intramuscular formulation), for example, has been used at more than the usual dose range (20–30 mg monthly) without additional toxicity.[15]

SST analogues may also have an antiproliferative effect on GEP-NETs. Endogenous SST has a well-documented inhibitory effect on gastrointestinal cell physiology and an antiproliferative effect on type II and III gastric carcinoids.[16] The PROMID study randomized 85 patients with well-differentiated midgut NETs to receive long acting octreotide (intramuscular formulation) or placebo.[17] Almost all patients (95%) had tumors with a Ki-67 of less than 2% positive cells, and 39% of patients had symptoms of the carcinoid syndrome. The time to progression (TTP) was 6 months in the placebo group compared with 14 months in the group given octreotide LAR. This effect was most marked in the subgroup with low-volume liver metastases (<10% of liver volume), in which TTP was 29 months. This study has been criticized because despite multicenter participation, it was slow to recruit (8 years), had a small sample size, and the intervention and placebo groups were not identical.[18] The intervention group had a significantly longer period between diagnosis and commencing octreotide, raising a concern that the group that received octreotide included more indolent tumors. Furthermore, there was no difference in median overall survival, although all patients in the placebo group were allowed to cross over to octreotide LAR at progression. This study exemplifies the difficulty in conducting NET research, and the authors are left with an appealing but uncertain conclusion that has excited much debate. Although some groups have adopted the PROMID data as providing the basis for a paradigm shift in therapeutic strategy (all NETs should be treated with an effective antiproliferative therapy), significant reservations have been expressed and it seems likely that more data (especially survival improvement) to validate SST as an antiproliferative agent are required before the matter is satisfactorily resolved.

The promising novel SST analogue pasireotide, a pan-receptor SST agonist, has been proposed as possessing the biologic credentials to outperform octreotide and lanreotide. There are 5 types of SST receptors (SSTRs). Pasireotide has a far higher affinity for SSTRs 1, 3, and 5 than octreotide or lanreotide. This broader specificity has been touted to likely provide an antiproliferative advantage. For example, the stimulation of SSTR1 is associated with reduced vascular endothelial growth factor (VEGF) and VEGF receptor (VEGFR) 2 expression, which may prevent tumor growth by reducing effective blood supply to the tumor. Also, receptor subtypes vary between and within tumor types, so a broad receptor subtype affinity might be an advantage. Pasireotide reduced the symptoms of hypersecretion in 27% of patients with carcinoid syndrome resistant to octreotide[19] and inhibited growth in carcinoid cell lines in vitro.[20] To date, no convincing data have been presented to indicate a major advantage for this pan-receptor agonist, and evidence of significant, unresolved issues relating to pasireotide-induced abnormalities in glucose metabolism continues to dominate clinical concerns.[19]

Therapy Targeting Cellular Pathways of Proliferation

NETs exhibit some differences in molecular profile to most other tumors. In contrast to many adenocarcinomas, they seldom express microsatellite instability and mutations in the Ras/Raf/MAP kinase or the transforming growth factor β pathway.[21,22] Molecular profiling of tumors instead shows overexpression of the phosphoinositide-3-kinase-Akt-mammalian target of rapamycin (PI3K-Akt-mTOR) pathway and the insulinlike growth factor 1 receptor.[23–25] Administering a pharmacologic agent that inhibits one or more of these proproliferative proteins provides a rationale for patient- or tumor-specific therapy and has been tested in early-stage clinical trials.

The most successful therapeutic agents for well-differentiated carcinoid tumors have targeted tumor angiogenesis. VEGF and VEGFR seem to be excellent targets based on clinical phenotype and cell line data. Carcinoid tumors are macroscopically vascular as evidenced by enhancement in the arterial phase of computed tomographic scanning, a characteristic often used to diagnose GEP-NETs radiologically. Carcinoid tumors express high levels of VEGF,[26] elevated expression of VEGF correlates with increased angiogenesis and decreased progression-free survival (PFS) among patients with low-grade NETs.[27] Bevacizumab is a monoclonal antibody that binds to VEGF and prevents activation of the VEGFR (**Fig. 2**). Bevacizumab has been evaluated in a phase 2 trial of 44 patients with unresectable or metastatic carcinoid tumors on a stable dose of SST analogue. Patients were randomized to 18 weeks of bevacizumab or pegylated interferon alfa-2b therapy before going on to receive both drugs. The group administered bevacizumab achieved radiologic reduction in tumor vascularity, tumor shrinkage in 18%, and a better 18-week PFS of 95% as compared with 67% in the pegylated interferon alfa-2b group.[28] Because of planned crossover at 18 weeks, no viable overall survival data were generated. Despite the small numbers, this promising finding warrants further investigation.

Two other tyrosine kinase inhibitors (TKIs) (sorafenib and sunitinib) have anti-VEGF or anti-VEGFR properties as part of their targeting arsenal; however, they exhibit only modest in vivo activity in carcinoid tumors. The oral multi-TKI sorafenib inhibits VEGFRs 2 and 3, platelet-derived growth factor receptor (PDGFR) β, RAF, FLT-3, and c-kit. Of 41 patients with carcinoid tumor, 4 had a radiologic response based on the response evaluation criteria in solid tumors (RECIST) and 3 had a smaller non-RECIST response.[29] Of concern is that approximately 40% of patients experienced grade 3 toxicity. Sunitinib is an oral multi-TKI that targets VEGFRs 1, 2, and 3; PDGFR α and β; stem cell factor receptor; glial cell line–derived neurotrophic factor receptor; and FMS-like tyrosine kinase 3 (FLT-3). Forty-one patients with well-differentiated metastatic carcinoid tumor received sunitinib as part of a nonrandomized phase 2 study.[30] Only 1 of 41 patients achieved a radiologic response, so further accrual was abandoned. Tumor differentiation in the participants is not described, although small cell carcinoma was excluded. Sunitinib caused significant adverse events, with more than 50% of patients needing a dose reduction or treatment delay.

Vatalanib, an oral TKI that targets multiple VEGFRs and PDGFRs, did not achieve any radiologic response in 2 small studies, and the drug was moderately toxic.[31,32] Given the failure of the VEGFR inhibitors sunitinib and vatalanib and the relative success of bevacizumab and sorafenib, it seems likely that targeting VEGF is more effective than targeting its receptor, VEGFR, in well-differentiated carcinoid tumors.

Two other drugs with antiangiogenic properties have had a minimal effect on carcinoid tumors. Thalidomide has an antiangiogenic and immune-modulating effect by inhibiting tumor necrosis factor α. No radiologic responses were seen in 18 patients with carcinoid, and grade 3 toxicities were common, with 4 patients stopping treatment because of the toxicity.[33] Endostatin is an endogenous inhibitor of vascular endothelial migration and proliferation. No patients (0/40) achieved a measurable tumor response when given a recombinant version of endostatin.[34] The experience

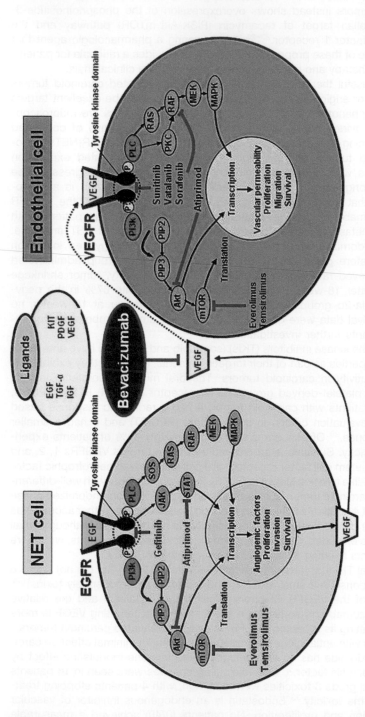

Fig. 2. Overview of the novel therapeutic targets for GEP-NETs. Neuroendocrine tumors are highly angiogenic and depend on endothelial growth factor (EGF)/endothelial growth factor receptor (EGFR) and VEGF/VEGFR activation to initiate and maintain proliferation, survival, and invasion. Intracellular targeting of the mTOR pathway (everolimus, temsirolimus), Akt/STAT (atiprimod), or growth factor receptors (eg, gefitinib or sorafenib) have some therapeutic efficacy in individual tumors. Targeting VEGF with bevacizumab inhibits crosstalk between tumor cells and endothelial cells in the tumor microenvironment. This is a critical relationship in metastatic development. IGF, insulinlike growth factor; JAK, Janus kinase; KIT, stem cell factor receptor; MAPK, mitogen-activated protein kinase; MEK, mitogen activated protein kinase; PDGF, platelet-derived growth factor; PIP, phosphatidylinositol 4,5-bisphosphate; PKC, protein kinase C, PLC, phospholipase C; SOS, son of sevenless protein.

with these 5 drugs represents the practical clinical difficulties encountered when seeking to inhibit a rational biochemical selected target.

Although the PI3K-Akt-mTOR pathway is upregulated in carcinoid cell lines and mammalian target of rapamycin (mTOR) inhibitors reduce proliferation of cell lines,[20] the in vivo response has been disappointing. The intravenous mTOR inhibitor temsirolimus achieved only 5% radiologic response rate in progressive carcinoid tumors in a small phase 2 trial.[35] Similarly, experience with the small molecule endothelial growth factor receptor (EGFR) TKI, gefitinib, is an example of thwarted rational target choice. EGFR is overexpressed in NETs, and EGFR inhibitors reduce growth in carcinoid cell lines.[23] A phase 2 study of gefitinib, including 57 patients with carcinoid tumors, reported that only 1 of 40 evaluable patients achieved a radiologic response, although 32% had a longer period of stability (TTP) than they had experienced before study entry (determined if TTP on study was 4 months longer than TTP before study).[36] This overall poor response might reflect the observation that NETs lack either of the 2 facilitating EGFR tyrosine kinase mutations associated with gefitinib activity in non–small cell lung cancer.[37] Therefore, although EGFR remains a rational target, the current agents might not be able to adequately inhibit the receptor.

Other targeted agents have been disappointing. A trial of the c-kit and PDGFR inhibitor imatinib showed minimal activity in a group of patients with endocrine tumors, including 2 patients with carcinoid and 1 with a pancreatic NET.[38] There were no objective responses in these 3 patients.

Cytotoxic Chemotherapy

A maxim of the medical oncologist is that slow-growing tumors seldom respond to traditional cytotoxic chemotherapy. The clinical determination of slow growth can be quantified using indices of proliferation, such as the number of mitoses per high-power field or the percentage of cells expressing Ki-67. Higher indices of proliferation (Ki-67>20%) are associated with significant but short-lived responses to chemotherapy, whereas very low indices of proliferation (Ki-67<2%) tend to infer resistance to cytotoxic chemotherapy.[10] It is now accepted that there is virtually no role for cytotoxics in well-differentiated carcinoid tumors, and response rates are less than 15%.[5,39,40] Similarly, adjuvant chemotherapy after resection of liver metastases does not reduce the rate of relapse.[41] Former enthusiasm for agents such as streptozotocin, 5-fluorouracil (5-FU), doxorubicin, and cyclophosphamide has abated given their toxicity and limited efficacy. The real advance in cytotoxic chemotherapy is the realization that it has no role in carcinoid tumors with low indices of proliferation. Cytotoxic chemotherapy takes primacy in the aggressive, poorly differentiated carcinoid tumors and is described later.

Summary

Overall, therapy targeting cellular pathways of proliferation has been ineffective for most patients with well-differentiated carcinoid tumors. Radiologic responses were seen in only 2% to 18% of patients in each series. There might be a role in well-differentiated carcinoid tumors for agents that target VEGF directly. Although response rates were low, most drugs had activity in some tumors. The real challenge is to identify and predict which tumors will respond to a specific therapy. For example, although treatment with VEGF inhibitors was successful in a few patients, it is well recognized that the level of VEGF expression is highly variable among different carcinoid tumors.[26] Delineation of specific levels would identify patients likely to be responsive to VEGF inhibition. Similarly, expressions of VEGF and VEGFR are lower in liver metastases than in the primary tumor,[42] suggesting that VEGFR inhibition might be a better strategy when disease is unresectable but not yet metastatic. And finally, if a cytostatic response is achieved in uncontrolled phase 2 trials, the activity of such agents may be undetected by measuring the response rate, unless a randomized controlled trial is undertaken.

WELL-DIFFERENTIATED PANCREATIC NETS

Therapy targeting cellular pathways of proliferation has been more effective in pancreatic NETs than in carcinoid tumors. Pancreatic NETs are a heterogenous group of tumors that includes the functioning tumors insulinoma, gastrinoma, glucagonoma, VIPoma, and rarer cases of pancreatic NETs secreting SST, adrenocorticotrophic hormone, and parathyroid hormone–related hormone.[3] They differ by the type of endocrine cell that undergoes neoplastic transformation; for example, the α, β, and δ cells are progenitors of glucagonoma, insulinoma, and somatostatinoma, respectively. A group of so-called nonfunctioning pancreatic NETs, although biologically indistinguishable, secrete neurotensin, chromogranin A, or several other hormones but do not produce clinically evident symptoms. The symptoms associated with bioactive peptide hypersecretion can be controlled by tumor resection, SST analogues, or occasionally exogenous counterhormones (eg, insulin in glucagonomas). Overall, the SST analogue class of agents, particularly the long-acting moieties (octreotide LAR and lanreotide autogel) have been effective at achieving a reduction in secreted products as measured in plasma.[43] SST analogues have even shown some paradoxic efficacy in somatostatinomas.[44]

Therapy Targeting Cellular Pathways of Proliferation

Inherited diseases that carry a predisposition to pancreatic NETs, such as neurofibromatosis, tuberous sclerosis, and Cowden syndrome, are associated with loss of the tumor suppressor genes NF-1, TSC2, and PTEN, respectively. Because these genes usually act as tumor suppressor genes by inhibiting the PI3K-Akt-mTOR pathway, there is considerable rationale for exploring therapy directed at the Akt/mTOR pathway in pancreatic NETs. Expression profiling of 72 primary pancreatic NETs showed underexpression of PTEN and TSC2.[45] The subsequent overactivity in this pathway results in angiogenesis and tumor cell proliferation. Therefore, inhibiting the downstream protein in this pathway, mTOR, seems to be a rational strategy to control the growth of pancreatic NETs.

Everolimus is an oral mTOR inhibitor and had an antitumor effect in the RADIANT-1 (RAD001 in Advanced Neuroendocrine Tumors) nonrandomized phase 2 trial of patients with well to moderately differentiated metastatic pancreatic NETs.[46] A stratum of patients given single-agent everolimus achieved a radiologic response rate of 10% and a PFS of about 10 months. A stratum of patients already on octreotide when everolimus was started achieved a radiologic response of 17% and a PFS of about 17 months. This might be explained by a synergistic effect of mTOR inhibition and SST analogues, which has been observed in NET cell lines.[20] Alternatively, the patients already on octreotide might have represented a more indolent group.

In contrast to NETs of the gut (carcinoid), the multi-TKI sunitinib has clear activity in pancreatic NETs. Sunitinib achieved a radiologic response of 17% and a TTP of 8 months when given to 66 patients with pancreatic NETs.[30] A subsequent multicenter, randomized, placebo-controlled, double-blind trial in advanced pancreatic NETs using sunitinib resulted in early study cessation because of differences in efficacy after 171 patients had been randomized.[47] Despite a radiologic response rate of only 9%, the median PFS of 11 months in the sunitinib arm was significantly longer than the 6 months in the group that received placebo. This result illustrates the difficulty in phase 2 trial design to detect activity in potentially cytostatic agents, and in this case, the real benefit was evident only when sunitinib was moved to a controlled trial.

The multi-TKI sorafenib also demonstrated some activity against pancreatic NETs. Sorafenib achieved a 10% radiologic response, increasing to 32% if smaller non-RECIST (20%–29% reduction) responses were included.[25] Toxicity was an issue as previously described. The EGFR inhibitor gefitinib may have had even less effect on pancreatic NETs than on gut neuroendocrine (carcinoid) tumors, with only a 6% response rate and 10% achieving a longer TTP than their previous TTP.[36] Atiprimod exhibits an antiangiogenic and proapoptotic effect by deactivating the Akt and STAT3 signaling pathways. The agent was well tolerated and may have stabilized low to intermediate grade neuroendocrine carcinomas in 23 patients in a phase 2 trial.[48]

Cytotoxic Chemotherapy

Well-differentiated advanced pancreatic NETs sometimes respond to cytotoxic chemotherapy; however, radiologic response rates vary widely. For the past 2 decades, the cytotoxic standard of care for well-differentiated pancreatic NETs has been streptozotocin with 5-FU, doxorubicin, or both.[49] Trials without placebo control suggested response rates as high as 69%,[50,51] but subsequent clinical experience failed to substantiate this level of benefit.[52] The studies with positive results did not describe indices of proliferation in their inclusion criteria, and the high response rates may relate to a high proportion of patients with more aggressive tumors. There is now consensus that cytotoxic chemotherapy has moderate utility in pancreatic NETs with higher indices of proliferation (Ki-67 and mitoses per high-power field) more aligned with the WHO grade 2 class of well-differentiated neuroendocrine carcinoma.[53]

The most recent combination of an alkylator and a fluoropyrimidine uses the oral agents temozolomide (oral equivalent of dacarbazine) and capecitabine (the oral equivalent of 5-FU). The oral administration of cytotoxic agents enhances the convenience of drug delivery, especially in the case of a slow-growing tumor in which administration is prolonged. Temozolomide might be effective in combination with capecitabine. In a small retrospective review, 10 of 17 patients achieved a radiologic response (partial response or complete response) despite progression on at least 1 previous line of chemotherapy.[54] It is too early to be certain as to whether this oral combination can supplant the intravenous equivalent, but there is a biologic rationale in support of the increased efficacy of temozolomide as opposed to the intravenous alkylators, dacarbazine and streptozotocin. Temozolomide is more effective in tumors with lower levels of the DNA repair enzyme methylguanine DNA methyltransferase (MGMT), and as a group, pancreatic NETs are often MGMT deficient on immunohistochemical staining.[55]

Combination of Targeted and Cytotoxic Agents

Temozolomide has also been combined with the mTOR inhibitor everolimus in patients with advanced pancreatic NETs.[56] There was a radiologic response in 6 of the 17 (35%) evaluable patients in this phase 1/2 trial. Tolerability was not obviously different when using single cytotoxic agents. Temozolomide has also been combined with thalidomide, with a 45% radiologic response in a small group of pancreatic NETs, but the combination had little activity in patients with gut neuroendocrine (carcinoid) tumors in the same trial.[57–59] Based on current data, it seems that a combination of cytotoxic and targeted agents has synergistic activity in pancreatic NETs.

Summary

The response to targeted agents and cytotoxic chemotherapy exhibited by pancreatic NETs differs from that of gut neuroendocrine (carcinoid) tumors. As a class, pancreatic NETs are more responsive to pharmacotherapy, particularly to mTOR and multi-TKI inhibition. The activity of cytotoxic chemotherapy might be limited to the WHO grade 2 tumors with slightly higher indices of proliferation, and trials of these agents in therapeutic doublets need to carefully describe the proliferative indices of tumors of trial participants.

POORLY DIFFERENTIATED CARCINOMAS

Cytotoxic chemotherapy is the only active therapy for poorly differentiated GEP-NETs (corresponding to WHO grade 3), but chemotherapy rarely achieves prolonged remission. The mainstay of chemotherapy is a platinum agent, for example, cisplatin coupled with the topoisomerase II inhibitor etoposide. Typical response rates range from 42% to 67% but only last for a median of around 6 months.[58,59]

Recent trials of new cytotoxic combinations in high-grade NETs do not seem likely to improve this prognosis. One phase 2 study substituted the topoisiomerase I inhibitor irinotecan in place of etoposide. A similar trial had suggested parity in small cell lung cancer,[60] the equivalent of a poorly differentiated NET in the lung. Noting the danger of intertrial comparisons, the cisplatin-and-irinotecan regimen achieved a radiologic response of 58%, and the median TTP among responders was 6 months.[61] The study was closed early because of slow accrual. A phase 2 study of the oxaliplatin, capecitabine, and bevacizumab regimen commonly used in colorectal cancer was recruiting in 2008 with an early signal of activity, but it is not possible to determine the histologic group from the abstract.[62] There is little role for SST analogues in poorly differentiated tumors because a high percentage of these lesions exhibit diminished SSTR expression with the aggressive phenotype.[63] Nevertheless, if severe symptoms are evident, an SST analogue may have some utility.

SUMMATION

GEP-NETs are heterogeneous tumors, but their pharmacologic treatment is governed by several unifying themes (see **Fig. 1**). SST analogues are effective in ameliorating symptoms, but their role in reducing tumor proliferation of low-grade GEP-NETs is thought by many to lack robust data support. Similarly, although the combinations of SST analogues and kinase inhibitors are biologically appealing, they are unsupported by rigorous long-term data. Novel agents that target proproliferative cellular proteins seem to have some promise in well-differentiated pancreatic NETs, but to date have been disappointing in well-differentiated carcinoid tumors. The newer oral cytotoxics, temozolamide and capecitabine, may prove to be more effective than traditional agents in pancreatic NETs and could conceivably be used in combination with targeted therapies. There have been no recent advances in systemic therapy for poorly differentiated GEP-NETs. All trials continue to be limited by small sample sizes, poor delineation of tumor types and grade, lack of a globally acceptable classification and staging system, and paucity of control group data. Future strategies should focus on not only developing new drugs but also identifying patient- or tumor-specific molecular profiles that provide predictive information necessary to align a targeted agent with a specific tumor in an individual patient.

REFERENCES

1. Hauso O, Gustafsson BI, Kidd M, et al. Neuroendocrine tumor epidemiology: contrasting Norway and North America. Cancer 2008;113(10):2655–64.
2. Yao JC, Hassan M, Phan A, et al. One hundred years after "carcinoid": epidemiology of and prognostic factors for neuroendocrine tumors in 35,825 cases in the United States. J Clin Oncol 2008;26(18):3063–72.
3. Modlin IM, Oberg K, Chung DC, et al. Gastroenteropancreatic neuroendocrine tumors. Lancet Oncol 2008;9:61–72.
4. Modlin IM, Moss SF, Chung DC, et al. Priorities for improving the management of gastroenteropancreatic neuroendocrine tumors. J Natl Cancer Inst 2008;100(18): 1282–9.
5. Eriksson B, Klöppel G, Krenning E, et al. Consensus guidelines for the management of patients with digestive neuroendocrine tumors – well-differentiated jejunal-ileal tumor/carcinoma. Neuroendocrinology 2008;87:8–19.
6. Ramage JK, Davies AHG, Ardill J, et al. Guidelines for the management of gastroenteropancreatic neuroendocrine (including carcinoid) tumours. Gut 2005;54: 1–16.
7. Clark OH, Benson AB 3rd, Berlin JD, et al. NCCN clinical practice guidelines in oncology: neuroendocrine tumors. J Natl Compr Canc Netw 2009;7(7): 712–47.
8. Oberg K, Jelic S, ESMO Guidelines Working Group. Neuroendocrine gastroenteropancreatic tumors: ESMO clinical recommendation for diagnosis, treatment and follow-up. Ann Oncol 2009;20(Suppl 4):150 3.
9. Williams E, Sandler M. The classification of carcinoid tumors. Lancet 1963;1: 238–9.
10. DeLellis RA, Lloyd RV, Heitz PU, et al. World health organization classification of tumors, pathology and genetics of tumors of endocrine organs. Lyon (France): IARC Press; 2004.
11. Rindi G, Kloppel G, Couvelard A, et al. TNM staging of midgut and hindgut (neuro) endocrine tumors: a consensus proposal including a grading system. Virchows Arch 2007;451:757–62.
12. Klimstra DS, Modlin IR, Adsay NV, et al. Pathology reporting of neuroendocrine tumors: application of the Delphic consensus process to the development of a minimum pathology data set. Am J Surg Pathol 2010;34(3):300–13.
13. Modlin IM, Kidd M, Latich I, et al. Current status of gastrointestinal carcinoids. Gastroenterology 2005;128:1717–51.
14. Moertel CG, Kvols LK, Rubin J. A study of cyproheptadine in the treatment of metastatic carcinoid tumor and the malignant carcinoid syndrome. Cancer 1991;67:33–6.
15. Chadha MK, Lombardo J, Mashtare T, et al. High-dose octreotide acetate for management of gastroenteropancreatic neuroendocrine tumors. Anticancer Res 2009;29(10):4127–30.
16. Tomasetti P, Migliori M, Caletti GC, et al. Treatment of type II gastric carcinoid tumors with somatostatin analogues. N Engl J Med 2000;343(8):551–4.
17. Rinke A, Müller HH, Schade-Brittinger C, et al. Placebo-controlled, double-blind, prospective, randomized study on the effect of octreotide LAR in the control of tumor growth in patients with metastatic neuroendocrine midgut tumors: a report from the PROMID study group. J Clin Oncol 2009;27(28):4656–63.
18. Chua YJ, Michael M, Zalcberg JR, et al. Anti-tumor effects of somatostatin analogues in neuroendocrine tumors [letter]. J Clin Oncol 2010;28(3):e41–2.

19. Kvols L, Wiedenmann B, Oberg K, et al. Safety and efficacy of pasireotide (SOM230) in patients with metastatic carcinoid tumors refractory or resistant to octreotide LAR: results of a phase II study. J Clin Oncol 2006;24:198s.

20. Kidd M, Svejda B, Giovinazzo F, et al. Effective inhibition of human neuroendocrine tumor cell proliferation by a TOR kinase inhibitor and a novel somatostatin receptor agonist, pasireotide [abstract: 174]. Proc Am Soc Clin Oncol Gast Intest 2010.

21. Tannapfel A, Vomschloss S, Karhoff D, et al. BRAF gene mutations are rare events in gastroenteropancreatic neuroendocrine tumors. Am J Clin Pathol 2005;123(2): 256–60.

22. Kidd M, Eick G, Shapiro MD, et al. Microsatellite instability and gene mutations in transforming growth factor-beta type II receptor are absent in small bowel carcinoid tumors. Cancer 2005;103(2):229–36.

23. Stilling GA, Zhang H, Ruebel KH, et al. Characterization of the functional and growth properties of cell lines established from ileal and rectal carcinoid tumors. Endocr Pathol 2007;18(4):223–32.

24. Pitt SC, Davis R, Kunnimalaiyaan M, et al. AKT and PTEN expression in human gastrointestinal carcinoid tumors. Am J Transl Res 2009;1(3):291–9.

25. Bowen KA, Silva SR, Johnson JN, et al. An analysis of trends and growth factor receptor expression of GI carcinoid tumors. J Gastrointest Surg 2009 Oct;13(10): 1773–80.

26. Oxboel J, Binderup T, Knigge U, et al. Quantitative gene-expression of the tumor angiogenesis markers vascular endothelial growth factor, integrin alphaV and integrin beta3 in human neuroendocrine tumors. Oncology Reports 2009;21(3): 769–75.

27. Zhang J, Jia Z, Li Q, et al. Elevated expression of vascular endothelial growth factor correlates with increased angiogenesis and decreased progression-free survival among patients with low-grade neuroendocrine tumors. Cancer 2007; 109:1478–86.

28. Yao JC, Ng C, Hoff PM, et al. Improved progression free survival (PFS), and rapid, sustained decrease in tumor perfusion among patients with advanced carcinoid treated with bevacizumab. Proc Am Soc Clin Oncol 2005;23:309.

29. Hobday TJ, Rubin J, Holen K, et al. MC044h, a phase II trial of sorafenib in patients (pts) with metastatic neuroendocrine tumors (NET): a phase II consortium (P2C) study. J Clin Oncol 2007;25(18S):4504.

30. Kulke MH, Lenz H, Meropol NJ, et al. Activity of sunitinib in patients with advanced neuroendocrine tumors. J Clin Oncol 2008;26(20):3403–10.

31. Anthony LB, McCall J, Nunez J, et al. An open-label phase II clinical trial of PTK787 in patients with progressive neuroendocrine cancer. J Clin Oncol 2007;25(18S):14127.

32. Pavel ME, Bartel C, Heuck F, et al. Open-label, non-randomized, multicenter phase II study evaluating the angiogenesis inhibitor PTK787/ZK222584 (PTK/ZK) in patients with advanced neuroendocrine carcinomas (NEC) [abstract: 14684]. J Clin Oncol 2008;26(Suppl).

33. Varker KA, Campbell J, Shah MH. Phase II study of thalidomide in patients with metastatic carcinoid and islet cell tumors. Cancer Chemother Pharmacol 2008; 61(4):661–8.

34. Kulke MH, Bergsland EK, Ryan DP, et al. Phase II study of recombinant human endostatin in patients with advanced neuroendocrine tumors. J Clin Oncol 2006;24(22):3555–61.

35. Duran I, Kortmansky J, Singh D, et al. A phase II clinical and pharmacodynamic study of temsirolimus in advanced neuroendocrine carcinomas. Br J Cancer 2006;95:1148–54.

36. Hobday T, Holen K, Donehower R, et al. A phase II trial of gefitinib in patients (pts) with progressive metastatic neuroendocrine tumors (NET): a phase II consortium (P2C) study. J Clin Oncol 2006;24(18s):189s. ASCO Annual Meeting Proceedings.
37. Gilbert JA, Lloyd RV, Ames MM. Lack of mutations in EGFR in gastroenteropancreatic neuroendocrine tumors. N Engl J Med 2005;353(2):209–10.
38. Gross DJ, Munter G, Bitan M, et al. The role of imatinib mesylate (Glivec) for treatment of patients with malignant endocrine tumors positive for c-kit or PDGF-R. Endocr Relat Cancer 2006;13(2):535–40.
39. Sun W, Lipsitz S, Catalano P, et al. Phase II/III study of doxorubicin with fluorouracil compared with streptozotocin with fluorouracil or dacarbazine in the treatment of advanced carcinoid tumors: eastern cooperative oncology group study E1281. J Clin Oncol 2005;23(22):4897–904.
40. Kulke MH, Wu B, Ryan DP, et al. A phase II trial of irinotecan and cisplatin in patients with metastatic neuroendocrine tumors. Dig Dis Sci 2006;51(6):1033–8.
41. Maire F, Hammel P, Kianmanesh R, et al. Is adjuvant therapy with streptozotocin and 5-fluorouracil useful after resection of liver metastases from digestive endocrine tumors? Surgery 2009;1451:69–75.
42. Besig S, Voland P, Baur DM, et al. Vascular endothelial growth factors, angiogenesis, and survival in human ileal enterochromaffin cell carcinoids. Neuroendocrinology 2009;90(4):402–15.
43. Modlin IM, Pavel M, Kidd M, et al. Review article: somatostatin analogues in the treatment of gastroenteropancreatic neuroendocrine (carcinoid) tumours. Aliment Pharmacol Ther 2010;31(2):169–88.
44. Arnold R, Trautmann ME, Creutzfeld W, et al. Somatostatin analogue octreotide and inhibition of tumor growth in metastatic endocrine gastroenteropancreatic tumors. Gut 1996;38:430–8.
45. Missiaglia E, Dalai I, Barbi S, et al. Pancreatic endocrine tumors: expression profiling evidences a role for AKT-mTOR pathway. J Clin Oncol 2010;28(2):245–55.
46. Yao JC, Lombard-Bohas C, Baudin E, et al. Daily everolimus activity in patients with metastatic pancreatic neuroendocrine tumors after failure of cytotoxic chemotherapy: a phase II trial. J Clin Oncol 2010;281:69–76.
47. Raymond E, Niccoli-Sire P, Bang Y, et al. Updated results of the phase III trial of sunitib (SU) versus placebo (PBO) for treatment of advanced pancreatic neuroendocrine tumors [abstract: 127]. Proc Am Soc Clin Oncol Gast Int 2010.
48. Sung M, Kvois L, Wolin E, et al. Phase II proof-of-concept study of atiprimod in patients with advanced low- to intermediate-grade neuroendocrine carcinoma [abstract: 4611]. J Clin Oncol 2008;26(Suppl).
49. Granberg D. Investigational drugs for neuroendocrine tumors. Expert Opin Investig Drugs 2009;18(5):601–8.
50. Kouvaraki M, Ajani JA, Hoff P, et al. Fluorouracil, doxorubicin, and streptozotocin in the treatment of patients with locally advanced and metastatic pancreatic endocrine carcinomas. J Clin Oncol 2004;22(23):4762–71.
51. Moertel CG, Lefkopoulo M, Lipsitz S, et al. Streptozotocin-doxorubicin, streptozotocin-fluorouracil or chlorozotocin in the treatment of advanced islet-cell carcinoma. N Engl J Med 1992;326(8):519–23.
52. Cheng PN, Saltz LB. Failure to confirm major objective antitumor activity for streptozotocin and doxorubicin in the treatment of patients with advanced islet cell carcinoma. Cancer 1999;86(6):944–8.
53. Ahlman H, Nilsson O, McNicol AM, et al. Poorly differentiated endocrine carcinomas of midgut and hindgut origin. Neuroendocrinology 2008;87:40–6.

54. Isacoff WH, Moss RA, Pecora AL, et al. Temozolomide/capecitabine therapy for metastatic neuroendocrine tumors of the pancreas. A retrospective review. J Clin Oncol 2006;247(18S):14023.

55. Kulke MH, Hornick JL, Frauenhoffer C, et al. O6-methylguanine DNA methyltransferase deficiency and response to temozolomide-based therapy in patients with neuroendocrine tumors. Clin Cancer Res 2009;15(1):338–45.

56. Kulke M, Blaszkowsky LS, Zhu AX, et al. Phase I/II study of everolimus (RAD001) in combination with temozolamide (TMZ) in patients (pts) with advanced pancreatic neuroendocrine tumors (NET) [abstract: 223]. Proc Am Soc Clin Oncol Gast Int 2010.

57. Kulke MH, Stuart K, Enzinger PC, et al. Phase II study of temozolomide and thalidomide in patients with metastatic neuroendocrine tumors. J Clin Oncol 2006;24(3):401–6.

58. Moertel CG, Kvols LK, O'Connell MJ, et al. Treatment of neuroendocrine carcinomas with combined etoposide and cisplatin. Evidence of major therapeutic activity in the anaplastic variants of these neoplasms. Cancer 1991;68(2):227–32.

59. Mitry E, Baudin E, Ducreux M, et al. Treatment of poorly differentiated neuroendocrine tumors with etoposide and cisplatin. Br J Cancer 1999;81(8):1351–5.

60. Lara PN Jr, Natale R, Crowley J, et al. Phase III trial of irinotecan/cisplatin compared with etoposide/cisplatin in extensive-stage small-cell lung cancer: clinical and pharmacogenomic results from SWOG S0124. J Clin Oncol 2009;27(15): 2530–5.

61. Mani MA, Shroff RT, Jacobs C, et al. A phase II study of irinotecan and cisplatin for metastatic or unresectable high grade neuroendocrine carcinoma [abstract: 15550]. J Clin Oncol 2008;26(Suppl).

62. Kunz PL, Kuo T, Kaiser HL, et al. A phase II study of capecitabine, oxaliplatin, and bevacizumab for metastatic or unresectable neuroendocrine tumors: preliminary results [abstract: 15502]. J Clin Oncol 2008;26(Suppl).

63. Reubi JC, Kvols LK, Waser B, et al. Detection of somatostatin receptors in surgical and percutaneous needle biopsy samples of carcinoids and islet cell carcinomas. Cancer Res 1990;50(18):5969–77.

The Gastrointestinal Complications of Oncologic Therapy

Mehnaz A. Shafi, MD, Robert S. Bresalier, MD*

KEYWORDS

- Drug-induced diarrhea • Neutropenic enterocolitis
- Graft-versus-host disease
- Chemotherapy-induced nausea and vomiting • Liver injury

A spectrum of oncologic treatments including chemotherapy, radiotherapy, and molecular targeted therapies is available to combat cancer. These treatments are associated with adverse effects in several organ systems including the gastrointestinal (GI) tract. Any part of the GI tract can be affected including the upper GI tract (esophagitis due to bacterial, viral, and fungal infections; mucositis due to chemotherapy or radiation; GI bleeding; nausea and vomiting), colon (diarrhea, graft-vs-host disease [GVHD], and constipation), liver (drug toxicity and GVHD), and pancreas (pancreatitis). Adverse effects range from mild to life threatening. The primary goal of cancer treatment is to administer the most effective therapy while minimizing potential toxicity. This review discusses common GI complications that can result from cancer therapy. The pathologic mechanisms underlying each complication and the pharmacology of the agents used to treat these complications are discussed.

ESOPHAGITIS

Esophagitis in patients with cancer may be caused either by the direct cytotoxic effects of chemotherapy or radiation or by the infections caused by immunosuppressive effects of cancer therapy (**Table 1**).[1] Treatment with chemotherapy or radiotherapy destroys rapidly dividing cells, such as those in the epithelial cell layer. Cell death decreases the renewal rate of the basal epithelium, causing mucosal atrophy, ulceration, and initiation of the inflammatory response. Synergy between chemotherapy and radiotherapy may increase the severity and extent of esophagitis

Financial disclosure: The authors have nothing to disclose.
Department of Gastroenterology, Hepatology and Nutrition, The University of Texas, MD Anderson Cancer Center, Houston, TX 77030-4009, USA
* Corresponding author. Department of Gastroenterology, Hepatology and Nutrition, The University of Texas, MD Anderson Cancer Center, Unit 1466, Houston, TX 77030-4009.
E-mail address: rbresali@mdanderson.org

Gastroenterol Clin N Am 39 (2010) 629–647
doi:10.1016/j.gtc.2010.08.004
0889-8553/10/$ – see front matter © 2010 Published by Elsevier Inc.

Table 1
Common causes of esophagitis in patients receiving oncologic therapy

Infectious Agent or Injury	Endoscopic Appearance	Treatment
Candida albicans	White plaquelike lesions with surrounding erythema on the esophageal mucosa	Systemic antifungal treatment with fluconazole, itraconazole, voriconazole, or echinocandins)
Herpes Simplex Virus	Small vesicles, coalescing to form ulcers	Acyclovir, foscarnet sodium
Cytomegalovirus	Linear or serpiginous ulcers	Ganciclovir, foscarnet sodium
Varicella-Zoster Virus	Small vesicles, similar to herpes simplex virus ulcers	Intravenous acyclovir
Polymicrobial Oral Flora	Bacteria mixed with necrotic epithelial cells in biopsy samples	Broad-spectrum antibiotics
Radiation Injury	Friable mucosa with erythema and edema	Lidocaine hydrochloride, proton pump inhibitors, endoscopic dilation, or stents

Data from Davila M, Bresalier RS. Gastrointestinal complications of oncologic therapy. Nat Clin Pract Gastroenterol Hepatol 2008;5(12):682–96.

observed with combined therapy.[2] Esophagitis may also be caused by pill-induced injury, acid reflux disease, and GVHD in hematopoietic stem cell transplant recipients.

Fungal Infections

Esophageal candidiasis is common in immunocompromised patients, with *Candida albicans* being the most frequent causative organism for esophageal and oropharyngeal candidiasis (OPC). Patients complain of odynophagia and/or dysphagia. On endoscopy, esophageal candidiasis is identified by white plaquelike lesions with surrounding erythema. Esophageal biopsies or brushings may confirm the presence of invasive yeast or hyphal forms of *C albicans*.

An empirical course of antifungal therapy is recommended in immunocompromised patients with odynophagia or dysphagia. Endoscopy should be performed if symptoms do not improve within 72 hours.[3] The general duration of antifungal treatment is 14 to 21 days. Candida esophagitis in immunocompromised patients requires systemic antifungal therapy and cannot be treated with topical agents.[4] Patients unable to tolerate oral agents require intravenous therapy.

The treatment of esophageal candidiasis includes agents such as azoles, echinocandins, or amphotericin B. Azoles inhibit cell membrane formation by inhibiting the synthesis of ergosterol, a principal component of fungal cell membranes.[5] Fluconazole is the recommended first line agent because of its efficacy, ease of administration, and low cost.[4] For patients with fluconazole-refractory esophageal candidiasis who can tolerate oral therapy, newer azoles (voriconazole and posaconazole) are available **(Table 2)**.[6,7] Itraconazole has been found to be as effective as fluconazole for the treatment of esophageal candidiasis, however, its use is limited by significant nausea and the potential for drug interactions because of the inhibition of cytochrome P-450.[8,9]

Patients requiring intravenous therapy should be treated with one of the echinocandins (caspofungin, micafungin, or anidulafungin), rather than amphotericin B, because of their better toxicity profiles.[10,11] Echinocandins inhibit synthesis of $\beta(1,3)$-D-glucan,

Table 2
Treatment of mucocutaneous candidiasis

	First Line Therapy	Alternative Therapy	Comments
Oropharyngeal Candidiasis	Clotrimazole troches; nystatin suspension or fluconazole	Itraconazole solution; or posaconazole or voriconazole or AmB-d oral suspension; IV echinocandin or AmB-d	Fluconazole is recommended for moderate to severe disease, and topical therapy with clotrimazole or nystatin is recommended for mild disease. Uncomplicated disease is treated for 7–14 d. For refractory disease, itraconazole, voriconazole, posaconazole, or AmB-d suspension is recommended
Esophageal Candidiasis	Fluconazole an echinocandin; or AmB-d	Itraconazole oral solution; or posaconazole or voriconazole	Oral fluconazole is preferred. For patients unable to tolerate an oral agent, IV fluconazole, an echinocandin, or AmB-d is appropriate. Treatment is for 14–21 d. For patients with refractory disease, the alternative therapy as listed or AmB-d or an echinocandin is recommended

Abbreviations: Amb-d, amphotericin B deoxycholate; IV, intravenous.

Data from Pappas PG, Kauffman CA, Andes D, et al. Clinical practice guidelines for the management of candidiasis: 2009 update by the Infectious Diseases Society of America. Clin Infect Dis 2009;48(5):503–35.

an essential component of the fungal cell wall. Mammalian cells do not require β(1,3)-D-glucan, thereby limiting potential toxicity.[10] Relapse rates are higher with echinocandins when compared with azoles, and echinocandins are used as second line therapeutic agents if treatment with azoles has failed. Amphotericin B is reserved for esophageal candidiasis during pregnancy and in patients with drug-resistant candidiasis.

OPC is a local infection. Risk factors include radiation, chemotherapy, antibiotics, and corticosteroids. Treatment is with local agents such as nystatin or clotrimazole.

Prophylaxis

Patients at risk of developing OPC may be given antifungal prophylaxis with topical antifungals, such as clotrimazole or miconazole.[4]

Viral Infections

Viral infections of the esophagus are caused by herpes simplex virus (HSV), cytomegalovirus (CMV), and uncommonly by, varicella-zoster virus (VZV). Diagnosis can be established by endoscopic biopsy.[3,12] In advanced stages, all 3 viruses may cause small mucosal ulcerations. Biopsies taken from the edge of an HSV-related ulcer show intranuclear inclusions and multinucleated giant cells. Inclusions can also be detected by immunohistochemistry, using monoclonal antibodies to HSV. Biopsies of CMV lesions show intranuclear inclusions in fibroblasts and endothelial cells.

For patients with HSV esophagitis, acyclovir (400 mg orally 5 times daily for 14–21 days or 5 mg/kg intravenously every 8 hours for 7–14 days) is the therapeutic agent of choice. Acyclovir resistance in HSV results from mutations in the thymidine kinase (TK) gene of HSV.[13] Viruses with TK mutations are generally cross-resistant to valacyclovir but remain susceptible to drugs that act directly on DNA polymerase, such as foscarnet.[14] Cases of severe persistent infection with acyclovir-resistant HSV occur almost exclusively in immunocompromised patients. Famciclovir or valacyclovir can be considered in patients able to tolerate oral therapy, although there is limited clinical experience with these drugs in the treatment of HSV-associated esophagitis.

VZV esophagitis is initially treated with intravenous acyclovir because these patients usually have disseminated infection. After clinical improvement, treatment may be changed to an oral agent as used for HSV esophagitis.

CMV esophagitis is treated with intravenous ganciclovir (5 mg/kg twice daily) or foscarnet sodium (90 mg/kg twice daily) for 3 to 6 weeks.[15,16] The role of maintenance treatment after the clearance of infection is not well defined. Valganciclovir is an oral precursor of ganciclovir. Although valganciclovir has been approved for treatment of CMV retinitis in patients with AIDS and is used for prophylaxis against CMV infection in solid-organ transplant recipients, its role in CMV GI disease has not been studied. At a dose of 900 mg daily, valganciclovir produces systemic drug exposure equivalent to 5 mg/kg of intravenous ganciclovir.[15]

Bacterial Infections

Bacterial esophagitis can occur in immunocompromised patients and is usually polymicrobial, derived from oral flora.[3] Diagnosis is made by endoscopic biopsies that demonstrate the presence of bacterial clusters mixed with necrotic epithelial cells. Treatment with broad-spectrum antibiotics is usually successful.

Radiation-Induced Esophagitis

Radiation-induced esophagitis can occur during external beam radiotherapy of lung, head and neck, and esophageal cancers. Acute radiation esophagitis is primarily caused by injury to the rapidly dividing cells of the basal epithelial layer, with subsequent thinning and denudation of esophageal mucosa. The severity of esophagitis depends on radiation dose and is exacerbated by concurrent use of chemotherapeutic agents such as cisplatin. Patients complain of odynophagia, dysphagia, and chest pain. Endoscopic findings include erythema, edema friable mucosa, ulcerations, or strictures.

Treatment includes use of local anesthetics such as viscous lidocaine hydrochloride and systemic narcotic analgesics and acid suppression with proton pump inhibitors and H_2 receptor antagonists. Esophageal strictures are treated by endoscopic dilation and refractory strictures may require placement of plastic stents. In patients with tracheoesophageal fistula due to esophageal cancer, self-expanding metal or plastic stents are the treatment of choice and they can achieve fistula closure in 70% to 100% of patients.[17]

DIARRHEA

Diarrhea is associated with several chemotherapeutic agents, particularly fluoropyrimidines such as 5-fluorouracil (5-FU) and capecitabine; irinotecan; and abdominal or pelvic radiotherapy. Other causes include small-molecule therapy, monoclonal antibodies, neutropenic enterocolitis, and *Clostridium difficile* infection (CDI).

Chemotherapy-Induced Diarrhea

Both 5-FU and irinotecan cause acute damage to intestinal mucosal epithelium leading to clinically significant diarrhea.[18] The severity of chemotherapy-induced diarrhea is determined by the frequency and volume of stool output. Diarrhea is reported in up to 50% of patients receiving weekly 5-FU/leucovorin combined treatment. It tends to be worse in patients receiving irinotecan hydrochloride, 5-FU, and leucovorin than in those receiving 5-FU and leucovorin without irinotecan.[19] Other factors that can increase the risk of 5-FU–induced diarrhea include female sex, the presence of an unresected primary tumor, and previous chemotherapy-induced diarrhea.[20]

Irinotecan can cause early-onset diarrhea, which is mediated via cholinergic receptors, and can be effectively treated with atropine and loperamide hydrochloride. In contrast, late-onset diarrhea associated with irinotecan hydrochloride is unpredictable and occurs at all doses. It is seen less frequently when irinotecan is given every 3 weeks rather than weekly. Diarrhea also occurs frequently with regimens that combine 5-FU, leucovorin, and oxaliplatin.[21]

Diarrhea commonly occurs in patients receiving small-molecule epidermal growth factor receptor–tyrosine kinase inhibitors. Grade 1 to 2 diarrhea, as defined by the National Cancer Institute's common toxicity criteria, has been reported in up to 56% of patients receiving erlotinib.[22] Another small-molecule inhibitor, sorafenib, is associated with diarrhea in approximately 34% of patients.[23]

Radiation-Induced Diarrhea

Radiotherapy causes injury to the GI mucosa. Pelvic or abdominal radiotherapy can lead to acute enteritis, characterized by abdominal cramping and diarrhea in approximately 50% of patients. These symptoms are made worse by concomitant chemotherapy.[24] Symptoms typically occur during the third week of fractionated radiotherapy.

Treatment of Chemotherapy- and Radiation-Induced Diarrhea

In 1998, Wadler and colleagues[25] published guidelines on the treatment of chemotherapy-induced diarrhea. These guidelines were revised by an expert panel in

2004.[26] The panel stressed the need for close monitoring of patients receiving a combination of irinotecan, 5-FU, and leucovorin and other intensive combination regimens, including weekly assessment of GI toxicity, particularly for older patients.

Opioid agonists are the cornerstone of therapy for chemotherapy-induced diarrhea. Loperamide and diphenoxylate are both widely used and are approved by the US Food and Drug Administration (FDA) for this indication; loperamide is more effective. For mild to moderate diarrhea, an initial dose of 4 mg of loperamide hydrochloride may be given, followed by a further 2-mg dose every 4 hours or after every stool discharge. Severe diarrhea often requires a more aggressive regimen, with an initial dose of 4 mg of loperamide hydrochloride followed by a further 2-mg dose every 2 hours or 4-mg dose every 4 hours until the patient is diarrhea-free for 12 hours.[26,27]

This high-dose loperamide has been used effectively for the control of irinotecan-induced diarrhea. Octreotide, a synthetic long-acting somatostatin analogue, has been used as a second line therapeutic agent in opioid-resistant patients. It decreases the secretion of vasoactive intestinal peptide, prolongs intestinal transit time, and reduces secretion of intestinal fluid and electrolytes. The recommended initial dose of octreotide is 100 to 150 mcg given subcutaneously 3 times daily or 25 to 50 mcg/h every hour if given as an intravenous infusion. Sucralfate, a nonsystemic aluminum hydroxide complex, has been studied for control of radiotherapy-induced diarrhea and mucosal injury, with only limited, if any, benefit. In fact, sucralfate may aggravate GI symptoms such as rectal bleeding.[28]

Other drugs used as adjunctive therapeutic agents in chemotherapy- or radiation-induced diarrhea include absorbents such as kaolin and charcoal, deodorized tincture of opium, paregoric, and codeine phosphate. **Fig. 1** shows an algorithm for the management of chemotherapy-induced diarrhea.

Optimal dose of octreotide
Octreotide can be titrated to higher doses (500–2500 mcg 3 times daily) for the treatment of those who do not respond to lower doses.[29] Early studies of octreotide for chemotherapy-induced diarrhea investigated subcutaneous doses ranging from 50 to 100 μg twice or thrice daily.[26] Recent data suggest that higher doses may be more effective. Goumas and colleagues[30] compared 100-μg octreotide with 500 μg administered 3 times a day in 59 patients with grade 3 or higher grade of chemotherapy-induced diarrhea who failed to respond to loperamide (4 mg 3 times a day) for at least 48 hours. Treatment with 500-μg octreotide was significantly more effective than with 100 μg (90% vs 61% of patients had complete resolution of diarrhea; $P<.05$), and both doses were well tolerated, suggesting that 500-μg octreotide given 3 times a day may be more effective than lower doses in patients who fail to respond to loperamide.

Role of prophylactic antidiarrheal therapy
Because of the well-recognized risk of diarrhea associated with irinotecan, recent studies have investigated prophylactic regimens for chemotherapy-induced diarrhea. Long-acting slow-release formulations of octreotide long acting release (octreotide LAR) can be administered by an intramuscular injection once a month. Once steady state has been achieved, administration of a 20-mg intramuscular dose of octreotide LAR every 4 weeks produces the same pharmacologic effects as 150-μg octreotide given thrice a day by subcutaneous injection[31] and dramatically reduces fluctuations in peak and trough octreotide concentrations. Octreotide LAR, at a starting dose of 20 mg, effectively controls diarrhea associated with carcinoid syndrome,[31] and monthly doses of 20 to 30 mg of octreotide LAR are currently being investigated for the treatment and prevention of chemotherapy-induced diarrhea.

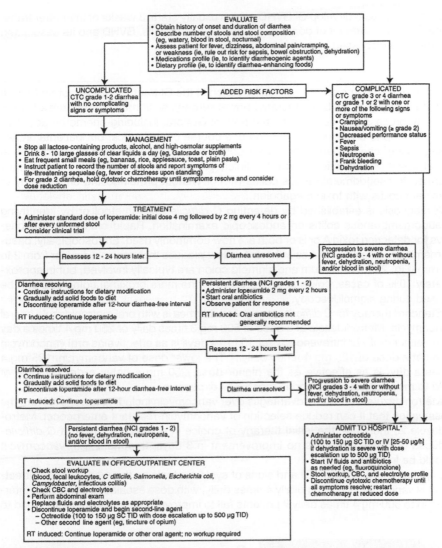

EVALUATE
- Obtain history of onset and duration of diarrhea
- Describe number of stools and stool composition (eg, watery, blood in stool, nocturnal)
- Assess patient for fever, dizziness, abdominal pain/cramping, or weakness (ie, rule out risk for sepsis, bowel obstruction, dehydration)
- Medications profile (ie, to identify diarrheogenic agents)
- Dietary profile (ie, to identify diarrhea-enhancing foods)

UNCOMPLICATED
CTC grade 1-2 diarrhea with no complicating signs or symptoms

ADDED RISK FACTORS

COMPLICATED
CTC grade 3 or 4 diarrhea or grade 1 or 2 with one or more of the following signs or symptoms
- Cramping
- Nausea/vomiting (≥ grade 2)
- Decreased performance status
- Fever
- Sepsis
- Neutropenia
- Frank bleeding
- Dehydration

MANAGEMENT
- Stop all lactose-containing products, alcohol, and high-osmolar supplements
- Drink 8 - 10 large glasses of clear liquids a day (eg, Gatorade or broth)
- Eat frequent small meals (eg, bananas, rice, applesauce, toast, plain pasta)
- Instruct patient to record the number of stools and report symptoms of life-threatening sequelae (eg, fever or dizziness upon standing)
- For grade 2 diarrhea, hold cytotoxic chemotherapy until symptoms resolve and consider dose reduction

TREATMENT
- Administer standard dose of loperamide: initial dose 4 mg followed by 2 mg every 4 hours or after every unformed stool
- Consider clinical trial

Reassess 12 - 24 hours later

Diarrhea unresolved

Progression to severe diarrhea (NCI grades 3 - 4 with or without fever, dehydration, neutropenia, and/or blood in stool)

Diarrhea resolving
- Continue instructions for dietary modification
- Gradually add solid foods to diet
- Discontinue loperamide after 12-hour diarrhea-free interval

RT induced: Continue loperamide

Persistent diarrhea (NCI grades 1 - 2)
- Administer loperamide 2 mg every 2 hours
- Start oral antibiotics
- Observe patient for response

RT induced: Oral antibiotics not generally recommended

Reassess 12 - 24 hours later

Diarrhea unresolved

Progression to severe diarrhea (NCI grades 3 - 4 with or without fever, dehydration, neutropenia, and/or blood in stool)

Diarrhea resolved
- Continue instructions for dietary modification
- Gradually add solid foods to diet
- Discontinue loperamide after 12-hour diarrhea-free interval

RT induced: Continue loperamide

Persistent diarrhea (NCI grades 1 - 2) (no fever, dehydration, neutropenia, and/or blood in stool)

EVALUATE IN OFFICE/OUTPATIENT CENTER
- Check stool workup (blood, fecal leukocytes, C difficile, Salmonella, Escherichia coli, Campylobacter, infectious colitis)
- Check CBC and electrolytes
- Perform abdominal exam
- Replace fluids and electrolytes as appropriate
- Discontinue loperamide and begin second-line agent
  – Octreotide (100 to 150 μg SC TID with dose escalation up to 500 μg TID)
  – Other second line agent (eg, tincture of opium)

RT induced: Continue loperamide or other oral agent; no workup required

ADMIT TO HOSPITAL*
- Administer octreotide (100 to 150 μg SC TID or IV [25-50 μg/h] if dehydration is severe with dose escalation up to 500 μg TID)
- Start IV fluids and antibiotics as needed (eg, fluoroquinolone)
- Stool workup, CBC, and electrolyte profile
- Discontinue cytotoxic chemotherapy until all symptoms resolve; restart chemotherapy at reduced dose

Fig. 1. Assessment and management of diarrhea complicating chemotherapy. Abbreviations: CBC, complete blood count; CTC, common toxicity criteria; IV, intravenous; NCI, National Cancer Institute; RT, radiotherapy; SC, subcutaneous. (*From* Benson AB 3rd, Ajani JA, Catalano RB, et al. Recommended guidelines for the treatment of cancer treatment-induced diarrhea. J Clin Oncol 2004;22:2918–26; with permission.)

Stem Cell Transplantation–Associated Diarrhea

Patients undergoing stem cell transplantation (SCT) can suffer from diarrhea caused by the conditioning regimen consisting of high-dose chemotherapy or radiotherapy, GVHD of the GI tract, or infection related to immunosuppressive therapy. Pretransplant conditioning regimens (including total body irradiation and/or combination chemotherapy) can injure the intestinal mucosa, as discussed earlier, causing secretory diarrhea that resolves after mucosal restitution. Transplant recipients of allogeneic stem cells can also develop GI GVHD, which usually starts 3 weeks or later after transplant, after engraftment of donor hematopoietic stem cells. GVHD and its associated diarrhea are discussed in a separate section later.

CDI

CDI is the most common nosocomial infection of the GI tract.[32,33] Risk factors for CDI include a history of antibiotic therapy, bowel surgery, an immunocompromised state, and any process that suppresses the normal GI flora, including chemotherapy. CDI can occur up to 8 weeks after the end of a course of antibiotics, but patients undergoing cancer chemotherapy are predisposed to *C difficile*-induced diarrhea even in the absence of antibiotic therapy.[34] Clinical presentation of CDI can vary from mild diarrhea to pseudomembranous colitis with or without protein-losing enteropathy to fulminant colitis with toxic megacolon.

A diagnosis is established by detecting *C difficile* toxin in stool or by identifying pseudomembranous colitis on endoscopic examination. Rapid enzyme immunoassays for detecting toxin A or B or both are now commonly used. Endoscopically, pseudomembranes can be seen as adherent yellow plaques that vary in diameter from 2 to 10 mm (**Fig. 2**).[32] The rectum and sigmoid colon are typically involved, but in approximately 10% of cases, colitis is only present in the more proximal colon and can be missed during sigmoidoscopy.

Standard therapy for *C difficile*-associated diarrhea is with oral metronidazole or oral vancomycin. Metronidazole at a dose of 500 mg 3 times daily or 250 mg 4 times a day given either orally or intravenously for 10 to 14 days is as effective as oral vancomycin given at a dose of 125 mg 4 times daily.[35] The lower dose of vancomycin, 125 mg 4 times a day, is as effective as the higher dose, 250 mg 4 times a day, in case of mild to moderate diarrhea and is much less expensive.

Metronidazole has some advantages over vancomycin including lower cost and the observation that it can reduce selection of vancomycin-resistant enterococci. Metronidazole is, therefore, the initial therapy of choice in nonsevere cases of *C difficile*-induced diarrhea. If there is no improvement in 3 days, treatment with vancomycin should be initiated.

In patients with severe CDI and signs of systemic toxicity, the recommended treatment is vancomycin 125 mg orally 4 times daily, with dose escalation at 48-hour intervals up to 500 mg 4 times daily if patients fail to improve. If patients do not respond to

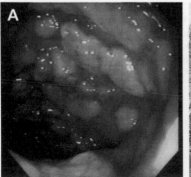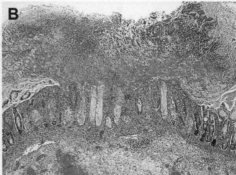

Fig. 2. Pseudomembranous colitis. (*A*) Plaquelike pseudomembranes adherent to the colonic mucosa observed endoscopically. (*B*) Typical lesion with luminal inflammatory exudates (hematoxylin-eosin).

oral vancomycin, the addition of intravenous metronidazole 500 mg every 8 hours or vancomycin retention enemas (0.5–1 g vancomycin dissolved in 1–2 L of normal saline every 4–12 hours) should be considered.[36]

The use of antidiarrheal agents is not recommended because the decreased transit time can lead to complications and lengthen the duration of illness.

Relapse of CDI is common, occurring in up to 10% to 25% of all patients with CDI. Relapses usually occur within 1 to 3 weeks after ending initial therapy and are probably caused by failure to eradicate the organism rather than by antibiotic resistance.[32] These patients are likely to relapse repeatedly. First relapses should be treated with a second 10- to 14-day course of oral metronidazole or vancomycin. If a patient relapses after taking a second course of antibiotics, different approaches have been suggested including tapered or pulsed antibiotic therapy, longer duration of treatment (several weeks), and the use of toxin-binding resins such as cholestyramine or colestipol hydrochloride alone or in combination with vancomycin.[37] In a small series, 2 weeks of vancomycin administration followed by 2 weeks of rifaximin administration has proved successful in controlling recurrent disease.[38] A recent study used 2 neutralizing human monoclonal antibodies against *C difficile* toxins A and B (CDA1 and CDB1, respectively) in 101 symptomatic patients, who were receiving either metronidazole or vancomycin. The rate of recurrence was significantly lower among patients treated with the monoclonal antibodies.[39]

NEUTROPENIC ENTEROCOLITIS

Neutropenic enterocolitis is characterized by fever and right lower quadrant pain in neutropenic patients. It is seen in children and adults with hematologic malignancies, with aplastic anemia, and after myelosuppressive therapy for solid malignancies.[40] In a systematic review of 145 published articles, a 5.3% pooled incidence was reported in adults hospitalized for the treatment of hematologic malignancies, aplastic anemia, or solid tumors.[33]

Histologic examination of biopsy samples from patients with neutropenic enterocolitis is characterized by a thickened bowel wall, edema, mucosal ulcerations, focal hemorrhage, and mucosal or transmural necrosis. Numerous bacterial and/or fungal species have been identified in surgical specimens and peritoneal fluid from patients with neutropenic enterocolitis.[41] The diagnosis is usually established by computed tomography, when findings include a fluid-filled and dilated cecum, a right lower quadrant inflammatory mass, and pericecal fluid or inflammatory changes in the pericecal soft tissues.[41]

Treatment consists of bowel rest, intravenous fluids and broad-spectrum antibiotics. Cytopenia and coagulopathy associated with oncologic treatment should be treated, because neutropenia contributes to the pathogenesis of the disease and coagulopathy can be associated with blood loss from mucosal hemorrhage. Recombinant granulocyte colony-stimulating factor may hasten leukocyte recovery, which contributes to the resolution of neutropenic enterocolitis.[42] Surgery has been recommended for patients with persistent GI bleeding, despite treatment of cytopenia and coagulopathy, and for patients with perforation or clinical deterioration, despite pharmacologic therapy.[43]

GVHD

GVHD is classified as either acute or chronic based on the time of disease onset after allogeneic SCT. Acute GVHD generally occurs within the first 100 days of SCT, whereas chronic GVHD generally occurs more than 100 days after allogeneic SCT.

This classification is somewhat arbitrary because a continuum of clinical findings can be observed in patients with acute or chronic GVHD. Acute GVHD results from donor T lymphocytes recognizing and mounting an immune response against minor antigens present on the recipient cells.

Acute GVHD

The incidence of acute GVHD varies from 10% to 50% in patients undergoing allogeneic SCT from an HLA antigen–identical sibling or unrelated donor. The most common sites of involvement include skin, GI tract, and liver. Involvement of the GI tract is characterized by profuse watery diarrhea and abdominal cramping. The diarrhea can frequently become bloody.[44] Less commonly, patients may also present with upper GI symptoms, such as nausea, vomiting, and anorexia. Factors that increase the risk of developing GVHD include histoincompatibility, advanced age of the donor and/or recipient, sex mismatch, the use of peripheral stem cells rather than bone marrow stem cells, greater intensity of the conditioning regimen, and suboptimal prophylactic therapy with immunosuppressants.

The most consistent histologic feature of acute GVHD is the presence of apoptotic bodies,[45] although this feature is not specific to acute GVHD.

Use of methylprednisolone, 2 mg/kg, is the first line treatment of acute GVHD. Complete response can be seen in about 50% of patients. Those not responding to this dose by 5 days improve with higher dose of steroids (10 mg/kg). A durable response from steroid therapy occurs in only 25% to 40% of patients. Oral beclomethasone with prednisone may show a better response in treating GI GVHD. Steroid-refractory acute GVHD is usually defined as progression of GVHD in the first 72 hours of steroid therapy or a lack of improvement after 3 to 7 days of steroid therapy.

Steroid-refractory patients may require additional immunosuppressive agents, including mycophenolate mofetil, antithymocyte globulin (ATG; Thymoglobulin), or infliximab. ATG has been commonly used as an initial salvage therapy in steroid-refractory acute GVHD, even though its effect on patient survival is limited. McCaul and colleagues[46] studied ATG in patients with steroid-refractory acute GVHD. Antithymocyte globulin, 2.5 mg/kg/d, was given intravenously for 4 to 6 days or on days 1, 3, 5, and 7. Of 36 patients, 2 withdrew from the study due to adverse reactions (hypoxemia and hypotension) and 34 were evaluated. Response rates were highest in patients with skin involvement (96%) and lowest in those with liver involvement (36%). The most common adverse events were infections (82%), leucopenia (25%), hepatic dysfunction (25%), posttransplant lymphoproliferative disease, and infusion-related reactions (19%). Only 2 patients (6%) were alive at 15 months. Cyclophosphamide is an alkylating agent that exhibits potent immunosuppressant activities and is effective in acute GVHD of the skin and liver, but response to cyclophosphamide has been poor in those with advanced GI tract involvement. Mycophenolate mofetil is a fungus-derived antibiotic that exhibits immunosuppressant activities. A 60% response rate to mycophenolate therapy is reported in patients with acute GVHD. Infliximab is a chimeric monoclonal antibody that binds to tumor necrosis factor α (TNF-α), thereby interfering with endogenous TNF-α activity. A multicenter retrospective study evaluated the efficacy of infliximab in patients with steroid-refractory acute GVHD.[47] The overall response rate was 59%, with a favorable outcome in younger (<35 years) male patients with GI involvement.

Chronic GVHD

Chronic GVHD is seen in up to 50% of patients after sibling or unrelated-donor SCT, generally occurring more than 100 days after transplantation.[48] The pathogenesis of chronic GVHD involves immunodysregulation, resulting from both autoimmune and alloimmune reactions. It may only affect skin or mucosal surface (mucocutaneous chronic GVHD) or visceral organs, such as liver or lungs. Chronic GI GVHD primarily affects the upper GI tract and may present as dry mouth or oral ulcers. Esophageal involvement may lead to formation of painful esophageal ulcers, webs, rings, and strictures. The small bowel and colon are less frequently involved. Patients present with diarrhea, malabsorption, submucosal fibrosis, and sclerosis of the intestine.[49]

The liver is commonly involved in acute and chronic GVHD. Pathologic examination reveals extensive bile duct damage with bile duct atypia and degeneration, epithelial cell dropout, and lymphocytic infiltration of small bile ducts leading to cholestasis.[50]

Initial therapy for chronic GVHD includes administration of corticosteroids at a dose of 1 mg/kg/d unless contraindicated by a comorbid disease. Infection is the primary cause of death. Patient education, infection prophylaxis, and supportive care are important components of chronic GVHD management.[51] Symptomatic relief rather than resolution of chronic GVHD can provide great benefits by improving patients' functional status and quality of life.

RADIATION PROCTITIS

Patients receiving radiation for the treatment of gynecologic, genitourinary, GI, and other malignancies are at risk of developing acute or chronic intestinal injury. Acute radiation injury in the rectum and distal colon usually occurs within 6 weeks of therapy and is characterized by diarrhea, rectal urgency, tenesmus, and, occasionally, rectal bleeding. These symptoms usually resolve within 6 months without the need for therapy.[52]

Chronic radiation proctitis or coloproctitis has a delayed onset, occurring approximately 1 year or later after exposure to radiation. It is caused by obliterative endarteritis and chronic mucosal ischemia, resulting in epithelial atrophy and fibrosis. It may end in stricture formation and bleeding within the colon and rectum. Patients with radiation proctitis often present with diarrhea, bleeding, tenesmus, urgency, difficulties with defecation, and less commonly, fecal incontinence.

The diagnosis of radiation proctitis is made by colonoscopy or sigmoidoscopy when mucosal edema, erythema, friability, and telangiectasias may be seen. In severe cases, mucosal ulcerations and strictures can be observed.[28]

Treatment of radiation proctitis depends on symptoms. Sucralfate is largely ineffective and according to some studies, may increase the risk of rectal bleeding.[28] Other treatments that have shown some benefit in small clinical trials include hyperbaric oxygen[53] and short-chain fatty acid enemas.[54]

Various thermal endoscopic interventions have also been used successfully to treat bleeding associated with radiation proctitis, including argon plasma coagulation, argon and Nd:YAG lasers, bipolar electrocoagulation, and heater probes.[55,56] Surgery should be considered in patients with intractable symptoms such as strictures, pain, or bleeding.[57] The selection of treatment of radiation proctitis should be based on the type and severity of symptoms as well as local expertise.

CONSTIPATION

Constipation is a common problem in patients undergoing cancer treatment and is usually caused by a combination of poor oral intake, decreased physical activity, and drugs such as opioid analgesics or antiemetic agents including ondansetron. These agents slow intestinal transit time. Constipation has also been reported in patients taking vinca alkaloids, in particular vincristine and thalidomide.[58]

Impaction, bowel obstruction, and colonic pseudo-obstruction must be ruled out before starting therapy for constipation, which should be anticipated in the patient with cancer, and general steps should be taken to avoid this complication. Electrolyte abnormalities and other reversible causes of constipation should be treated. Drugs that cause constipation should be discontinued if possible. Laxatives, with or without stool softeners, can be used initially, including stimulant laxatives, such as bisacodyl and senna, which alter electrolyte transport by the intestinal mucosa and increase intestinal motor activity. If these laxatives are not effective, osmotic agents such as lactulose or sorbitol can be effective at improving stool frequency and consistency. Polyethylene glycol solutions are available in powder form and improve chronic constipation. Drugs to improve colonic transit have been disappointing. Metoclopramide is ineffective, and tegaserod (a 5-hydroxytryptamine receptor agonist) has significant cardiovascular adverse effects. Tegaserod is still available in the United States under an emergency investigational new drug protocol from the FDA. It is contraindicated in women older than 55 years and has not been studied well in men and therefore, its availability and clinical application are limited.

Lubiprostone, a chloride channel activator, is FDA approved for the treatment of chronic idiopathic constipation. It is a bicyclic acid that works locally on the apical aspect of the intestinal epithelial cell and increases fluid secretion and intestinal motility. It may be useful in patients with opioid- and chemotherapy-induced constipation.

In April 2008, the US FDA granted approval to methylnaltrexone, the first peripheral micro-opioid–receptor antagonist for the treatment of opioid-induced constipation in advanced-illness patients. Methylnaltrexone, a derivative of naltrexone, selectively antagonizes the peripheral microreceptors in the GI tract without central effects. Subcutaneous methylnaltrexone reversed opioid-induced constipation after the first dose in approximately 50% to 60% of the patients.[59] In most of the cases, the benefit was seen within an hour. Methylnaltrexone does not affect opioid analgesic effects or induce opioid symptoms.

DRUG-INDUCED HEPATOTOXICITY

Patients undergoing chemotherapy require careful assessment of liver function both before and during therapy. If liver function test results are abnormal, the cause must be defined promptly. In addition to drug reactions, there are multiple possible causes of abnormal liver function test results in patients undergoing chemotherapy, including tumor progression, infection, or the presence of coexisting hepatic disease.

Hepatitis

Patients with a preexisting liver disease can be more susceptible to drug-induced hepatotoxicity. Chemotherapy (including the use of monoclonal antibodies) can reactivate hepatitis B virus (HBV) and associated diseases,[60,61] and risk factors include HBV surface antigen and HBV envelope antigen seropositivity, detectable HBV DNA before chemotherapy, male sex, diagnosis of lymphoma or breast cancer, and use of steroids.[62,63]

Prophylactic treatment with lamivudine seems to be beneficial in preventing HBV reactivation or reducing the severity of HBV-related diseases in patients on cytotoxic chemotherapy.[64] For short-term prophylaxis (<6 months), lamivudine is a reasonable choice because the risk of lamivudine resistance is extremely low. If treatment is required for more than 6 months, the use of either adefovir dipivoxil or entecavir instead of lamivudine is recommended.[65]

The relationship between chemotherapy and hepatitis C virus (HCV) reactivation is less clear. It seems that HCV infection increases the risk of abnormal liver function tests[66]; however, severe flares of clinical hepatitis are extremely rare.

Idiosyncratic Hepatotoxicities

Most hepatotoxic drug reactions are idiosyncratic and caused by hypersensitivity mechanisms or host metabolic idiosyncrasy.[67] Treatment is largely supportive by monitoring liver function and discontinuation of the drug.

Alkylating agents

Alkylating agents are not commonly associated with hepatotoxicity, and with the exception of cyclophosphamide and ifosfamide, patients receiving alkylating agents generally do not require any dose reduction. Cyclophosphamide is rarely hepatotoxic, probably due to an idiosyncratic reaction, if it occurs. On rare occasions, diffuse hepatocellular destruction and massive hepatic necrosis have been described with cyclophosphamide.[68] Other alkylating agents, including melphalan, chlorambucil, nitrogen mustards, and busulfan, do not depend on the liver for metabolism and are not frequently associated with hepatotoxicity.

Antimetabolites

The antimetabolites include cytarabine, 5-FU, 6-mercaptopurine (6-MP), azathioprine, 6-thioguanine, and methotrexate. Hepatic metabolism is important in the processing of these drugs, and dose reductions are usually necessary in patients developing liver dysfunction.

Cytarabine is used for the treatment of acute myelogenous leukemia and has rarely been associated with cholestasis, which seems reversible. There are rare reports of hepatotoxicity with intravenous 5-FU; however, hepatotoxicity is more common when 5-FU is administered in combination with ascaricides.[69] Intra-arterial administration of the 5-FU metabolite floxuridine (fluorodeoxyuridine) has been associated with 2 types of toxicity one is suggestive of hepatocellular injury and the other consistent with sclerosing cholangitis.[70] 6-MP is often used in the maintenance therapy for acute lymphoblastic leukemia, and 2 patterns of toxicity have been reported: hepatocellular injury and cholestasis. Hepatotoxicity caused by 6-MP occurs more commonly when a daily dose of 2 mg/kg is exceeded. Toxicity with azathioprine, a nitroimidazole derivative of 6-MP, is less common and less dose dependent than with 6-MP. High-dose methotrexate has been associated with reversible elevation in levels of aminotransferases.[71] Patients taking long-term low-dose methotrexate therapy are at risk of developing hepatic fibrosis and cirrhosis; however, the risk is low in patients who receive less than 1.5 g of methotrexate as a cumulative dose.

Antitumor antibiotics

The antitumor antibiotics, which include doxorubicin hydrochloride and daunorubicin, can cause hepatocellular injury and steatosis. With doxorubicin, dose reduction has been recommended in patients with cholestasis to avoid further toxicity.[72] Similar guidelines are recommended for daunorubicin.

Neoadjuvant regimens

Combinations of 5-FU and oxaliplatin or irinotecan hydrochloride are used as agents of neoadjuvant therapy in patients with colorectal cancer, before resection of liver metastases. These regimens have been associated with steatosis, hepatic vascular injury, and nodular regenerative hyperplasia.[73] Venoocclusive disease has also been seen with many chemotherapeutic agents including dacarbazine, 6-MP,[74] cyclophosphamide, and busulfan.[75]

OTHER COMPLICATIONS
Nausea and Vomiting

Nausea and vomiting frequently occur after administration of chemotherapeutic agents. The likelihood of developing nausea and vomiting after chemotherapy depends on several factors including the dose and the intrinsic emetogenicity of a given agent.[76] The emetogenic potential of intravenously administered antineoplastic agents is assigned to 5 levels, ranging from minimal or less than 10% risk (eg, bevacizumab) to high or greater than 90% risk (eg, cisplatin). Emesis can be acute (occurring within the first 24 hours) or delayed.

Various antiemetic agents are now available for the prevention and treatment of chemotherapy-induced nausea and vomiting. These agents include drugs with a high therapeutic index such as 5-hydroxytryptamine 3 receptor antagonists (eg, ondansetron, granisetron, dolasetron, tropisetron, palonosetron), neurokinin 1 receptor antagonists (eg, aprepitant), and corticosteroids (usually used in combination with other agents). Agents with a low therapeutic index are also used, such as metoclopramide hydrochloride, butyrophenones, phenothiazines, cannabinoids, and olanzapine. The preferred agent and regimen depend on the emetogenic level of a given chemotherapeutic drug. For drugs with a low emetogenic risk, antiemetics are given only before chemotherapy, whereas for drugs with a high emetogenic risk (level 3 or higher), antiemetics are provided before and after chemotherapy.

GI Perforation, Fistula Formation, Arterial Thrombosis, and Bleeding

GI perforation, fistula formation, arterial thrombosis, and bleeding have been reported with bevacizumab, a monoclonal antibody against vascular endothelial growth factor,[77] with perforation reported in 1% to 2% of patients treated for metastatic colorectal cancer.[78] Risk for perforation includes an intact primary tumor, prior irradiation, acute diverticulitis, intra-abdominal abscess, and GI obstruction.

Acute Pancreatitis

Acute pancreatitis in patients with cancer or in those who have undergone hematopoietic SCT can be caused by conditions present in the general population, including gallstones and alcohol consumption. However, other causes should be considered when managing patients with cancer with acute pancreatitis, including medications and chemotherapeutic agents.

Drug-induced pancreatitis has no distinguishing features, and therefore taking a careful drug history and excluding other causes are essential to diagnosis. Drugs known to cause acute pancreatitis include metronidazole, sulfonamides, tetracycline, furosemide, thiazides, estrogen, and tamoxifen.[79] During chemotherapy, pancreatitis has been reported with azathioprine, prednisone, cytosine arabinoside, and various regimens of combination chemotherapy, including vinca alkaloids, methotrexate, mitomycin, 5-FU, cyclophosphamide, cisplatin, and bleomycin.[80]

Oral Mucositis or Ulceration of the Oropharynx

Oral mucositis occurs frequently in patients undergoing radiotherapy and chemotherapy for solid malignancies and in up to 98% of those undergoing hematopoietic SCT.[81] Palifermin, a recombinant human keratinocyte growth factor, decreases the incidence and duration of mucositis in patients with hematologic malignancies, who are receiving chemotherapy and requiring the support of SCT. Use of palifermin is approved by the FDA for this indication. Results from phase I and II trials in patients receiving chemotherapy for solid tumors are also encouraging.[81]

SUMMARY

Cancer therapy can frequently cause a host of adverse GI events. Chemotherapy and radiotherapy have increased in complexity, with greater therapeutic effectiveness achieved from combination therapies. These therapies often result in more severe complications, including esophagitis, diarrhea, and drug-induced hepatotoxicity, which reduce quality of life and can be life threatening. The immunocompromised state induced by oncologic therapy is also an important contributing factor underlying GI complications.

The gastroenterologist has an important role in managing the GI complications associated with various cancer treatments. A growing number of pharmacologic agents designed to address the pathophysiology of complications related to oncologic therapies are becoming available. These agents are leading to a mechanism-based approach to treating these often life-threatening situations.

REFERENCES

1. Benson CA, Kaplan JE, Masur H, et al. Treating opportunistic infections among HIV-infected adults and adolescents: recommendations from CDC, the National Institutes of Health, and the HIV Medicine Association/Infectious Diseases Society of America. MMWR Recomm Rep 2004;53(RR-15):1–112.
2. Choy H, LaPorte K, Knill-Selby E, et al. Esophagitis in combined modality therapy for locally advanced non-small cell lung cancer. Semin Radiat Oncol 1999;9(2 Suppl 1):90–6.
3. McDonald GB, Sharma P, Hackman RC, et al. Esophageal infections in immunosuppressed patients after marrow transplantation. Gastroenterology 1985; 88(5 Pt 1):1111–7.
4. Pappas PG, Kauffman CA, Andes D, et al. Clinical practice guidelines for the management of candidiasis: 2009 update by the Infectious Diseases Society of America. Clin Infect Dis 2009;48(5):503–35.
5. Kaplan JE, Benson C, Holmes KH, et al. Guidelines for prevention and treatment of opportunistic infections in HIV-infected adults and adolescents: recommendations from CDC, the National Institutes of Health, and the HIV Medicine Association of the Infectious Diseases Society of America. MMWR Recomm Rep 2009; 58(RR-4):1–207, quiz CE201–4.
6. Hegener P, Troke PF, Fatkenheuer G, et al. Treatment of fluconazole-resistant candidiasis with voriconazole in patients with AIDS. AIDS 1998;12(16):2227–8.
7. Skiest DJ, Vazquez JA, Anstead GM, et al. Posaconazole for the treatment of azole-refractory oropharyngeal and esophageal candidiasis in subjects with HIV infection. Clin Infect Dis 2007;44(4):607–14.
8. Ally R, Schurmann D, Kreisel W, et al. A randomized, double-blind, double-dummy, multicenter trial of voriconazole and fluconazole in the treatment of esophageal candidiasis in immunocompromised patients. Clin Infect Dis 2001; 33(9):1447–54.
9. Wilcox CM, Darouiche RO, Laine L, et al. A randomized, double-blind comparison of itraconazole oral solution and fluconazole tablets in the treatment of esophageal candidiasis. J Infect Dis 1997;176(1):227–32.

10. Villanueva A, Arathoon EG, Gotuzzo E, et al. A randomized double-blind study of caspofungin versus amphotericin for the treatment of candidal esophagitis. Clin Infect Dis 2001;33(9):1529–35.

11. Villanueva A, Gotuzzo E, Arathoon EG, et al. A randomized double-blind study of caspofungin versus fluconazole for the treatment of esophageal candidiasis. Am J Med 2002;113(4):294–9.

12. Reed EC, Wolford JL, Kopecky KJ, et al. Ganciclovir for the treatment of cytomegalovirus gastroenteritis in bone marrow transplant patients. A randomized, placebo-controlled trial. Ann Intern Med 1990;112(7):505–10.

13. Frobert E, Ooka T, Cortay JC, et al. Herpes simplex virus thymidine kinase mutations associated with resistance to acyclovir: a site-directed mutagenesis study. Antimicrob Agents Chemother 2005;49(3):1055–9.

14. Malvy D, Treilhaud M, Bouee S, et al. A retrospective, case-control study of acyclovir resistance in herpes simplex virus. Clin Infect Dis 2005;41(3):320–6.

15. Biron KK. Antiviral drugs for cytomegalovirus diseases. Antiviral Res 2006; 71(2–3):154–63.

16. Blanshard C, Benhamou Y, Dohin E, et al. Treatment of AIDS-associated gastrointestinal cytomegalovirus infection with foscarnet and ganciclovir: a randomized comparison. J Infect Dis 1995;172(3):622–8.

17. Raijman I, Siddique I, Ajani J, et al. Palliation of malignant dysphagia and fistulae with coated expandable metal stents: experience with 101 patients. Gastrointest Endosc 1998;48(2):172–9.

18. Benson AB 3rd, Schrag D, Somerfield MR, et al. American Society of Clinical Oncology recommendations on adjuvant chemotherapy for stage II colon cancer. J Clin Oncol 2004;22(16):3408–19.

19. Sargent DJ, Niedzwiecki D, O'Connell MJ, et al. Recommendation for caution with irinotecan, fluorouracil, and leucovorin for colorectal cancer. N Engl J Med 2001; 345(2):144–5 [author reply: 146].

20. Sloan JA, Goldberg RM, Sargent DJ, et al. Women experience greater toxicity with fluorouracil-based chemotherapy for colorectal cancer. J Clin Oncol 2002; 20(6):1491–8.

21. Kuebler JP, Wieand HS, O'Connell MJ, et al. Oxaliplatin combined with weekly bolus fluorouracil and leucovorin as surgical adjuvant chemotherapy for stage II and III colon cancer: results from NSABP C-07. J Clin Oncol 2007;25(16): 2198–204.

22. Perez-Soler R, Chachoua A, Hammond LA, et al. Determinants of tumor response and survival with erlotinib in patients with non–small-cell lung cancer. J Clin Oncol 2004;22(16):3238–47.

23. Strumberg D, Clark JW, Awada A, et al. Safety, pharmacokinetics, and preliminary antitumor activity of sorafenib: a review of four phase I trials in patients with advanced refractory solid tumors. Oncologist 2007;12(4):426–37.

24. Miller RC, Martenson JA, Sargent DJ, et al. Acute treatment-related diarrhea during postoperative adjuvant therapy for high-risk rectal carcinoma. Int J Radiat Oncol Biol Phys 1998;41(3):593–8.

25. Wadler S, Benson AB 3rd, Engelking C, et al. Recommended guidelines for the treatment of chemotherapy-induced diarrhea. J Clin Oncol 1998;16(9): 3169–78.

26. Benson AB 3rd, Ajani JA, Catalano RB, et al. Recommended guidelines for the treatment of cancer treatment-induced diarrhea. J Clin Oncol 2004;22(14): 2918–26.

27. Abigerges D, Armand JP, Chabot GG, et al. Irinotecan (CPT-11) high-dose escalation using intensive high-dose loperamide to control diarrhea. J Natl Cancer Inst 1994;86(6):446–9.

28. Kneebone A, Mameghan H, Bolin T, et al. The effect of oral sucralfate on the acute proctitis associated with prostate radiotherapy: a double-blind, randomized trial. Int J Radiat Oncol Biol Phys 2001;51(3):628–35.

29. Barbounis V, Koumakis G, Vassilomanolakis M, et al. Control of irinotecan-induced diarrhea by octreotide after loperamide failure. Support Care Cancer 2001;9(4):258–60.

30. Goumas P, Naxakis S, Christopoulou A, et al. Octreotide acetate in the treatment of fluorouracil-induced diarrhea. Oncologist 1998;3(1):50–3.

31. Rubin J, Ajani J, Schirmer W, et al. Octreotide acetate long-acting formulation versus open-label subcutaneous octreotide acetate in malignant carcinoid syndrome. J Clin Oncol 1999;17(2):600–6.

32. Kelly CP, Pothoulakis C, LaMont JT. Clostridium difficile colitis. N Engl J Med 1994;330(4):257–62.

33. Gorschluter M, Mey U, Strehl J, et al. Neutropenic enterocolitis in adults: systematic analysis of evidence quality. Eur J Haematol 2005;75(1):1–13.

34. Anand A, Glatt AE. Clostridium difficile infection associated with antineoplastic chemotherapy: a review. Clin Infect Dis 1993;17(1):109–13.

35. Bartlett JG. Clinical practice. Antibiotic-associated diarrhea. N Engl J Med 2002; 346(5):334–9.

36. Apisarnthanarak A, Razavi B, Mundy LM. Adjunctive intracolonic vancomycin for severe Clostridium difficile colitis: case series and review of the literature. Clin Infect Dis 2002;35(6):690–6.

37. Tedesco FJ, Gordon D, Fortson WC. Approach to patients with multiple relapses of antibiotic-associated pseudomembranous colitis. Am J Gastroenterol 1985; 80(11):867–8.

38. Johnson S, Schriever C, Galang M, et al. Interruption of recurrent Clostridium difficile-associated diarrhea episodes by serial therapy with vancomycin and rifaximin. Clin Infect Dis 2007;44(6):846–8.

39. Lowy I, Molrine DC, Leav BA, et al. Treatment with monoclonal antibodies against Clostridium difficile toxins. N Engl J Med 2010;362(3):197–205.

40. Urbach DR, Rotstein OD. Typhlitis. Can J Surg 1999;42(6):415–9.

41. Sloas MM, Flynn PM, Kaste SC, et al. Typhlitis in children with cancer: a 30-year experience. Clin Infect Dis 1993;17(3):484–90.

42. Kouroussis C, Samonis G, Androulakis N, et al. Successful conservative treatment of neutropenic enterocolitis complicating taxane-based chemotherapy: a report of five cases. Am J Clin Oncol 2000;23(3):309–13.

43. Wade DS, Nava HR, Douglass HO Jr. Neutropenic enterocolitis. Clinical diagnosis and treatment. Cancer 1992;69(1):17–23.

44. Schwartz JM, Wolford JL, Thornquist MD, et al. Severe gastrointestinal bleeding after hematopoietic cell transplantation, 1987–1997: incidence, causes, and outcome. Am J Gastroenterol 2001;96(2):385–93.

45. Snover DC, Weisdorf SA, Vercellotti GM, et al. A histopathologic study of gastric and small intestinal graft-versus-host disease following allogeneic bone marrow transplantation. Hum Pathol 1985;16(4):387–92.

46. McCaul KG, Nevill TJ, Barnett MJ, et al. Treatment of steroid-resistant acute graft-versus-host disease with rabbit antithymocyte globulin. J Hematother Stem Cell Res 2000;9(3):367–74.

47. Patriarca F, Sperotto A, Damiani D, et al. Infliximab treatment for steroid-refractory acute graft-versus-host disease. Haematologica 2004;89(11):1352–9.
48. Carlens S, Ringden O, Remberger M, et al. Risk factors for chronic graft-versus-host disease after bone marrow transplantation: a retrospective single centre analysis. Bone Marrow Transplant 1998;22(8):755–61.
49. Akpek G, Chinratanalab W, Lee LA, et al. Gastrointestinal involvement in chronic graft-versus-host disease: a clinicopathologic study. Biol Blood Marrow Transplant 2003;9(1):46–51.
50. Shulman HM, Sharma P, Amos D, et al. A coded histologic study of hepatic graft-versus-host disease after human bone marrow transplantation. Hepatology 1988; 8(3):463–70.
51. Couriel D, Carpenter PA, Cutler C, et al. Ancillary therapy and supportive care of chronic graft-versus-host disease: national institutes of health consensus development project on criteria for clinical trials in chronic Graft-versus-host disease: V. Ancillary Therapy and Supportive Care Working Group Report. Biol Blood Marrow Transplant 2006;12(4):375–96.
52. Babb RR. Radiation proctitis: a review. Am J Gastroenterol 1996;91(7):1309–11.
53. Mayer R, Klemen H, Quehenberger F, et al. Hyperbaric oxygen–an effective tool to treat radiation morbidity in prostate cancer. Radiother Oncol 2001;61(2): 151–6.
54. al-Sabbagh R, Sinicrope FA, Sellin JH, et al. Evaluation of short-chain fatty acid enemas: treatment of radiation proctitis. Am J Gastroenterol 1996;91(9):1814–6.
55. Fantin AC, Binek J, Suter WR, et al. Argon beam coagulation for treatment of symptomatic radiation-induced proctitis. Gastrointest Endosc 1999;49(4 Pt 1): 515–8.
56. Taieb S, Rolachon A, Cenni JC, et al. Effective use of argon plasma coagulation in the treatment of severe radiation proctitis. Dis Colon Rectum 2001;44(12): 1766–71.
57. Lucarotti ME, Mountford RA, Bartolo DC. Surgical management of intestinal radiation injury. Dis Colon Rectum 1991;34(10):865–9.
58. Singhal S, Mehta J, Desikan R, et al. Antitumor activity of thalidomide in refractory multiple myeloma. N Engl J Med 1999;341(21):1565–71.
59. Portenoy RK, Thomas J, Moehl Boatwright ML, et al. Subcutaneous methylnaltrexone for the treatment of opioid-induced constipation in patients with advanced illness: a double-blind, randomized, parallel group, dose-ranging study. J Pain Symptom Manage 2008;35(5):458–68.
60. Liang R, Lau GK, Kwong YL. Chemotherapy and bone marrow transplantation for cancer patients who are also chronic hepatitis B carriers: a review of the problem. J Clin Oncol 1999;17(1):394–8.
61. Aksoy S, Harputluoglu H, Kilickap S, et al. Rituximab-related viral infections in lymphoma patients. Leuk Lymphoma 2007;48(7):1307–12.
62. Yeo W, Chan PK, Zhong S, et al. Frequency of hepatitis B virus reactivation in cancer patients undergoing cytotoxic chemotherapy: a prospective study of 626 patients with identification of risk factors. J Med Virol 2000;62(3):299–307.
63. Yeo W, Zee B, Zhong S, et al. Comprehensive analysis of risk factors associating with hepatitis B virus (HBV) reactivation in cancer patients undergoing cytotoxic chemotherapy. Br J Cancer 2004;90(7):1306–11.
64. Yeo W, Chan PK, Ho WM, et al. Lamivudine for the prevention of hepatitis B virus reactivation in hepatitis B s-antigen seropositive cancer patients undergoing cytotoxic chemotherapy. J Clin Oncol 2004;22(5):927–34.

65. Keeffe EB, Dieterich DT, Han SH, et al. A treatment algorithm for the management of chronic hepatitis B virus infection in the United States: an update. Clin Gastroenterol Hepatol 2006;4(8):936–62.
66. Kawatani T, Suou T, Tajima F, et al. Incidence of hepatitis virus infection and severe liver dysfunction in patients receiving chemotherapy for hematologic malignancies. Eur J Haematol 2001;67(1):45–50.
67. Lee WM. Drug-induced hepatotoxicity. N Engl J Med 1995;333(17):1118–27.
68. Goldberg JW, Lidsky MD. Cyclophosphamide-associated hepatotoxicity. South Med J 1985;78(2):222–3.
69. Moertel CG, Fleming TR, Macdonald JS, et al. Hepatic toxicity associated with fluorouracil plus levamisole adjuvant therapy. J Clin Oncol 1993;11(12):2386–90.
70. Kemeny N, Daly J, Reichman B, et al. Intrahepatic or systemic infusion of fluorodeoxyuridine in patients with liver metastases from colorectal carcinoma. A randomized trial. Ann Intern Med 1987;107(4):459–65.
71. Berkowitz RS, Goldstein DP, Bernstein MR. Ten year's experience with methotrexate and folinic acid as primary therapy for gestational trophoblastic disease. Gynecol Oncol 1986;23(1):111–8.
72. Johnson PJ, Dobbs N, Kalayci C, et al. Clinical efficacy and toxicity of standard dose adriamycin in hyperbilirubinaemic patients with hepatocellular carcinoma: relation to liver tests and pharmacokinetic parameters. Br J Cancer 1992;65(5): 751–5.
73. Vauthey JN, Pawlik TM, Ribero D, et al. Chemotherapy regimen predicts steatohepatitis and an increase in 90-day mortality after surgery for hepatic colorectal metastases. J Clin Oncol 2006;24(13):2065–72.
74. Stoneham S, Lennard L, Coen P, et al. Veno-occlusive disease in patients receiving thiopurines during maintenance therapy for childhood acute lymphoblastic leukaemia. Br J Haematol 2003;123(1):100–2.
75. Vassal G, Hartmann O, Benhamou E. Busulfan and veno-occlusive disease of the liver. Ann Intern Med 1990;112(11):881.
76. Hesketh PJ. Chemotherapy-induced nausea and vomiting. N Engl J Med 2008; 358(23):2482–94.
77. Gordon MS, Cunningham D. Managing patients treated with bevacizumab combination therapy. Oncology. 2005;69(Suppl 3):25–33.
78. Badgwell BD, Camp ER, Feig B, et al. Management of bevacizumab-associated bowel perforation: a case series and review of the literature. Ann Oncol 2008; 19(3):577–82.
79. Runzi M, Layer P. Drug-associated pancreatitis: facts and fiction. Pancreas 1996; 13(1):100–9.
80. Davila M, Bresalier RS. Gastrointestinal complications of oncologic therapy. Nat Clin Pract Gastroenterol Hepatol 2008;5(12):682–96.
81. Beaven AW, Shea TC. The effect of palifermin on chemotherapy and radiation therapy-induced mucositis: a review of the current literature. Support Cancer Ther 2007;4(4):188–97.

Pharmacokinetics and Pharmacodynamics of Peginterferon and Ribavirin: Implications for Clinical Efficacy in the Treatment of Chronic Hepatitis C

Mazen Noureddin, MD, Marc G. Ghany, MD, MHSc*

KEYWORDS

- Pharmacokinetics • Pharmacodynamics
- Peginterferon alfa-2a • Peginterferon alfa-2b • Ribavirin
- Chronic hepatitis C

More than 3.2 million people in the United States and more than 200 million people worldwide are chronically infected with hepatitis C virus (HCV) and are at risk for the development of cirrhosis, decompensated liver disease, and hepatocellular carcinoma.[1] The efficacy of therapy for chronic hepatitis C has improved from 10% to 20% with regimens using standard interferon-alfa monotherapy[2–4] to 54% to 56% with regimens using peginterferon in combination with ribavirin.[5–7] Thus, the current standard of treatment of chronic hepatitis C is the combination of a peginterferon with ribavirin administered for 24 or 48 weeks, depending on the HCV genotype.[8] Two pegylated interferons are approved for the treatment of chronic hepatitis C: peginterferon alfa-2a and peginterferon alfa-2b. These compounds differ in size and the type of pegylation, resulting in different pharmacokinetics and pharmacodynamics. This article focuses on how the different properties of these compounds affect their in vivo performance and clinical efficacy.

Financial Support: This work was supported by the intramural program of the National Institute of Diabetes and Digestive and Kidney Diseases, National Institutes of Health.
Liver Diseases Branch, National Institute of Diabetes and Digestive and Kidney Diseases, National Institutes of Health, Building 10, Room 9B-16, 10 Center Drive, MSC 1800, Bethesda, MD 20892-1800, USA
* Corresponding author.
E-mail address: marcg@intra.niddk.nih.gov

FORMULATION OF PEGINTERFERON ALFA-2A AND PEGINTERFERON ALFA-2B

Pegylation is the process of covalent attachment of polyethylene glycol (PEG) polymer chains to another molecule, normally a drug or therapeutic protein. In general, pegylation results in improved pharmacokinetic and pharmacodynamic properties, increased drug stability, overall half-life and changes in tissue distribution pattern and elimination pathways.[9] Molecular weight, configuration (llnear or branched), and means of attachment of the PEG moiety are the primary contributors to the physicochemical properties of the PEG-peptide conjugate. Attachment of PEG at multiple sites can lead to steric interference between the compound and its receptor, which reduces the biologic activity of the conjugate.[9] Pegylated interferon alfa-2a consists of a 40-kDa branched PEG moiety covalently attached to an interferon alfa-2a molecule.[10] Pegylated interferon alfa-2b consists of a 12-kDa linear PEG molecule covalently attached to an interferon alfa-2b molecule.[11] The branched PEG formulation has many advantages compared with the linear one. Although the 2 PEG molecules are of the same molecular mass, the branched PEG molecule acts as if it were much larger than the corresponding linear molecule. In addition, the branched-chain PEG conjugates have greater thermal and pH stability, are more resistant to proteolytic degradation, and are less antigenic because of the shielding of the attached polypeptide from the immune system.[9] Key differences in the formulation of peginterferon alfa-2a and peginterferon alfa-2b are summarized in **Table 1**.

PHARMACOKINETICS OF PEGINTERFERON

The difference in pegylation between the 2 peginterferons has a significant effect on their pharmacokinetic properties. Peginterferon alfa-2b has a relatively rapid

Table 1
Comparison of the formulation of peginterferon alfa-2b and peginterferon alfa-2a

Characteristic	Peginterferon Alfa-2b	Peginterferon Alfa-2a
PEG Structure	Small, linear, 12-kDa mPEG	Two 20-kDa mPEG chains, linked to form a large, branched, 40-kDa mPEG
PEG Conjugation	mPEG activated with succinimidyl carbonate, resulting in potential reactions with several amino acids	mPEG activated with N-hydroxysuccinimide, which attaches to Lys residues
Positional Isomers	13	6
Protein Bond	Major positional isomer (12-kDa PEG attached to His) has a hydrolytically unstable urethane (carbonyl) bond	Stable amide bond between mPEG and Lys residues on protein chain
Monopegylation (%)	95	95
Stability	Stored as a powder; must be reconstituted immediately before injection	Stored as a solution, which is stable for at least 2 y

Abbreviation: mPEG, methoxy polyethylene glycol.

absorption rate, with a half-life of 4.6 hours and a volume of distribution of 0.99 L/kg, which are not significantly different from those of standard interferon alfa-2b (2.3 hours and approximately 1.4 L/kg, respectively).[11] Maximum serum concentrations are achieved between 15 and 44 hours postdosing and are maintained for 48 to 72 hours, with a peak to trough ratio of greater than 10 after multiple doses.[11] However, mean apparent clearance for pegylated interferon alfa-2b (22 mL/h/kg) is approximately one-tenth of that of nonpegylated interferon alfa-2b (231 mL/h/kg).[11] Thus, the observed increase in the clinical efficacy of peginterferon alfa-2b is principally the result of reduced renal clearance rather than of the effects of pegylation on the rate of absorption or distribution.

Peginterferon alfa-2a is absorbed more slowly than peginterferon alfa-2b and has a restricted volume of distribution (confined largely to the vasculature and liver). In healthy volunteers, a single dose of 180 μg of peginterferon alfa-2a produced a mean maximum serum concentration of 14.2 μg/L in a mean time of 78 hours.[12] After administration of multiple doses of peginterferon alfa-2a (180 μg weekly) to patients with chronic hepatitis C, the mean maximum serum concentration was 25.6 μg/L in a mean time of 45 hours.[12] Peginterferon alfa-2a has a lower peak to trough ratio (1.5:2) than peginterferon alfa-2b, indicating less fluctuation in the serum concentration of the drug during the 1-week dosing interval. Peginterferon alfa-2a is cleared by both the kidney and the liver. Because of its relatively large size, peginterferon alfa-2a has more than a 100-fold reduction in renal clearance than interferon alfa-2b. The pharmacokinetics of the drug is unaffected by renal failure, and hence, no dose modifications are necessary in the setting of renal impairment, as opposed to peginterferon alfa-2b.[13]

Head-to-head comparison of the 2 peginterferons indicated that peginterferon alfa-2b has a shorter half-life in serum than peginterferon alfa-2a. A significant proportion of patients who received peginterferon alfa-2b had levels of drug less than the limits of detection by the end of day 7.[14,15] Low serum concentrations toward the end of the dosing schedule may be associated with viral rebound. These observations suggest that a shorter dosing interval is necessary for peginterferon alfa-2b. Indeed, one study has reported improved viral kinetics with a twice-weekly regimen, but SVR rates were not reported and a formal study has not been conducted.[16]

PHARMACOKINETICS OF RIBAVIRIN

Bioavailability of ribavirin was assessed in 6 healthy volunteers by administering an intravenous dose of $^{13}C3$-ribavirin, 150 mg, followed 1 hour later by an oral dose of ribavirin, 400 mg. Intravenous and oral ribavirin produced mean maximum plasma concentrations of 4187 and 638 ng/mL, respectively.[17] The mean bioavailability was 51.8% ± 21.8%, and the mean γ-phase half-life was 37.0 ± 14.2 hours. The mean renal clearance, metabolic clearance, and volume of distribution of the central compartment were 6.94 L/h, 18.1 L/h, and 17.8 L, respectively.[17] There is no evidence that peginterferons alter the pharmacokinetics of ribavirin.[18] After the administration of ribavirin, 600, 800, and 1000 to 1200 mg/d, in combination with peginterferon alfa-2b, the mean peak plasma ribavirin concentrations at week 1 were 741, 799, and 1101 ng/mL, respectively. The mean peak plasma ribavirin concentrations at week 4 were 1770, 2297, and 2750 ng/mL, respectively, for patients treated with 600, 800, and 1000 to 1200 mg of ribavirin daily in combination with peginterferon alfa-2b ribavirin. The mean time to the mean peak plasma levels occurred between 1 and 2 hours after dosing at weeks 1 and 4.[18]

PHARMACODYNAMICS OF PEGINTERFERON

Interferon has both direct and indirect antiviral actions against HCV, but the mechanism of eradication of HCV infection by interferon-alfa is not certain. Interferon mediates its antiviral effect by inducing interferon-stimulated genes (ISGs), which encode for several effector proteins with antiviral effects, such as protein kinase, $2',5'$ oligoadenylate synthetase ($2',5'$ OAS), adenosine deaminase, and protein GTPase MX, leading to the inhibition of messenger RNA (mRNA) translation, RNA degradation and editing, and production of nitric oxide.[19,20] Interferon-alfa also acts indirectly via upregulation of major histocompatibility complex class I genes in antigen-presenting cells, promoting the cytotoxic T-cell clearance of virally infected cells.[20]

Peginterferon alfa-2b is considered a prodrug of interferon alfa-2b. The urethane bond linking the 12-kDa PEG chain to interferon in peginterferon alfa-2b is unstable and susceptible to hydrolysis such that after injection, native interferon alfa-2b is released and circulates in the body. In contrast, the amide bond linking the PEG chain to interferon alfa-2a is not subject to hydrolysis. Overall, the in vitro antiviral activity of peginterferon alfa-2a is approximately 7% of that of interferon alfa-2a,[10] whereas the antiviral activity of peginterferon alfa-2b is approximately 28% of that of interferon alfa-2b.[21] This difference may be, in part, a result of the reduced affinity of peginterferon alfa-2a for its receptor in vitro because of the more stable covalent linkage of the PEG moiety.

The biologic activity of interferon-alfa is estimated by measuring the serum levels of ISGs or known endogenous proteins induced by interferon, such as $2',5'$ OAS, neopterin, and β_2-microglobulin. Serum levels of $2',5'$ OAS increased rapidly following single doses of standard interferon alfa-2a and peginterferon alfa-2a and peaked 24 or 48 hours after the administration.[22] $2',5'$ OAS levels declined rapidly in recipients of standard interferon alfa-2a but remained near peak levels for 1 week in recipients of pegylated interferon alfa-2a.[22] Similarly, the administration of peginterferon alfa-2b was associated with dose-related increases in serum neopterin levels and non–dose-related increases in serum $2',5'$ OAS levels in patients with chronic hepatitis C.[11]

Pharmacodynamic studies comparing the 2 peginterferon preparations have yielded conflicting results. In a small study, 22 patients were randomized to receive either peginterferon alfa-2a (180 μg weekly) or peginterferon alfa-2b (1.0 μg weekly).[23] The enzymatic activity of $2',5'$ OAS and the levels of neopterin and β_2-microglobulin were measured over a 7-day period. $2',5'$ OAS activity and the serum concentrations of neopterin and β_2-microglobulin did not differ significantly between the 2 patient groups at any time point, and there was no significant correlation between the serum area under the concentration-time curve of either peginterferon and that of $2',5'$ OAS, neopterin, and β_2-microglobulin.[23] In contrast, in another study, 36 patients were randomized to receive either peginterferon alfa-2b (1.5 μg/kg/wk) or peginterferon alfa-2a (180 μg/wk) for 4 weeks and then in combination with ribavirin (13 mg/kg/d) for an additional 4 weeks.[24] The pharmacokinetic profile of both peginterferons, mRNA expression of a selected group of ISG transcripts, and serum HCV RNA levels were assessed. Patients who received peginterferon alfa-2b had a significantly greater upregulation of interferon-alfa response genes than those who received peginterferon alfa-2a. Correspondingly, patients treated with peginterferon alfa-2b also had a significantly greater $\log_{10}$ maximum and $\log_{10}$ time-weighted average decrease in serum HCV RNA levels. The differences in the test to measures interferon's effectiveness enzymatic assays compared with mRNA levels, and the study design account for the differences in the results. The pharmacodynamics of peginterferon alfa-2a is not affected by race.[25]

SAFETY OF PEGINTERFERONS

Interferon alfa-2a or alfa-2b is associated with a range of side effects. The early side effects include influenza like symptoms (fever, chills, myalgia, fatigue, and arthralgia), dermatologic problems (rash), and bone marrow suppression (neutropenia, anemia, and thrombocytopenia).The later complications include infections and neuropsychiatric, cardiovascular, and autoimmune side effects. Peginterferons have similar side-effect profiles as standard interferons. Several head-to-head studies have demonstrated similar safety and tolerability profiles between the 2 peginterferons.[26–28] One of the larger trials, the Individualized Dosing Efficacy versus Flat Dosing to Assess Optimal Pegylated Interferon Therapy (IDEAL) study, reported discontinuation rates of peginterferon alfa-2a and alfa-2b for adverse events of 13% and 12.7%, respectively.[26] The rates of grade 2 (hemoglobin <10 g/dL) and grade 3 (hemoglobin <8.5 g/dL) anemia were similar between peginterferon alfa-2a and alfa-2b (29.6% vs 30.7% and 3.8% vs 2.5%, respectively).[26] The rates of mild (<750/µL) and moderate (<500/µL) neutropenia were significantly different between the 2 preparations (27% vs 22.2% and 5.9% vs 2.8%) in the IDEAL study[26] but not in the 2 randomized Italian studies.[27,28] Although patients receiving peginterferon alfa-2a were more likely to require dose reduction for neutropenia in the later studies, a recent meta-analysis of adverse events leading to treatment discontinuation in 11 head-to-head trials comparing peginterferon alfa-2a and alfa-2b revealed no significant differences between the 2 peginterferons.[29]

CLINICAL EFFICACY OF PEGINTERFERON AND RIBAVIRIN COMBINATION
Week 4 and 12 Viral Kinetics

The rate of clearance of virus from serum during therapy is a strong predictor of the treatment response.[30] Patients who achieve a rapid virological response (RVR), defined as undetectable HCV RNA by week 4 of the treatment, have a high likelihood of obtaining a sustained virological response (SVR) (>80%). In contrast, the absence of an early virological response (EVR), defined as greater than or equal to 2 log reduction in HCV RNA from baseline or testing HCV RNA negative by week 12 of the treatment, is the best predictor of a lack of SVR.[8] Thus, the comparison of week 4 and 12 viral kinetics provides a means of comparing the clinical efficacy of the 2 peginterferon preparations. RVR rates are similar for the 2 peginterferon preparations.[27,28,31] In one study, RVR rates were reported as 29% and 24% for patients treated with peginterferon alfa-2b and alfa-2a, respectively.[31] In the IDEAL study (see later discussion), RVR rates did not differ between the standard-dose peginterferon alfa-2b and alfa-2a arms (12.2% vs 12.1%, respectively). In contrast, EVR rates were significantly higher with peginterferon alfa-2a. In the IDEAL trial, EVR rates were 45% in the peginterferon alfa-2a arm and 39.9% in the peginterferon alfa-2b arm.[26] In another trial of 320 consecutive, treatment-naive subjects with chronic hepatitis C randomly assigned to once-weekly peginterferon alfa-2a (180 µg, group A) or peginterferon alfa-2b (1.5 µg/kg, group B) plus ribavirin 1000 mg/d (body weight <75 kg) or 1200 mg/d (body weight ≥75 kg) for 48 weeks (genotype 1 or 4) or 24 weeks (genotype 2 or 3), significantly higher EVR and complete EVR rates were reported in patients with HCV genotype 1 infection treated with peginterferon alfa-2a compared with peginterferon alfa-2b.[28] Thus, the emerging data suggest that the branched peginterferon formulation seems to be associated with better viral clearance by week 12.

SVR

The IDEAL study was designed to compare standard- and low-dose regimens of peginterferon alfa-2b plus ribavirin after it was observed that both dose levels yielded similar SVR rates in the absence of ribavirin. A third treatment group, peginterferon alfa-2a plus ribavirin, was added to the study because it was the other approved regimen. Patients with HCV genotype 1 infection who had not previously been treated were randomly assigned to undergo 48 weeks of treatment with 1 of the 3 regimens: peginterferon alfa-2b at a standard dose of 1.5 μg/kg/wk or a low dose of 1.0 μg/kg/wk, peginterferon alfa-2b plus ribavirin at a dose of 800 to 1400 mg/d, or peginterferon alfa-2a at a dose of 180 μg/wk plus ribavirin at a dose of 1000 to 1200 mg/d.[26] Among 3070 patients, SVR rates were similar among the regimens: 39.8% with standard-dose peginterferon alfa-2b, 38.0% with low-dose peginterferon alfa-2b, and 40.9% with peginterferon alfa-2a ($P = .20$ for standard- vs low-dose peginterferon alfa-2b and $P = .57$ for standard-dose peginterferon alfa-2b vs peginterferon alfa-2a). The end-of-treatment response was significantly higher for peginterferon alfa-2a (64.4%) compared with standard-dose peginterferon alfa-2b (53.2%).[26] However, relapse rates were significantly higher among patients receiving peginterferon alfa-2a compared with standard-dose peginterferon alfa-2b (31.5% vs 23.5%). Different ribavirin doses and dose-reduction schedules may have influenced the relapse rates.

The results of the IDEAL study are convincing and supported by several other studies. However, 5 recent studies, including a meta-analysis, suggested that peginterferon alfa-2a is associated with a significantly higher SVR rate compared with peginterferon alfa-2b plus ribavirin (**Table 2**).[27–29,32,33] In an Italian study, 447 treatment-naive patients with chronic hepatitis C were randomly assigned to receive either 1.5 μg/kg/wk peginterferon alfa-2b plus ribavirin 800 to 1200 mg/d or 180 μg/wk peginterferon alfa-2a plus ribavirin 800 to 1200 mg/d for 24 or 48 weeks, according to the HCV genotype.[27] By intention to treat, the SVR rate was higher in patients assigned to peginterferon alfa-2a than in those assigned to peginterferon alfa-2b (66% vs 54%, respectively; $P = .02$). In another Italian study, 320 consecutive treatment-naive patients with chronic hepatitis C were randomly assigned to once-weekly peginterferon alfa-2a, 180 μg, or peginterferon alfa-2b, 1.5 μg/kg, plus weight-based ribavirin. The SVR rate was greater in the patients receiving peginterferon alfa-2a than in those receiving peginterferon alfa-2b (68.8% vs 54.4%; $P = .008$). Subanalysis by genotype demonstrated that the higher SVR rate associated with peginterferon alfa-2a was observed across all genotypes,[28] but this was not confirmed in another study.[27] A third observational study, PRACTICE study, involving 23 German centers, evaluated the efficacy and tolerability of peginterferon alfa-2a compared with peginterferon alfa-2b plus weight-based ribavirin for the treatment of chronic hepatitis C in routine clinical practice.[33] No difference in SVR rates was noted in the intent-to-treat cohort (n = 3414) between peginterferon alfa-2a and peginterferon alfa-2b (52.9% vs 50.5%, respectively). However, in a subanalysis of patients infected with genotype 1 matched by baseline parameters and cumulative ribavirin dose, SVR rates were 49.6% and 43.7% for those receiving peginterferon alfa-2a and peginterferon alfa-2b, respectively ($P \leq .047$).[33] In addition, another retrospective observational study of a large cohort (n = 9544) of US veterans reported that the treatment of genotype 1 patients with peginterferon alfa-2a was associated with an almost 50% higher likelihood of SVR than the treatment with peginterferon alfa-2b. Finally, a recent meta-analysis of 12 randomized clinical trials (n = 5008) that directly compared peginterferon

Table 2
Comparison of clinical efficacy of peginterferon alfa-2a and peginterferon alfa-2b in patients with HCV genotype 1

Author, Year	Trial Design	Treatment Regimen	Number of Patients	ETR	SVR	RR
McHutchison et al,[26] 2009	RCT	PegIFN α-2a, 180 μg	1035	64.4	40.9	31.5
		PegIFN α-2b, 1.5 μg/kg	1019	53.2	39.8	23.5
Rumi et al,[27] 2010	RCT	PegIFN α-2a, 180 μg	91	65	48	22
		PegIFN α-2b, 1.5 μg/kg	87	44	32	26
Ascione et al,[28] 2010	RCT	PegIFN α-2a, 180 μg	93[a]	75.3	54.8	20.4
		PegIFN α-2b, 1.5 μg/kg	93	49.5	39.8	9.7
Mangia et al,[31] 2008	RCT	PegIFN α-2a, 180 μg	334	61	49.1	19.6
		PegIFN α-2b, 1.5 μg/kg	362	56.6	45.6	19.6
Backus et al,[32] 2007	Retrospective	PegIFN α-2a, 180 μg	2091	—	25[b]	—
		PegIFN α-2b, 1.5 μg/kg	3853	—	18	—
Witthoeft et al,[33] 2010	Retrospective	PegIFN α-2a, 180 μg	1784	—	49.6[c]	—
		PegIFN α-2b, 1.5 μg/kg	1686	—	43.7	—

Abbreviations: ETR, end of treatment response; IFN, interferon; RCT, randomized controlled trial; RR, relapse rate; SVR, sustained virological response.
[a] Includes 4 and 1 patients with HCV genotype 4 randomized to peginterferon alfa-2a and alfa-2b, respectively.
[b] Overall SVR rates for all HCV genotypes were 31% and 25% for peginterferon alfa-2a and alfa-2b, respectively.
[c] Overall SVR rates for all HCV genotypes were 52.3% and 50.5% for peginterferon alfa-2a and alfa-2b, respectively.

alfa-2a plus ribavirin with peginterferon alfa-2b plus ribavirin reported higher SVR rates with peginterferon alfa-2a than with peginterferon alfa-2b (47% vs 41%, respectively).[29] Peginterferon alfa-2a and peginterferon alfa-2b generally have similar clinical efficacy; however, several recent trials suggest that peginterferon alfa-2a is associated with higher SVR rates than peginterferon alfa-2b. Further studies controlling for baseline features using similar ribavirin dosing regimens will be needed to determine if there is a difference in clinical efficacy.

The pharmacokinetics and pharmacodynamics of standard interferon alfa-2a and interferon alfa-2b are substantially altered by pegylation. The size, geometry, and site of attachment of the PEG moiety affect the pharmacokinetics and pharmacodynamics as evidenced by the different absorption, volume of distribution, and clearance of the linear 12-kDa peginterferon alfa-2b and the branched 40-kDa peginterferon alfa-2a. Despite these differences, the clinical efficacy, safety, and tolerability of the 2 peginterferons are similar. However, tantalizing evidence from recent studies suggests that peginterferon alfa-2 plus ribavirin is associated with small but significantly higher SVR rates compared with peginterferon alfa-2b. Carefully designed studies are necessary to confirm whether a true difference exists between the 2 peginterferon preparations. This may be moot once the direct acting antiviral agents become available.

REFERENCES

1. Williams R. Global challenges in liver disease. Hepatology 2006;44:521–6.
2. McHutchison JG, Gordon SC, Schiff ER, et al. Interferon alfa-2b alone or in combination with ribavirin as initial treatment for chronic hepatitis C. Hepatitis Interventional Therapy Group. N Engl J Med 1998;339:1485–92.
3. Davis GL, Esteban-Mur R, Rustgi V, et al. Interferon alfa-2b alone or in combination with ribavirin for the treatment of relapse of chronic hepatitis C. International Hepatitis Interventional Therapy Group. N Engl J Med 1998;339:1493–9.
4. Poynard T, Marcellin P, Lee SS, et al. Randomised trial of interferon alpha2b plus ribavirin for 48 weeks or for 24 weeks versus interferon alpha2b plus placebo for 48 weeks for treatment of chronic infection with hepatitis C virus. International Hepatitis Interventional Therapy Group (IHIT). Lancet 1998;352:1426–32.
5. Manns MP, McHutchison JG, Gordon SC, et al. Peginterferon alfa-2b plus ribavirin compared with interferon alfa-2b plus ribavirin for initial treatment of chronic hepatitis C: a randomised trial. Lancet 2001;358:958–65.
6. Fried MW, Shiffman ML, Reddy KR, et al. Peginterferon alfa-2a plus ribavirin for chronic hepatitis C virus infection. N Engl J Med 2002;347:975–82.
7. Hadziyannis SJ, Sette H Jr, Morgan TR, et al. Peginterferon-alpha2a and ribavirin combination therapy in chronic hepatitis C: a randomized study of treatment duration and ribavirin dose. Ann Intern Med 2004;140:346–55.
8. Ghany MG, Strader DB, Thomas DL, et al. Diagnosis, management, and treatment of hepatitis C: an update. Hepatology 2009;49:1335–74.
9. Harris JM, Chess RB. Effect of pegylation on pharmaceuticals. Nat Rev Drug Discov 2003;2:214–21.
10. Bailon P, Palleroni A, Schaffer CA, et al. Rational design of a potent, long-lasting form of interferon: a 40 kDa branched polyethylene glycol-conjugated interferon alpha-2a for the treatment of hepatitis C. Bioconjug Chem 2001;12:195–202.
11. Glue P, Fang JW, Rouzier-Panis R, et al. Pegylated interferon-alpha2b: pharmacokinetics, pharmacodynamics, safety, and preliminary efficacy data. Hepatitis C Intervention Therapy Group. Clin Pharmacol Ther 2000;68:556–67.

12. Algranati NE, Sy S, Modi M. A branched methoxy 40 kDa polyethylene glycol (PEG) moiety optimizes the pharmacokinetics (PK) of peginterferon alfa-2a (PEG-IFN) and may explain its enhanced efficacy in chronic hepatitis C (CHC). Hepatology 1999;30(Suppl):130A.

13. Martin NE, Mitra S, Farrington K, et al. Pegylated (40 kDa) interferon alfa-2a is unaffected by renal impairment. Hepatology 2000;32(Suppl):370A.

14. Bruno R, Sacchi P, Ciappina V, et al. Viral dynamics and pharmacokinetics of peginterferon alpha-2a and peginterferon alpha-2b in naive patients with chronic hepatitis C: a randomized, controlled study. Antivir Ther 2004;9:491–7.

15. Di Bisceglie AM, Ghalib RH, Hamzeh FM, et al. Early virologic response after peginterferon alpha-2a plus ribavirin or peginterferon alpha-2b plus ribavirin treatment in patients with chronic hepatitis C. J Viral Hepat 2007;14:721–9.

16. Formann E, Jessner W, Bennett L, et al. Twice-weekly administration of peginterferon-alpha-2b improves viral kinetics in patients with chronic hepatitis C genotype 1. J Viral Hepat 2003;10:271–6.

17. Preston SL, Drusano GL, Glue P, et al. Pharmacokinetics and absolute bioavailability of ribavirin in healthy volunteers as determined by stable-isotope methodology. Antimicrob Agents Chemother 1999;43:2451–6.

18. Glue P, Rouzier-Panis R, Raffanel C, et al. A dose-ranging study of pegylated interferon alfa-2b and ribavirin in chronic hepatitis C. The Hepatitis C Intervention Therapy Group. Hepatology 2000;32:647–53.

19. Feld JJ, Hoofnagle JH. Mechanism of action of interferon and ribavirin in treatment of hepatitis C. Nature 2005;436:967–72.

20. Samuel CE. Antiviral actions of interferons [table of contents]. Clin Microbiol Rev 2001;14:778–809.

21. Youngster S, Wang YS, Grace M, et al. Structure, biology, and therapeutic implications of pegylated interferon alpha-2b. Curr Pharm Des 2002;8:2139–57.

22. Xu ZX, Patel I, Joubert P. Single-dose safety/tolerability and pharmacokinetics/pharmacodynamics (PK/PD) following administration of ascending subcutaneous doses of pegylated interferon (PEG-IFN) and interferon alfa-2a (IFN-2a) to healthy subjects. Hepatology 1998;28(Suppl):702A.

23. Bruno R, Sacchi P, Scagnolari C, et al. Pharmacodynamics of peginterferon alpha-2a and peginterferon alpha-2b in interferon-naive patients with chronic hepatitis C: a randomized, controlled study. Aliment Pharmacol Ther 2007;26:369–76.

24. Silva M, Poo J, Wagner F, et al. A randomised trial to compare the pharmacokinetic, pharmacodynamic, and antiviral effects of peginterferon alfa-2b and peginterferon alfa-2a in patients with chronic hepatitis C (COMPARE). J Hepatol 2006;45:204–13.

25. Howell CD, Dowling TC, Paul M, et al. Peginterferon pharmacokinetics in African American and Caucasian American patients with hepatitis C virus genotype 1 infection. Clin Gastroenterol Hepatol 2008;6:575–83.

26. McHutchison JG, Lawitz EJ, Shiffman ML, et al. Peginterferon alfa-2b or alfa-2a with ribavirin for treatment of hepatitis C infection. N Engl J Med 2009;361:580–93.

27. Rumi MG, Aghemo A, Prati GM, et al. Randomized study of peginterferon-alpha2a plus ribavirin vs peginterferon-alpha2b plus ribavirin in chronic hepatitis C. Gastroenterology 2010;138:108–15.

28. Ascione A, De Luca M, Tartaglione MT, et al. Peginterferon alfa-2a plus ribavirin is more effective than peginterferon alfa-2b plus ribavirin for treating chronic hepatitis C virus infection. Gastroenterology 2010;138:116–22.

29. Awad T, Thorlund K, Hauser G, et al. Peginterferon alpha-2a is associated with higher sustained virological response than peginterferon alfa-2b in chronic hepatitis C: systematic review of randomized trials. Hepatology 2010;51:1176–84.

30. Jessner W, Watkins-Riedel T, Formann E, et al. Hepatitis C viral dynamics: basic concept and clinical significance. J Clin Virol 2002;25(Suppl 3):S31–9.
31. Mangia A, Minerva N, Bacca D, et al. Individualized treatment duration for hepatitis C genotype 1 patients: a randomized controlled trial. Hepatology 2008;47: 43–50.
32. Backus LI, Boothroyd DB, Phillips BR, et al. Predictors of response of US veterans to treatment for the hepatitis C virus. Hepatology 2007;46:37–47.
33. Witthoeft T, Hueppe D, John C, et al. Efficacy and tolerability of peginterferon alfa-2a or alfa-2b plus ribavirin in the daily routine treatment of patients with chronic hepatitis C in Germany: the PRACTICE study. J Viral Hepat 2010;17(7):459–68.

New Pharmacologic Therapies in Chronic Hepatitis B

Chanunta Hongthanakorn, MD, Anna S.F. Lok, MD*

KEYWORDS

- Hepatitis B virus • Interferon • Nucleos(t)ide analogue
- Entecavir • Tenofovir

Approximately 350 million persons worldwide are chronically infected with hepatitis B, which can result in cirrhosis, liver failure, and hepatocellular carcinoma. Currently, 2 interferons (IFNs) and 5 nucleos(t)ide analogues have been approved for the treatment of chronic hepatitis B (CHB). This article discusses the mechanisms of action, pharmacokinetics, optimal dose, clinical efficacy, and side effects of medications used for the treatment of CHB.

REPLICATION CYCLE OF HEPATITIS B VIRUS

Hepatitis B virus (HBV) is a member of the family Hepadnaviridae, a small DNA-containing virus that replicates its DNA genome through reverse transcription of pregenomic RNA. The replication cycle of HBV starts with attachment of the virus to the hepatocyte membrane (**Fig. 1**). The virion is uncoated and the viral genome is transported to the hepatocyte nucleus and converted to covalently closed circular DNA (cccDNA). cccDNA has a long half-life, accounting for the difficulty in achieving viral clearance during treatment of CHB. The cccDNA serves as a template for transcription of the pregenomic RNA as well as the messenger RNAs. The pregenomic RNA is reverse transcribed to produce, first, a minus strand, and then a plus strand HBV DNA. Nucleocapsids with the partially double-stranded HBV DNA can reenter the hepatocyte nucleus to generate more cccDNA or be secreted as virions after coating with envelope proteins.[1] Recent studies suggest that turnover of infected hepatocytes is the major mechanism by which cccDNA is eliminated.[2]

Financial Disclosures: Chanunta Hongthanakorn, no conflict; Anna SF Lok, consulting for Roche, Gilead, Bristol-Myers Squibb, Merck/Schering, and Bayer, and grant/research support from Bristol-Myers Squibb, GlaxoSmithKline, Gilead, Innogenetics, Merck/Schering, and Roche.
Division of Gastroenterology, University of Michigan, 3110G Taubman Center, 1500 East Medical Center Drive, SPC 5362, Ann Arbor, MI 48109, USA
* Corresponding author.
E-mail address: aslok@med.umich.edu

Gastroenterol Clin N Am 39 (2010) 659–680
doi:10.1016/j.gtc.2010.08.012
0889-8553/10/$ – see front matter © 2010 Elsevier Inc. All rights reserved.

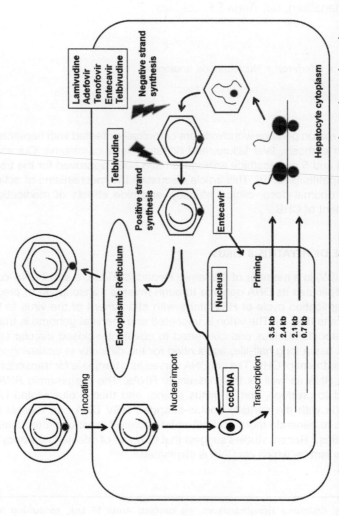

Fig. 1. HBV replication cycle. After entry into a hepatocyte, the uncoated HBV genome enters the nucleus where the second strand HBV DNA is completed. The covalently closed circular DNA (cccDNA) serves as a template for transcription of the pregenomic RNA as well as messenger RNAs. The pregenomic RNA is reverse transcribed into the first (−) and then the second (+) strand HBV DNA. Nucleocapsids with relaxed circular double stranded HBV DNA are coated and secreted or recycled back into the nucleus. The predominant site of action of approved nucleos(t)ide analogues (lamivudine, telbivudine, entecavir, adefovir, and tenofovir) is shown.

IFN
Mechanisms of Action

IFN was discovered as a substance that protects cells from viral infection. Two types of IFNs exist. Type I IFNs include IFN α (IFN-α), IFN β (IFN-β), and IFN ω (IFN-ω), whereas type II IFN includes only IFN γ (IFN-γ). There are at least 18 distinct genes encoding human IFN-α. Recently, 3 IFN-like cytokines in the interleukin (IL) 10 family designated as IL 28A, 28B, and 29 had been reported and termed IFN λ (IFN-λ). IFN-λ is similar to IFN-α and shares the same intracellular activation pathways. The recent discovery of IL-28B polymorphism as a genetic marker associated with spontaneous clearance of hepatitis C virus in patients with acute hepatitis C, as well as a sustained virological response (SVR) after pegylated IFN (PEG-IFN) and ribavirin treatment in patients with chronic hepatitis C, highlight the importance of IFN in immune recovery from viral hepatitis.[3,4]

All type I IFNs bind to the same cell surface receptor (IFNAR1/2), although they differ in affinities. Type I IFNs have antiviral, antiproliferative, and immunomodulatory activities. IFN plays a role in adaptive as well as innate immune responses (**Fig. 2**). IFN-α stimulates activity of T cells, natural killer cells, monocytes, macrophages, and dendritic cells. IFN-α also has antiviral activity. It induces IFN-stimulated genes (ISGs) resulting in a non–virus-specific antiviral state within the cell.[5] This process begins with circulating IFN-α binding to IFN receptors, leading to activation of Janus-activated kinase 1 (Jak1) and tyrosine kinase 2 (Tyk2). The activated kinases phosphorylate the signal transducer and activator of transcription proteins 1 and 2 (STAT1 and STAT2). The activated STAT complex is translocated to the cell nucleus, where it combines with IFN-regulatory factor 9 (IRF-9), and this complex in turn binds to IFN-stimulated response element on cellular DNA, leading to expression of multiple ISGs. IFN-α also affects the translation of viral proteins via the protein kinase R (PKR) gene, which blocks viral protein synthesis through inhibition of eukaryotic initiation factor 2 (eIF2). IFN-α can reduce viral RNA stability through 2′,5′-oligoadenylate synthetase (2′5′OAS) and trafficking or activity of viral polymerase via induction of Mx proteins.

IFN-β has similar activities to IFN-α. IFN-λ acts on the same target genes as the type I IFNs as well as increasing the antiviral activity of subsaturating doses of IFN-α. IFN-γ has a more marked immunoregulatory effect but less potent antiviral activity compared with IFN-α.

Most studies of IFN in hepatitis B have focused on IFN-α. IFN-α has less-potent antiviral activity compared with oral nucleos(t)ide analogues that directly inhibit HBV replication. Clinical trials comparing IFN with lamivudine have consistently shown a smaller decrease in serum HBV DNA in the IFN-treated patients.[6–9] Viral kinetic studies confirmed that the phase I decline of HBV DNA, which reflects the direct antiviral effect on virus production, was less steep in patients receiving IFN compared with those receiving lamivudine, with a mean HBV half-life of 1.6 ($\pm$1.1) days versus 9.5 ($\pm$3) hours, respectively.[6] IFN also has immunomodulatory effects. Flares in aminotransferases have been observed in 25% to 40% of patients during IFN treatment. Flares followed by a decrease in serum HBV DNA levels have been termed host-induced flares and are believed to reflect immune-mediated lysis of infected hepatocytes. In one study, host-induced flares were observed in 24 of 67 (36%) patients who were hepatitis B e antigen (HBeAg) positive and receiving PEG-IFN. Patients with host-induced flares had a higher rate of HBeAg loss: 58% compared with 20% in patients who did not have a host-induced flare.[10] Viral kinetic studies have shown that the second- (with PEG-IFN monotherapy) or third-phase

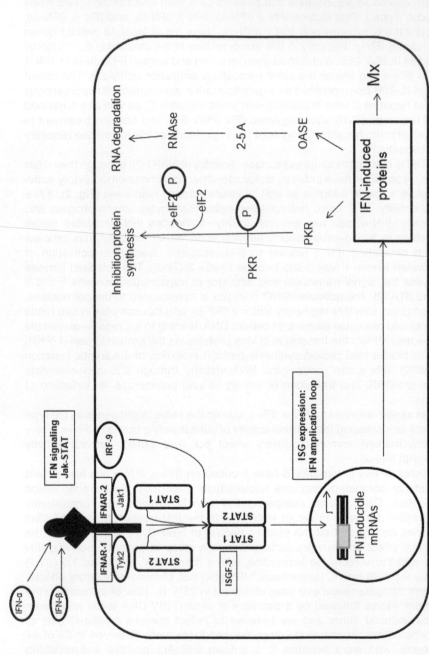

Fig. 2. Mechanisms of action of IFN. IFNs bind to cell surface receptors leading to activation of the Jak-STAT pathway. The activated complex is translocated to the cell nucleus, stimulating the expression of multiple ISGs. IFNs decrease the translation of viral protein synthesis by RNA degradation and induction of Mx proteins. eIF2, eukaryotic initiation factor; IFNAR, Interferon alpha/beta receptor; IRF, Interferon regulatory factor; ISG, IFN-stimulated gene; Jak, Janus kinase; Mx, Mx protein; OASE 2-5 A, 2′, 5′-oligoadenylate synthetase; RNAse, ribonuclease; STAT, signal transducer and activator of transcription; Tyk2, tyrosine kinase 2; PKR, dsRNA dependent protein kinase.

(with PEG-IFN and lamivudine combination or lamivudine alone) viral decline reflects clearance of infected hepatocytes.[6] These studies also suggest that PEG-IFN-α cleared infected cells to a greater extent than lamivudine, possibly reflecting its immunomodulatory activity, which is believed to be important in eliminating infected hepatocytes that harbor cccDNA.

Pharmacokinetics

Initial studies used IFN prepared from leukocytes or lymphoblastoid cell lines. IFNs used nowadays are manufactured using recombinant technology and PEG-IFN has superseded standard IFN.

Early studies on standard IFN and lymphoblastoid IFN involved a wide range of doses administered intravenously or as subcutaneous (SC) or intramuscular injections daily, every other day, or 3 times a week. The bioavailabilities of SC IFN-α2a and IFN-α2b are high, comparable to intravenous formulation. The mean terminal elimination half-life (t1/2β) of IFN-α2a and IFN-α2b following SC injection is 3.5 and 2.9 hours, respectively, but the duration of the biologic effects is likely much longer.[11,12] One study found that dosing on alternate days, or 3 times a week, was as effective in suppressing HBV DNA as daily dosing but an insensitive assay was used to determine this dose-response effect.[13]

PEG-IFN involves the conjugation of a polyethylene glycol molecule to IFN. Pegylation increases the molecular weight, thereby decreasing renal clearance and increasing the elimination half-life. PEG-IFN α-2a is conjugated with a single 40-kDa branched PEG moiety that consists of 2 monomethoxy PEG chains. PEG-IFN-α2b is conjugated with a linear 12-kDa PEG molecule.

PEG-IFN-α2a has a mean t1/2 of 77 hours after a single dose. At steady state, the ratio of serum peak to trough concentrations of PEG-IFN-α2a is about 1.5:2.0, indicating that serum concentrations of the drug are sustained during the 1-week dosing interval. The elimination half-life of PEG-IFN-α2b is 40 hours at week 1 and 58 hours at week 4. Previous studies showed that a significant proportion of chronic hepatitis C patients receiving PEG-IFN-α2b had a trough concentration less than the limits of detection by day 7 during once-weekly dosing.[14] Viral kinetic studies have also observed viral rebounds by day 3.[14] These data suggest that the optimal dosing interval of PEG-IFN-α2b should be shorter than 7 days.

PEG-IFN-α2a has a restricted volume of distribution, being distributed predominantly in the intravascular compartment, whereas PEG-IFN-α2b is distributed widely throughout the body fluids and tissues. The volume of distribution of PEG-IFN-α2b is dependent on the patient's body weight; therefore, weight-based dosing is recommended.[15] By contrast, PEG-IFN-α2a is administered as a fixed dose.

PEG-IFN-α2a is primarily metabolized by the liver and the metabolic products are subsequently excreted by the kidney,[16] whereas PEG-IFN-α2b is metabolized and cleared by the kidney. Compared with standard IFN-α, renal clearance of PEG-IFN-α2a and PEG-IFN-α2b is reduced more than 100-fold and tenfold, respectively.[17,18] There is a 25% to 45% reduction in clearance of PEG-IFN-α2a in patients undergoing chronic hemodialysis and a dose reduction from 180 μg/wk to 135 μg/wk is recommended for these patients. Maximum plasma concentration of PEG-IFN-α2b is increased by 90%, and half-life by up to 40% in patients with creatinine clearance (CrCl) less than 30 mL/min compared with those with normal renal function. It is recommended that the dose of PEG-IFN-α2b be reduced by 25% and 50% in patients with CrCl of 30 to 50 mL/min and less than 30 mL/min including those undergoing hemodialysis, respectively.

Optimal Dose and Duration of PEG-IFN

A phase II dose-ranging study that involved mainly Asian patients with HBeAg-positive CHB receiving PEG-IFN-α2a 90 μg, 180 μg, or 270 μg once weekly compared with standard IFN-α2a 4.5 MIU 3 times a week for 24 weeks, demonstrated an HBeAg clearance rate at week 48 of 37%, 35%, 29%, and 25%, respectively.[19] These data indicate that response to 90 μg and 180 μg of PEG-IFN-α2a was comparable with and superior to standard IFN-α2a. Phase III trials of PEG-IFN-α2a used 180-μg doses to conform to the dose approved for the treatment of hepatitis C and to ensure that all patients regardless of size received an adequate dose, and 48 weeks was chosen to synchronize with the comparator arm (lamivudine). The optimal dose and duration of PEG-IFN-α2a for HBeAg-positive chronic hepatitis is being evaluated in an ongoing study comparing 90- versus 180-μg doses and 24 versus 48 weeks treatment.

Dose-ranging studies in patients with CHB have not been performed for PEG-IFN-α2b. A phase II dose-ranging study of PEG-IFN-α2b in patients with chronic hepatitis C found that SVR rates were comparable in patients who received 1.0-μg/kg or 1.5-μg/kg doses and better than those who received 0.5-μg/kg doses.[15] The similarity in SVR rates in patients with hepatitis C receiving 1.0-μg/kg and 1.5-μg/kg doses of PEG-IFN-α2b was confirmed in the IDEAL study.[20] Clinical trials of PEG-IFN-α2b in CHB have used varying doses. In the 2 largest studies, doses of 100 μg/wk for 32 weeks followed by 50 μg/wk until week 52 were used in 1 study, whereas doses of 100 μg/wk for 32 weeks were used in the other study.[7,21] Weight-based dosing was not used in studies of PEG-IFN-α2b in CHB.

A longer duration of standard IFN therapy, 24 versus 12 months, had previously been shown to result in a higher rate of sustained response in patients with HBeAg-negative chronic hepatitis.[22] Studies are ongoing to determine whether a higher rate of sustained response can be achieved with a 24- versus 12-month course of PEG-IFN in patients with HBeAg-negative chronic hepatitis.

Clinical Efficacy of PEG-IFN

HBeAg-positive chronic hepatitis

Responses to PEG-IFN treatment with and without lamivudine are summarized in Table 1. In the phase III trial comparing PEG-IFN-α2a monotherapy, combination of PEG-IFN-α2a and lamivudine, and lamivudine monotherapy, serum HBV DNA decreased by 4.5, 7.2, and 5.8 $\log_{10}$ copies/mL, respectively at the end of 48 weeks of treatment. HBeAg seroconversion occurred in 27%, 24%, and 20% of patients, respectively, at week 48, and in 32%, 27%, and 19% ($P = .02$), respectively, 24 weeks after stopping treatment.[8] Studies of PEG-IFN-α2b showed similar results. One study found that HBeAg seroconversion rates 26 weeks after stopping treatment were similar in patients who received PEG-IFN-α2b with or without lamivudine (29.2% and 28.6%, respectively), whereas another study showed that HBeAg seroconversion rates 24 weeks after stopping treatment were higher in patients who received a combination of PEG-IFN-α2b and lamivudine than in patients who received lamivudine monotherapy: 36% and 14%, respectively.[7,21] These data showed that, although PEG-IFN has weaker antiviral activity compared with lamivudine, PEG-IFN with its immunomodulatory effect results in a higher rate of HBeAg seroconversion than lamivudine, and the difference is magnified during posttreatment follow-up. These studies also showed that addition of lamivudine to PEG-IFN did not increase the rate of HBeAg seroconversion, despite a greater decline in serum HBV DNA during treatment.

Factors associated with a higher rate of HBeAg seroconversion include high pretreatment alanine aminotransferase (ALT) and low HBV DNA, as well as HBV

Table 1
Efficacy of PEG-IFN-α therapies in patients with HBeAg-positive chronic hepatitis

	PEG-IFN-α2a	PEG-IFN-α2b	PEG-IFN-α + Lamivudine	Lamivudine
Responses at Week 48–52				
Log reduction in HBV DNA (copies/mL)	4.5	~2	~5–7.2	5.8
Undetectable HBV DNA (%)	25	10	33–69	40
ALT normalization (%)	39	34	46–51	62
Loss of HBeAg (%)	30	29	27–44	22
HBeAg seroconversion (%)	27	22	24–25	20
Loss of HBsAg (%)	NA	5	7	NA
Histologic improvement (%)	NA	22	33	NA
Responses at Week 72–78				
Undetectable HBV DNA (%)	14	7	9–14	5
ALT normalization (%)	41	32	25–39	28
HBeAg seroconversion (%)	32	29	27–29	19
HBsAg seroconversion (%)	3	5	3–7	0
Histologic improvement (%)	38	NA	41	34
Responses 3 Years After Completion of Treatment				
Undetectable HBV DNA (%)	NA	13	26	NA
HBeAg seroconversion (%)	NA	35	25	NA
Loss of HBsAg (%)	NA	8	15	NA

Abbreviations: ALT, alanine aminotransferase; HBsAg, hepatitis B surface antigen; NA, not available.
Data from Refs.[7,8,24]

genotypes A and B.[23] Retrospective analyses found that patients who experienced a greater decline in HBeAg titer or hepatitis B surface antigen (HBsAg) titer during treatment were more likely to undergo HBeAg seroconversion.[23] In a study of PEG-IFN-α2b, HBeAg loss and HBeAg seroconversion in patients who received PEG-IFN with or without lamivudine therapy were found in 36% versus 37%, and 25% versus 35% patients, respectively, 3.5 years after treatment was stopped.[24] Predictors associated with a higher rate of sustained response include HBV genotype A, high baseline ALT, and low baseline HBV DNA level.[24,25]

IFN treatment has been reported to be associated with a higher rate of HBsAg loss (the ultimate goal of CHB treatment) than nucleos(t)ide analogue treatment. The higher rate of HBsAg loss is likely related to IFN's immunomodulatory effect. In a study of PEG-IFN-α2a, HBsAg loss was observed in 3%, 3%, and 0% of patients who received PEG-IFN-α2a alone, PEG-IFN-α2a and lamivudine combination, and lamivudine alone, respectively, 24 weeks after treatment.[8] In another study of PEG-IFN-α2b, rates of HBsAg loss 26 weeks after stopping treatment were similar in patients who received PEG-IFN-α2b with or without lamivudine: 7% and 7%, respectively.[7] In this study, rates of HBsAg loss increased to 15% and 8%, respectively, during long-term follow-up of up to 3 years after stopping treatment.[24] HBsAg loss occurred almost exclusively in patients with HBV genotype A: 28% versus 3% in patients with other genotypes.

HBeAg-negative chronic hepatitis

In a large phase III trial comparing PEG-IFN-α2a monotherapy, combination of PEG-IFN-α2a and lamivudine, and lamivudine monotherapy, serum HBV DNA decreased to fewer than 20,000 copies/mL at the end of 48 weeks of treatment in 63%, 87%, and 73% of patients, respectively (**Table 2**). When response was assessed 24 weeks after treatment, the percentage of patients with serum HBV DNA of fewer than 20,000 copies/mL were 43%, 44%, and 29%, respectively, whereas the percentage of patients with undetectable serum HBV DNA (<400 copies/mL) were 19%, 20%, and 7%, respectively. These data indicate that PEG-IFN-α2a resulted in a higher rate of sustained viral suppression compared with lamivudine alone, and combination with lamivudine did not increase the rate of sustained virological response.[9]

A follow-up report found that the percentage of patients with serum HBV DNA fewer than or equal to 10,000 copies/mL in these 3 treatment groups were 28%, 25%, and 15%, respectively, 3 years after completion of treatment, and the percentage of patients with undetectable serum HBV DNA were 18%, 13%, and 6%, respectively.[26] HBsAg loss was observed in 8%, 8%, and 0% in the groups that received PEG-IFN-α2a monotherapy, combination of PEG-IFN-α2a and lamivudine, and lamivudine monotherapy, respectively. Factors associated with a higher rate of sustained response include low pretreatment HBV DNA level, undetectable HBV DNA at the end of 48 weeks of treatment, and HBV genotype B or C compared with D.[27] A post-hoc study showed that less than a 1-log reduction in HBsAg concentration at treatment week 24 of PEG-IFN had a 97% negative predictive value for sustained viral suppression.[28] Another study found that HBsAg levels of less than 10 IU/mL at the end of treatment or a reduction in HBsAg levels of more than 1 $\log_{10}$ IU/mL during treatment was associated with sustained HBsAg loss 3 years after treatment.[29]

Side Effects

Standard IFN-α and PEG-IFN-α have a similar side effect profile. The most common side effects include headache, myalgia, fever, and flulike symptoms.[8,9,15] An important side effect is emotional lability that may manifest as anxiety, depression,

Table 2
Efficacy of PEG-IFN-α therapies in patients with HBeAg-negative chronic hepatitis

	PEG-IFN-α2a	PEG-IFN-α2a + Lamivudine	Lamivudine
Responses at Week 48			
Log reduction in HBV DNA (copies/mL)	4.1	5	4.2
Undetectable HBV DNA (%)	63	87	73
ALT normalization (%)	38	49	73
Responses at Week 72			
Undetectable HBV DNA (%)	19	20	7
ALT normalization (%)	59	60	44
Loss of HBsAg (%)	4	3	0
Histologic improvement (%)	48	38	40
Responses 3 Years After Completion of Treatment			
Undetectable HBV DNA (%)	18	13	6
Loss of HBsAg (%)	8	8	0

Data from Refs.[9,26]

insomnia, irritability, and suicidal ideation. It has been suggested that emotional side effects are less common in patients receiving PEG-IFN for CHB compared with those receiving PEG-IFN for chronic hepatitis C, but whether the difference is real or related to cultural differences between Asian people, who predominated in the studies of CHB, and white people, who predominated in the studies of chronic hepatitis C, is unclear. IFN has a myelosuppressive effect, which could result in neutropenia and thrombocytopenia. Recent studies in patients with hepatitis C found that patients with a greater degree of cytopenia had higher rates of SVR, suggesting that decreases in blood cell counts may be an indicator of the biologic effects of IFN.[8,9,15] ALT flares have been observed in 25% to 40% of patients during IFN treatment and may be a reflection of immune clearance if accompanied by a decrease in serum HBV DNA levels, but ALT flares can also result in hepatic decompensation in patients with cirrhosis.[8,9] Other side effects of IFN include exacerbation or unmasking of autoimmune diseases such as hypothyroidism and hyperthyroidism. Less common adverse effects include hearing loss, retinal disorders, and arrhythmia.

NUCLEOS(T)IDE ANALOGUES
Mechanisms of Action

Nucleos(t)ide analogues have to be phosphorylated by intracellular kinases to the active moiety (triphosphates) to exert an antiviral effect. Currently approved nucleos(t)ide analogues act primarily by inhibiting the reverse transcription of the pregenomic RNA to HBV DNA and do not have a direct effect on cccDNA; therefore, viral relapse is common when treatment is discontinued (see **Fig. 1**). The chemical structures of the 5 nucleos(t)ide analogues approved for treatment of CHB are shown in **Fig. 3**. Almost all nucleos(t)ide analogues can act as a chain terminator because of the lack of a 3'-hydroxyl group, which is necessary for the incorporation of the next nucleotide into viral DNA. In theory, the incorporation of a single-chain terminator would be enough to completely block reverse transcription.

Lamivudine and telbivudine are L-nucleosides. Lamivudine ([−]-β-L-stereoisomer of 2'3'-dideoxy-3'-thiacytidine [3TC]) is phosphorylated to 3TC-triphosphate, a competitive inhibitor of deoxycytidine triphosphate (dCTP). It can act as a chain terminator during HBV DNA synthesis. Telbivudine [1-(2 deoxy-β-L-ribofuranosyl)-5-methyluracil] can act as a chain terminator and a competitive inhibitor of natural thymidine 5'-triphosphate. Telbivudine triphosphate inhibits both the first- and second-strand HBV DNA synthesis.

Entecavir (2-amino-1,9-dihydro-9-[(1S,3R,4S)-4-hydroxy-3-(hydroxymethyl)-2 methylenecyclopentyl] -6H-purin-6-one, monohydrate) is a guanosine nucleoside. Entecavir triphosphate inhibits HBV replication at 3 steps: as a chain terminator 2 or 3 nucleotides downstream from its incorporation, an inhibitor in the priming of the HBV DNA polymerase, and a competitive inhibitor of natural deoxyguanosine triphosphate (dGTP) during HBV DNA synthesis.

Adefovir dipivoxil [9-(2-phosphonylmethoxyethyl) adenine; PMEA)] is a nucleotide. It is phosphorylated to PMEApp, which works as an obligatory chain terminator if incorporated into the DNA chain and/or a competitive inhibitor of deoxyadenosine triphosphate (dATP). Tenofovir disoproxil fumarate (9-[(R)-2-(phosphonomethoxy)prophy] adenine [PMPA]) is a nucleotide. It is phosphorylated to PMPApp, which works as a chain terminator if incorporated into the DNA chain and a competitive inhibitor of natural deoxyadenosine 5'-triphosphate.

Nucleos(t)ide analogue therapy results in biphasic decline of serum HBV DNA. One study of adefovir for 12 weeks showed that the first-phase decline, which reflects the

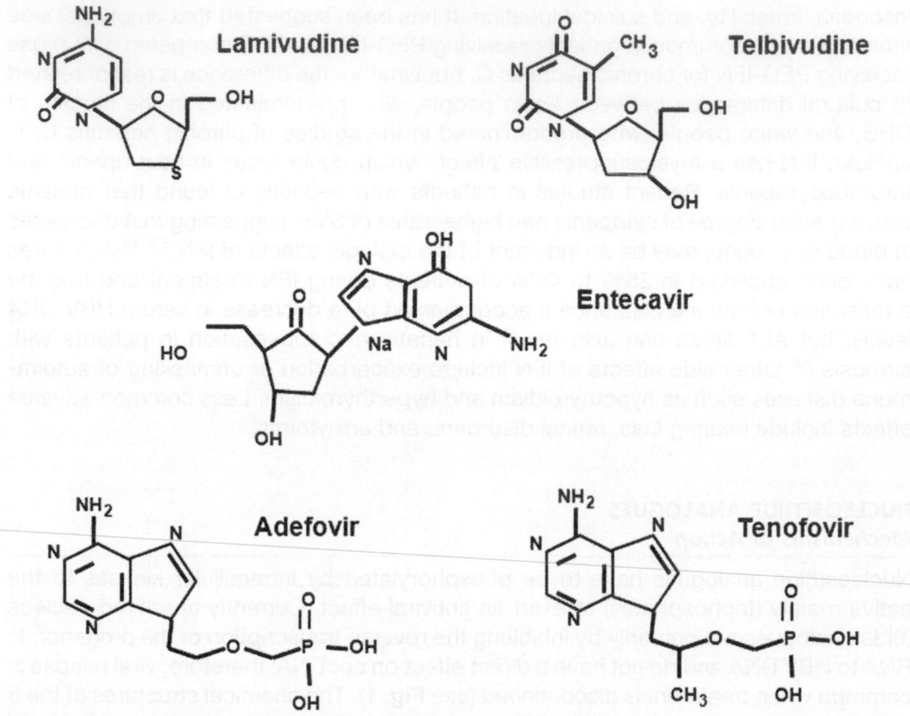

Fig. 3. Molecular structure of the 5 nucleos(t)ide analogues approved for the treatment of CHB.

clearance of HBV DNA from plasma, was more rapid with a half-life of 1.1 days, whereas the second phase of viral decline, which reflects the clearance of infected cells, was slower, with a half-life of 18 days.[30] A viral kinetic study comparing 12 weeks treatment of telbivudine and entecavir in patients who were HBeAg positive showed no difference in the rate of clearance of circulating virus or of infected cells, suggesting that these 2 drugs are equipotent.[31]

Pharmacokinetics

All 5 approved HBV nucleos(t)ide analogues are well absorbed orally, with bioavailability ranging from 25% to 100%. Administration of entecavir with a high-fat meal or a light meal resulted in a 0.25- to 0.75-hour delay in absorption, a decrease in maximum concentration of 44% to 46%, and a decrease in area under the curve of 18% to 20%; therefore, entecavir should be administrated on an empty stomach. Administration of tenofovir with a high-fat meal showed 40% higher oral bioavailability. Adefovir and tenofovir are administered as the prodrugs adefovir dipivoxil and tenofovir disoproxil fumarate. After oral administration, adefovir dipivoxil is hydrolyzed to adefovir and tenofovir disoproxil fumarate to tenofovir by plasma esterases.

Lamividine, telbivudine, entecavir, adefovir, and tenofovir are mainly eliminated in urine as unchanged drugs with elimination half-lives of approximately 5 to 7 hours, 2.5 to 5 hours, 77 to 149 hours, 7.5 hours, and 12 to 18 hours, respectively. Dose adjustments are recommended for all HBV nucleos(t)ide analogues in patients with moderate (CrCl 30–49 mL/min), or severe (CrCl<30 mL/min) renal impairment to achieve optimal plasma exposure; however, data on efficacy of these dose regimens in suppressing HBV replication are not available.

Optimal Dose

A dose-ranging study of lamivudine 25 mg, 100 mg, and 300 mg once daily found that serum HBV DNA became undetectable after 24 weeks of treatment in 58%, 93%, and 88% of patients, respectively.[32] A daily dose of 100 mg was chosen for the treatment of CHB based on these data; however, an insensitive HBV DNA assay, with a lower limit of detection of ~1 million copies/mL, was used in this study. It is possible that a difference in potency between the 100- and 300-mg dose groups was missed because the HBV DNA assay used was unable to detect differences in HBV DNA levels of less than 1 million copies/mL. A subsequent study used a semiquantitative polymerase chain reaction assay with a lower limit of detection of roughly 1000 copies/mL found that serum HBV DNA became undetectable after 24 weeks of treatment in 12%, 29%, and 37% of patients who received lamivudine doses of 25, 100, and 300 mg, respectively.[33] These data suggest that the 300-mg dose is more potent than the 100-mg dose. A higher dose (150 mg twice daily) is recommended for the treatment of human immunodeficiency virus (HIV) monoinfection as well as HIV and HBV coinfection, and this dose is well tolerated.

A dose-ranging study of 25 to 800 mg of telbivudine showed that maximum antiviral activity was achieved with doses of 400 mg or higher.[34] A phase IIb trial showed that median changes in serum HBV DNA concentrations at 52 weeks were -6.4, -6.1, and -4.7 $\log_{10}$ copies/mL in patients who received telbivudine 400 mg and 600 mg, and lamivudine 100 mg, respectively.[35] The recommended dose of telbivudine is 600 mg once daily. Combination of telbivudine and lamivudine was inferior to telbivudine alone, possibly because the 2 drugs are both L-nucleosides and compete for the same binding site in the reverse transcriptase.

A dose-ranging study of entecavir 0.01 to 0.5 mg once daily in nucleoside-naive patients with CHB showed that the 0.5-mg dose was associated with maximum viral suppression.[36] Another study comparing entecavir 0.1, 0.5, and 1 mg doses in lamivudine-refractory patients with CHB showed that mean reductions in serum HBV DNA level at 48 weeks were 5.1, 4.5, and 2.9 $\log_{10}$ copies/mL in patients who received entecavir 1 mg, 0.5 mg, and 0.1 mg daily, respectively.[37] The recommended dose of entecavir is 0.5 mg in patients who are nucleoside naive, and 1 mg in patients who are lamivudine refractory.

In a phase II trial of adefovir dipivoxil, 30- and 60-mg doses resulted in more marked reduction in serum HBV DNA than 5-mg doses. In the phase III trial in patients who were HBeAg positive, doses of 10 mg and 30 mg once daily were chosen because 5-mg doses had weak antiviral activity and 60-mg doses were associated with a high rate of nephrotoxicity. At week 48, mean serum HBV DNA decreased by 3.52 and 4.76 $\log_{10}$ copies/mL in patients who received 10-mg and 30-mg doses, respectively.[38] These data indicate that 30-mg doses had more potent antiviral activity than 10-mg doses of adefovir dipivoxil. The 10- dose was chosen for licensing because of safety concerns, because nephrotoxicity, defined as an increase in serum creatinine by 0.5 mg per dL or more, was observed in 8% of patients who received the 30-mg dose and in none of the patients who received the 10-mg dose.[38] The restriction on adefovir dipivoxil dosing based on safety concerns accounts for the high rate of suboptimal response. A post-hoc analysis of the phase III trial found that serum HBV DNA decreased by less than 2.22 $\log_{10}$ copies/mL in 25% of patients after 48 weeks of treatment.[39] None of these patients had adefovir-resistant HBV mutations before treatment or at the end of 48 weeks of treatment, suggesting that the poor response in these patients was related to the weak antiviral activity of the 10-mg dose and not adefovir resistance. The recommended dose of adefovir dipivoxil is 10 mg daily, and is the same for patients who are nucleoside naive as well as patients who are lamivudine refractory of tenofovir.

A dose-ranging study in patients infected with HIV-1 showed that the 300-mg dose resulted in a greater reduction in plasma HIV-1 RNA compared with 150-mg and 75-mg doses.[40] Dose-ranging studies have not been performed in patients with HBV infection. The recommended dose for tenofovir is 300 mg once daily in patients with CHB who are nucleoside naive. This same dose is used for patients who are lamivudine refractory.

Genetic Barrier to Resistance

The genetic barrier to resistance of an antiviral agent is defined as the number of mutations that the virus must accumulate to replicate efficiently in the presence of that drug. An antiviral agent with a higher genetic barrier to resistance is associated with a lower rate of drug resistance.

The most common mutation associated with resistance to lamivudine is a substitution of methionine in the tyrosine-methionine-aspartate-aspartate (YMDD) motif in the reverse transcriptase domain of the HBV DNA polymerase for valine or isoleucine (rtM204V/I). The rtM204V/I mutation decreases susceptibility of HBV to lamivudine by more than 10,000-fold.[41] HBV variants with the rtM204V/I mutation do not replicate as efficiently as wild-type HBV, but compensatory mutations that restore replication fitness are often selected during continued treatment with lamivudine. The most common compensatory mutations include valine-to-isoleucine substitution at position 173 (rtV173L), leucine-to-methionine substitution at 180 (rtL180M), and amino acid substitutions or a stop codon at position L80. Recent studies showed that, in a small percentage of patients, the primary mutation associated with lamivudine resistance is an alanine-to-threonine or valine substitution at position 181 (rtA181T/V).[42]

Telbivudine also selects for mutations in the YMDD motif. The predominant mutation is rtM204I, whereas rtM204V is rarely detected.[35] In vitro studies found that rtA181V mutation was associated with a slight reduction in antiviral activity. In phase III trials, rtA181T mutation was observed in some patients after 48 weeks of telbivudine therapy.[43]

Entecavir resistance occurs through a 2-hit mechanism with initial selection of an rtM204V/I mutation followed by amino acid substitutions at rtT184, rtS202, or rtM250. In vitro studies showed that the mutations at 184, 202, or 250 have minimal effect on susceptibility to entecavir, but susceptibility to entecavir is decreased by 10- to 250-fold when one of those mutations is present with rtM204V/I mutations, and by more than 500-fold when 2 or more of those mutations are present with rtM204V/I mutations.[44] The requirement for multiple mutations explains the low rate of resistance in patients who are nucleoside naive and receiving entecavir treatment, and the role of the rtM204V/I mutation as the first hit in the 2-hit mechanism explains the high rate of entecavir resistance in patients who are lamivudine refractory even when a higher dose of entecavir is used.

The mutations associated with primary resistance to adefovir include the rtA181V/T substitution that has also been associated with resistance to lamivudine and telbivudine, and a unique mutation involving the substitution of asparagine for threonine at position 236 (rtN236T).[45,46] In vitro studies showed that these mutations decrease susceptibility of adefovir by only 3- to 15–fold but selection of these mutations have been reported to be associated with virological rebound, hepatitis flares, and hepatic decompensation, possibly because of the weak antiviral activity of the 10-mg dose that is used in clinical practice.

The mutations associated with primary resistance to tenofovir have not been clearly defined. One study found that an alanine-to-threonine substitution at position 194 (rtA194T) was associated with tenofovir resistance in 2 patients with HBV and HIV coinfection. Another study showed that the rtA194T mutation was associated with partial resistance to tenofovir and lamivudine. HBV variants with the rtA194T mutation remain susceptible to entecavir and telbivudine.[47]

Clinical studies showed that lamivudine is associated with the highest rate of antiviral resistance, with rates of up to 70% after 5 years of treatment,[48] followed by telbivudine with resistance rates of 11% to 25% after 2 years of treatment,[43] and adefovir with a resistance rate of 29% after 5 years (**Fig. 4**).[49] By contrast, entecavir and tenofovir have been associated with very low rates of antiviral resistance. The rate of entecavir resistance after 5 years of treatment was reported to be only 1.2% in patients who are nucleoside naive, but as high as 51% in patients who are lamivudine refractory.[50] No confirmed tenofovir resistance after up to 3 years of treatment was reported in the phase III trials of tenofovir in patients with CHB,[51] but the study design allowed for the addition of emtricitabine at week 72 in patients who still had detectable serum HBV DNA. Therefore, the rate of resistance during tenofovir monotherapy beyond week 72 is unknown.

Clinical Efficacy

HBeAg-positive chronic hepatitis

All 5 approved nucleos(t)ide analogues have potent antiviral activity with a decrease in serum HBV DNA by 3.5 to 6.9 $\log_{10}$ copies/mL and undetectable serum HBV DNA in 13% to 76% of patients after 48 to 52 weeks of treatment (**Table 3**).[38,51–55] In phase III trials, lamivudine and adefovir dipivoxil were shown to be superior to placebo, telbivudine and entecavir were found to be superior to lamivudine, and tenofovir was shown to be superior to adefovir in suppressing HBV replication. Subsequent studies showed that both telbivudine and entecavir have more potent antiviral activity than adefovir dipivoxil.[56,57] Thus, although direct comparison is not available for all 5 approved nucleos(t)ide analogues, telbivudine, entecavir, and tenofovir disoproxil fumarate have similarly potent antiviral activity, followed by lamivudine and then adefovir dipivoxil. Continued treatment results in an increased percentage of patients with undetectable serum HBV DNA as well as HBeAg seroconversion (see **Table 3**).[43,55]

High pretreatment serum ALT is the strongest predictor of response in patients receiving lamivudine.[58] Post-hoc analysis of the phase III trial of entecavir showed that high ALT was also a predictor of response, and patients with ALT more than twice the upper limit of normal (ULN) had higher rates of HBeAg seroconversion and undetectable serum HBV DNA: 26% and 73% versus 8% and 48% in patients with pretreatment ALT less than 2 ULN.[59] Results of the phase III trial of adefovir dipivoxil showed that the reduction in serum HBV DNA was comparable across the 4 major HBV genotypes (A–D). Analyses of the data in the phase III clinical trial of telbivudine showed that rapid viral suppression (undetectable serum HBV DNA at 24 weeks) was associated with higher rates of response and lower rates of antiviral resistance at week 104.[60]

HBeAg-negative chronic hepatitis

Phase III clinical trials showed that 60% to 93% of patients had undetectable serum HBV DNA after 48 to 52 weeks treatment with the 5 approved nucleos(t)ide analogues **Table 4**.[51,55,61,62] The response was not sustained when treatment was stopped after

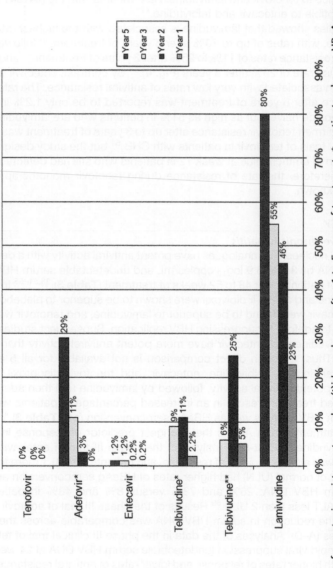

Fig. 4. Incidence of genotypic resistance to nucleos(t)ide analogues after 1 to 5 years of treatment. *, patients who are HBeAg negative; **, patients who are HBeAg positive. Data beyond 3 years are not available for telbivudine or tenofovir. Data from Refs. [43,50,51,55,64,72]

Table 3
Efficacy of nucleos(t)ide analogue therapies in nucleoside naive patients with HBeAg-positive chronic hepatitis

	Lamivudine	Telbivudine	Entecavir	Adefovir	Tenofovir
Responses at Week 48–52					
Log reduction in HBV DNA (copies/mL)	5.5	6.5	6.9	3.5	6.2
Undetectable HBV DNA (%)	36–44	60	67	13–21	76
ALT normalization (%)	41–75	77	68	48–61	77
Loss of HBeAg (%)	17–32	26	22	24	NA
HBeAg seroconversion (%)	16–21	22	21	12–18	21
Loss of HBsAg (%)	≤1	<1	2	0	3
Histologic improvement (%)	49–56	65	72	53	74
Responses at Year 2					
Undetectable HBV DNA (%)	39	56	80	40	89
HBeAg seroconversion (%)	25–29	30	31	29	27
Loss of HBsAg (%)	1–3	1	5	NA	6
Responses at Year 3					
Undetectable HBV DNA (%)	NA	75	82	48	95
HBeAg seroconversion (%)	43	39	NA	37	26
Loss of HBsAg (%)	NA	2	NA	NA	8
Responses at Year 5					
Undetectable HBV DNA (%)	NA	NA	94	NA	NA
HBeAg seroconversion (%)	50	NA	~42	48	NA
Loss of HBsAg (%)	NA	NA	~6	2	NA

Abbreviation: NA, not available.
Data from Refs.[38,51,52,53,54,55,65,73,74]

Table 4
Efficacy of nucleos(t)ide analogue therapies in patients with HBeAg-negative chronic hepatitis

	Lamivudine	Telbivudine	Entecavir	Adefovir	Tenofovir
Responses at Week 48–52					
Log reduction in HBV DNA (copies/mL)	4.4	5.2	5.0	3.9	4.6
Undetectable HBV DNA (%)	60–73	88	90	63	93
ALT normalization (%)	62–78	74	78	77	76
Loss of HBsAg (%)	≤1	<1	<1	0	0
Histologic improvement (%)	61–66	67	70	69	72
Responses at Year 2					
Undetectable HBV DNA (%)	57	82	94	60–80	90
Loss of HBsAg (%)	0.9	0.5	NA	NA	0

Abbreviation: NA, not available.
Data from Refs.[51,55,61,62]

1 year. Sustained HBV DNA suppression to fewer than 300 copies/mL and ALT normalization 24 weeks after completing a 1-year course of entecavir was only 3%,[63] and sustained viral suppression after a 1-year course of adefovir was 8%.[49] Continued treatment with adefovir dipivoxil increased the percentage of patients with undetectable serum HBV DNA from 51% after 1 year to 62% after 4 to 5 years, and the rate of HBsAg loss increased from 0% to 5%.[64] Preliminary data from the tenofovir trial showed that the percentage of patients with undetectable serum HBV DNA was 93% at year 1 and 88% at year 3, but none of the patients lost HBsAg.[51,65]

Side Effects

All 5 approved nucleos(t)ide analogues for CHB are well tolerated. Lamivudine and adefovir dipivoxil 10 mg have a side effect profile similar to placebo. The side effect profile of telbivudine and entecavir are comparable with that of lamivudine, and the side effect profile of tenofovir disoproxil fumarate is similar to that of adefovir dipivoxil. ALT flares have been observed in 1% to 6% of patients during the first year of nucleos(t)ide analogue treatment. These flares have been attributed to immune clearance when accompanied by HBeAg seroconversion or antiviral resistance when accompanied by virological breakthrough.[48] Although on-treatment ALT flares are largely asymptomatic, posttreatment ALT flares, which have been reported in 1% to 10% of patients when nucleos(t)ide analogues were withdrawn after 1 year, had been reported to be associated with liver failure leading to liver transplantation or death.

Although uncommon, a few side effects of HBV nucleos(t)ide analogues deserve attention. Telbivudine has been reported to be associated with myopathy and peripheral neuropathy. In the phase III trial, asymptomatic grade 3 or 4 increase in creatine kinase was observed in 12.9% versus 4.1% of patients after 1 year of telbivudine and lamivudine, respectively.[43] During continued treatment, grade 3 or 4 increase in creatine kinase was observed in 16% and myositis was observed in 0.5% after 4 years of telbivudine treatment.[66] Telbivudine combined with PEG-IFN therapy was associated with a higher rate and earlier onset of peripheral neuropathy than telbivudine monotherapy: 18.8% versus 0.28%, and median of 4.5 months versus 14 months, respectively.[67] Animal studies found that high doses (up to 40 times that used in humans) of entecavir were associated with various tumors, including lung adenomas and lung carcinomas. To date, there has been no evidence of entecavir-associated malignancies in humans. An observational study is ongoing to determine whether there is increased carcinogenesis during long-term treatment with entecavir.

Adefovir and tenofovir have both been reported to be associated with impaired renal function. Nephrotoxicity (defined as confirmed increase in serum creatinine by ≥0.5 mg/dL) has been observed in less than 1% and 3% of patients with CHB after 1 and 5 years of adefovir dipivoxil 10-mg doses, respectively.[51,64] The rate of nephrotoxicity was much higher in patients having liver transplants: 6%, 47%, and 21% of wait-listed patients, patients who underwent liver transplant during the study, and posttransplant recipients, respectively.[68] In these patients, other factors, such as concomitant use of diuretics or calcineurin inhibitors and hepatorenal syndrome, may have been responsible for, or contributed to, the impaired renal function. Adefovir and tenofovir have also been reported to be associated with renal tubular dysfunction including phosphate wasting and Fanconi syndrome.[69] Tenofovir has been reported to be associated with decreased bone mineral density in patients with HIV infection.[70]

Telbivudine and tenofovir are categorized as class B drugs regarding safety for use in pregnancy, whereas lamivudine, entecavir, adefovir, and PEG-IFNs are categorized as class C drugs. The Antiretroviral Pregnancy Registry has been tracking spontaneously reported maternal and fetal outcomes in women receiving oral nucleosides since 1989. As of July 2009, 10,803 pregnancies in which the mother had received an oral nucleoside analogue for HBV and/or HIV infection had been reported.[71] The prevalence of birth defects in babies who had been exposed to lamivudine in the first trimester was 2.9% (96 of 3314) and was 2.4% (18 of 756) in those exposed to tenofovir. These results were similar to population controls. However, only outcomes of live births were recorded. The frequency of spontaneous abortions and the effect of exposure to nucleos(t)ides on growth and development of the babies have not been studied. Data regarding the risk of birth defects associated with entecavir, adefovir, or telbivudine are limited because of the small number of live births reported.

SUMMARY

Substantial progress has been made in the treatment of CHB, with 5 new therapies approved in the past decade. IFNs have antiviral and immunomodulatory activities, whereas nucleos(t)ide analogues possess only antiviral activity. PEG-IFNs have weaker antiviral activity than nucleos(t)ide analogues but are associated with a higher rate of HBsAg loss and more durable viral suppression than nucleos(t)ide analogues. PEG-IFNs are administered for a finite duration, whereas nucleos(t)ide analogues are administered until therapeutic endpoint; HBeAg seroconversion in patients who are HBeAg positive, and HBsAg loss in patients who are HBeAg negative. New nucleos(t)ide analogues are more potent and less prone to resistance. Understanding the pharmacokinetics, optimal dose, clinical efficacy, and side effects of each medication is necessary to select the most appropriate treatment for each patient.

REFERENCES

1. Wu TT, Coates L, Aldrich CE, et al. In hepatocytes infected with duck hepatitis B virus, the template for viral RNA synthesis is amplified by an intracellular pathway. Virology 1990;175(1):255–61.
2. Summers J, Jilbert AR, Yang W, et al. Hepatocyte turnover during resolution of a transient hepadnaviral infection. Proc Natl Acad Sci U S A 2003;100(20): 11652–9.

3. Ge D, Fellay J, Thompson AJ, et al. Genetic variation in IL28B predicts hepatitis C treatment-induced viral clearance. Nature 2009;461(7262):399–401.

4. Thomas DL, Thio CL, Martin MP, et al. Genetic variation in IL28B and spontaneous clearance of hepatitis C virus. Nature 2009;461(7265):798–801.

5. Bekisz J, Schmeisser H, Hernandez J, et al. Human interferons alpha, beta and omega. Growth Factors 2004;22(4):243–51.

6. Colombatto P, Civitano L, Bizzarri R, et al. A multiphase model of the dynamics of HBV infection in HBeAg-negative patients during pegylated interferon-alpha2a, lamivudine and combination therapy. Antivir Ther 2006;11(2):197–212.

7. Janssen HL, van Zonneveld M, Senturk H, et al. Pegylated interferon alfa-2b alone or in combination with lamivudine for HBeAg-positive chronic hepatitis B: a randomised trial. Lancet 2005;365(9454):123–9.

8. Lau GK, Piratvisuth T, Luo KX, et al. Peginterferon alfa-2a, lamivudine, and the combination for HBeAg-positive chronic hepatitis B. N Engl J Med 2005; 352(26):2682–95.

9. Marcellin P, Lau GK, Bonino F, et al. Peginterferon alfa-2a alone, lamivudine alone, and the two in combination in patients with HBeAg-negative chronic hepatitis B. N Engl J Med 2004;351(12):1206–17.

10. Flink HJ, Sprengers D, Hansen BE, et al. Flares in chronic hepatitis B patients induced by the host or the virus? Relation to treatment response during Peg-interferon {alpha}-2b therapy. Gut 2005;54(11):1604–9.

11. Wills RJ, Dennis S, Spiegel HE, et al. Interferon kinetics and adverse reactions after intravenous, intramuscular, and subcutaneous injection. Clin Pharmacol Ther 1984;35(5):722–7.

12. Radwanski E, Perentesis G, Jacobs S, et al. Pharmacokinetics of interferon alpha-2b in healthy volunteers. J Clin Pharmacol 1987;27(5):432–5.

13. Lok AS, Weller IV, Karayiannis P, et al. Thrice weekly lymphoblastoid interferon is effective in inhibiting hepatitis B virus replication. Liver 1984;4(1):45–9.

14. Formann E, Jessner W, Bennett L, et al. Twice-weekly administration of peginterferon-alpha-2b improves viral kinetics in patients with chronic hepatitis C genotype 1. J Viral Hepat 2003;10(4):271–6.

15. Lindsay KL, Trepo C, Heintges T, et al. A randomized, double-blind trial comparing pegylated interferon alfa-2b to interferon alfa-2b as initial treatment for chronic hepatitis C. Hepatology 2001;34(2):395–403.

16. Modi M, Fulton JS, Buckmann DK, et al. Clearance of pegylated (40 kDa) interferon alfa-2a (Pegasys™) is primary hepatic [abstract]. Hepatology 2000;32(4): 371A.

17. Algranati NE, Sy S, Modi M. A branched methoxy 40 kDa polyethylene glycol (PEG) moiety optimizes the pharmacokinetic(PK) of peginterferon alfa-2a and may explain its enhanced efficacy in chronic hepatitis C [abstract]. Hepatology 1999;30(Suppl):190A.

18. Glue P, Fang JW, Rouzier-Panis R, et al. Pegylated interferon-alpha2b: pharmacokinetics, pharmacodynamics, safety, and preliminary efficacy data. Hepatitis C intervention therapy group. Clin Pharmacol Ther 2000;68(5): 556–67.

19. Cooksley WG, Piratvisuth T, Lee SD, et al. Peginterferon alpha-2a (40 kDa): an advance in the treatment of hepatitis B e antigen-positive chronic hepatitis B. J Viral Hepat 2003;10(4):298–305.

20. McHutchison JG, Lawitz EJ, Shiffman ML, et al. Peginterferon alfa-2b or alfa-2a with ribavirin for treatment of hepatitis C infection. N Engl J Med 2009;361(6): 580–93.

21. Chan HL, Leung NW, Hui AY, et al. A randomized, controlled trial of combination therapy for chronic hepatitis B: comparing pegylated interferon-alpha2b and lamivudine with lamivudine alone. Ann Intern Med 2005;142(4):240–50.
22. Lampertico P, Del Ninno E, Vigano M, et al. Long-term suppression of hepatitis B e antigen-negative chronic hepatitis B by 24-month interferon therapy. Hepatology 2003;37(4):756–63.
23. Perrillo RP, Schiff ER, Davis GL, et al. A randomized, controlled trial of interferon alfa-2b alone and after prednisone withdrawal for the treatment of chronic hepatitis B. The hepatitis interventional therapy Group. N Engl J Med 1990;323(5): 295–301.
24. Buster EH, Flink HJ, Cakaloglu Y, et al. Sustained HBeAg and HBsAg loss after long-term follow-up of HBeAg-positive patients treated with peginterferon alpha-2b. Gastroenterology 2008;135(2):459–67.
25. Buster EH, Hansen BE, Lau GK, et al. Factors that predict response of patients with hepatitis B e antigen-positive chronic hepatitis B to peginterferon-alfa. Gastroenterology 2009;137(6):2002–9.
26. Marcellin P, Bonino F, Lau GK, et al. Sustained response of hepatitis B e antigen-negative patients 3 years after treatment with peginterferon alpha-2a. Gastroenterology 2009;136(7):2169–79, e2161–4.
27. Bonino F, Marcellin P, Lau GK, et al. Predicting response to peginterferon alpha-2a, lamivudine and the two combined for HBeAg-negative chronic hepatitis B. Gut 2007;56(5):699–705.
28. Moucari R, Mackiewicz V, Lada O, et al. Early serum HBsAg drop: a strong predictor of sustained virological response to pegylated interferon alfa-2a in HBeAg-negative patients. Hepatology 2009;49(4):1151–7.
29. Brunetto MR, Moriconi F, Bonino F, et al. Hepatitis B virus surface antigen levels: a guide to sustained response to peginterferon alfa-2a in HBeAg-negative chronic hepatitis B. Hepatology 2009;49(4):1141–50.
30. Tsiang M, Rooney JF, Toole JJ, et al. Biphasic clearance kinetics of hepatitis B virus from patients during adefovir dipivoxil therapy. Hepatology 1999;29(6): 1863–9.
31. Suh DJ, Um SH, Herrmann E, et al. Early viral kinetics of telbivudine and entecavir: results of a 12-week randomized exploratory study in patients with HBeAg-positive chronic hepatitis B. Antimicrobial Agents Chemother 2010;54(3):1242–7.
32. Nevens F, Main J, Honkoop P, et al. Lamivudine therapy for chronic hepatitis B: a six-month randomized dose-ranging study. Gastroenterology 1997;113(3): 1258–63.
33. Honkoop P, de Man RA, Niesters HG, et al. Quantitative hepatitis B virus DNA assessment by the limiting-dilution polymerase chain reaction in chronic hepatitis B patients: evidence of continuing viral suppression with longer duration and higher dose of lamivudine therapy. J Viral Hepat 1998;5(5):307–12.
34. Zhou XJ, Lim SG, Lloyd DM, et al. Pharmacokinetics of telbivudine following oral administration of escalating single and multiple doses in patients with chronic hepatitis B virus infection: pharmacodynamic implications. Antimicrobial Agents Chemother 2006;50(3):874–9.
35. Lai CL, Leung N, Teo EK, et al. A 1-year trial of telbivudine, lamivudine, and the combination in patients with hepatitis B e antigen-positive chronic hepatitis B. Gastroenterology 2005;129(2):528–36.
36. Lai CL, Rosmawati M, Lao J, et al. Entecavir is superior to lamivudine in reducing hepatitis B virus DNA in patients with chronic hepatitis B infection. Gastroenterology 2002;123(6):1831–8.

37. Chang TT, Gish RG, Hadziyannis SJ, et al. A dose-ranging study of the efficacy and tolerability of entecavir in lamivudine-refractory chronic hepatitis B patients. Gastroenterology 2005;129(4):1198–209.
38. Marcellin P, Chang TT, Lim SG, et al. Adefovir dipivoxil for the treatment of hepatitis B e antigen-positive chronic hepatitis B. N Engl J Med 2003;348(9): 808–16.
39. Carrouee-Durantel S, Durantel D, Werle-Lapostolle B, et al. Suboptimal response to adefovir dipivoxil therapy for chronic hepatitis B in nucleoside-naive patients is not due to pre-existing drug-resistant mutants. Antivir Ther 2008;13(3):381–8.
40. Hammer SM, Saag MS, Schechter M, et al. Treatment for adult HIV infection: 2006 recommendations of the International AIDS Society-USA panel. Jama 2006; 296(7):827–43.
41. Allen MI, Deslauriers M, Andrews CW, et al. Identification and characterization of mutations in hepatitis B virus resistant to lamivudine. Lamivudine clinical investigation group. Hepatology 1998;27:1670–7.
42. Yatsuji H, Noguchi C, Hiraga N, et al. Emergence of a novel lamivudine-resistant hepatitis B virus variant with a substitution outside the YMDD motif. Antimicrobial Agents Chemother 2006;50(11):3867–74.
43. Liaw YF, Gane E, Leung N, et al. 2-Year GLOBE trial results: telbivudine is superior to lamivudine in patients with chronic hepatitis B. Gastroenterology 2009; 136(2):486–95.
44. Tenney DJ, Levine SM, Rose RE, et al. Clinical emergence of entecavir-resistant hepatitis B virus requires additional substitutions in virus already resistant to lamivudine. Antimicrobial Agents Chemother 2004;48(9):3498–507.
45. Angus P, Vaughan R, Xiong S, et al. Resistance to adefovir dipivoxil therapy associated with the selection of a novel mutation in the HBV polymerase. Gastroenterology 2003;125(2):292–7.
46. Villeneuve JP, Durantel D, Durantel S, et al. Selection of a hepatitis B virus strain resistant to adefovir in a liver transplantation patient. J Hepatol 2003;39(6): 1085–9.
47. Amini-Bavil-Olyaee S, Herbers U, Sheldon J, et al. The rtA194T polymerase mutation impacts viral replication and susceptibility to tenofovir in hepatitis B e antigen-positive and hepatitis B e antigen-negative hepatitis B virus strains. Hepatology 2009;49(4):1158–65.
48. Lok AS, Lai CL, Leung N, et al. Long-term safety of lamivudine treatment in patients with chronic hepatitis B. Gastroenterology 2003;125(6):1714–22.
49. Hadziyannis SJ, Tassopoulos NC, Heathcote EJ, et al. Long-term therapy with adefovir dipivoxil for HBeAg-negative chronic hepatitis B. N Engl J Med 2005; 352(26):2673–81.
50. Tenney DJ, Rose RE, Baldick CJ, et al. Long-term monitoring shows hepatitis B virus resistance to entecavir in nucleoside-naive patients is rare through 5 years of therapy. Hepatology 2009;49(5):1503–14.
51. Marcellin P, Heathcote EJ, Buti M, et al. Tenofovir disoproxil fumarate versus adefovir dipivoxil for chronic hepatitis B. N Engl J Med 2008;359(23):2442–55.
52. Dienstag JL, Schiff ER, Wright TL, et al. Lamivudine as initial treatment for chronic hepatitis B in the United States. N Engl J Med 1999;341(17):1256–63.
53. Zeng M, Mao Y, Yao G, et al. A double-blind randomized trial of adefovir dipivoxil in Chinese subjects with HBeAg-positive chronic hepatitis B. Hepatology 2006; 44(1):108–16.
54. Chang TT, Gish RG, de Man R, et al. A comparison of entecavir and lamivudine for HBeAg-positive chronic hepatitis B. N Engl J Med 2006;354(10):1001–10.

55. Lai CL, Gane E, Liaw YF, et al. Telbivudine versus lamivudine in patients with chronic hepatitis B. N Engl J Med 2007;357(25):2576–88.
56. Chan HL, Heathcote EJ, Marcellin P, et al. Treatment of hepatitis B e antigen positive chronic hepatitis with telbivudine or adefovir: a randomized trial. Ann Intern Med 2007;147(11):745–54.
57. Leung N, Peng CY, Hann HW, et al. Early hepatitis B virus DNA reduction in hepatitis B e antigen-positive patients with chronic hepatitis B: A randomized international study of entecavir versus adefovir. Hepatology 2009;49(1):72–9.
58. Perrillo RP, Lai CL, Liaw YF, et al. Predictors of HBeAg loss after lamivudine treatment for chronic hepatitis B. Hepatology 2002;36(1):186–94.
59. Wu I-C, Lai CL, Han SB, et al. Efficacy of entecavir in chronic hepatitis B patients with mildly elevated alanine aminotransferase and biopsy-proven histological damage. Hepatology 2010;51(4):1185–9.
60. Zeuzem S, Gane E, Liaw YF, et al. Baseline characteristics and early on-treatment response predict the outcomes of 2 years of telbivudine treatment of chronic hepatitis B. J Hepatol 2009;51(1):11–20.
61. Lai CL, Shouval D, Lok AS, et al. Entecavir versus lamivudine for patients with HBeAg-negative chronic hepatitis B. N Engl J Med 2006;354(10):1011–20.
62. Hadziyannis SJ, Tassopoulos NC, Heathcote EJ, et al. Adefovir dipivoxil for the treatment of hepatitis B e antigen-negative chronic hepatitis B. N Engl J Med 2003;348(9):800–7.
63. Shouval D, Lai CL, Chang TT, et al. Relapse of hepatitis B in HBeAg-negative chronic hepatitis B patients who discontinued successful entecavir treatment: the case for continuous antiviral therapy. J Hepatol 2009;50(2):289–95.
64. Hadziyannis SJ, Tassopoulos NC, Heathcote EJ, et al. Long-term therapy with adefovir dipivoxil for HBeAg-negative chronic hepatitis B for up to 5 years. Gastroenterology 2006;131(6):1743–51.
65. Marcellin P, Buti M, Krastev Z, et al. Three years of tenofovir disoproxil fumarate treatment in HBeAg-negative patients with chronic hepatitis B (study102); preliminary analysis. Hepatology 2009;50(S4):532A.
66. Wang Y, Thongsawat S, Gane EJ, et al. Efficacy and safety outcomes after 4 years of telbivudine treatment in patients with chronic hepatitis B(CHB). Hepatology 2009;50(S4):533A.
67. Fleischer RD, Lok AS. Myopathy and neuropathy associated with nucleos(t)ide analog therapy for hepatitis B. J Hepatol 2009;51(4):787–91.
68. Schiff E, Lai CL, Hadziyannis S, et al. Adefovir dipivoxil for wait-listed and post-liver transplantation patients with lamivudine-resistant hepatitis B: final long-term results. Liver Transpl 2007;13(3):349–60.
69. Malik A, Abraham P, Malik N. Acute renal failure and Fanconi syndrome in an AIDS patient on tenofovir treatment–case report and review of literature. J Infect 2005;51(2):E61–5.
70. Purdy JB, Gafni RI, Reynolds JC, et al. Decreased bone mineral density with off-label use of tenofovir in children and adolescents infected with human immunodeficiency virus. J Pediatr 2008;152(4):582–4.
71. Antiretroviral Pregnancy Registry Steering Committee. Antiretroviral Pregnancy Registry Steering Commitee. Antiretroviral pregnancy registry international interim report for 1 July 1989 through July 2009. Available at: http://www.apregistry.com/Interimreport.pdf. Accessed December 31, 2009.
72. Lai CL, Dienstag J, Schiff E, et al. Prevalence and clinical correlates of YMDD variants during lamivudine therapy for patients with chronic hepatitis B. Clin Infect Dis 2003;36(6):687–96.

73. Marcellin P, Chang TT, Lim SG, et al. Long-term efficacy and safety of adefovir dipivoxil for the treatment of hepatitis B e antigen-positive chronic hepatitis B. Hepatology 2008;48(S4):750–8.

74. Heathcote EJ, Gane EJ, De Man RA, et al. Three years of tenofovir disoproxil (TDF) treatment in HBeAg-positive patients with chronic hepatitis B (study 103), preliminary analysis. Hepatology 2009;50(S4):533A–4A.

Clinical Pharmacology of Portal Hypertension

Cecilia Miñano, MD, MPH[a,b], Guadalupe Garcia-Tsao, MD[a,b],*

KEYWORDS

• Portal hypertension • Cirrhosis • Varices
• Variceal hemorrhage • Hepatic venous pressure gradient
• Portal pressure

Portal hypertension is an increase in pressure in the portal vein and its tributaries. It is defined as a portal pressure gradient (the difference in pressure between the portal vein and the hepatic veins) greater than 5 mm Hg. Although this gradient defines portal hypertension, a gradient of 10 mm Hg or greater defines clinically significant portal hypertension, because this pressure gradient predicts the development of varices,[1] decompensation of cirrhosis,[2,3] and hepatocellular carcinoma.[4] The most direct consequence of portal hypertension is the development of gastroesophageal varices that may rupture and lead to the development of variceal hemorrhage. This article reviews the pathophysiologic bases of the different pharmacologic treatments for portal hypertension in patients with cirrhosis and places them in the context of the natural history of varices and variceal hemorrhage.

PATHOPHYSIOLOGY OF PORTAL HYPERTENSION

Anatomically, the portal vein is formed by the union of the superior mesenteric vein and the splenic vein. The mesenteric vein collects blood from the splanchnic circulation. Thus, portal venous inflow is determined by the state of constriction or dilatation of splanchnic arterioles.

The initial mechanism in the genesis of portal hypertension is an increase in vascular resistance that can occur at any level within the portal venous system. Portal hypertension is therefore classified as prehepatic (portal or splenic vein thrombosis); intrahepatic (cirrhosis), and posthepatic (Budd-Chiari syndrome). The most common cause of portal hypertension is cirrhosis. In cirrhosis, the increased resistance is mostly caused by hepatic architectural distortion (fibrosis and regenerative nodules) but about a third of the increased resistance is caused by intrahepatic

[a] Section of Digestive Diseases, Yale University School of Medicine, 333 Cedar Street, LMP 1080, New Haven, CT 06520, USA
[b] Section of Digestive Diseases, VA-Connecticut Healthcare System, 950 Campbell Avenue, West Haven, CT 06516, USA
* Corresponding author. Section of Digestive Diseases, Yale University School of Medicine, 333 Cedar Street, LMP 1080, New Haven, CT 06520.
E-mail address: guadalupe.garcia-tsao@yale.edu

Gastroenterol Clin N Am 39 (2010) 681–695
doi:10.1016/j.gtc.2010.08.015
0889-8553/10/$ – see front matter. Published by Elsevier Inc.

gastro.theclinics.com

vasoconstriction, amenable to vasodilators.[5] This is caused by the activation of stellate cells with active contraction of myofibroblasts and vascular smooth muscle cells in portal venules,[6] which in turn is caused by increased endogenous vasoconstrictors, such as endothelin, and reduced nitric oxide bioavailability.[7,8]

Portosystemic collaterals develop as a consequence of the high pressure in the portal vein and ameliorate the increased resistance. However, even when portal blood flow is entirely diverted through collaterals, portal hypertension persists because of a concomitant increase in portal venous inflow, which in turn is caused by splanchnic vasodilatation,[9] mostly mediated by an increase in nitric oxide.[7]

The most important collaterals are those that constitute gastroesophageal varices. Although the formation of collaterals had been assumed to be the result of dilatation of preexisting vascular channels, recent studies have implicated a process of neoangiogenesis. This process has been shown to contribute not only to portal-systemic collaterals but also to increased splanchnic blood flow (arteriolar-capillary network).[10]

MEASUREMENT OF PORTAL PRESSURE

Measurement of portal pressure in patients with portal hypertension is important in the evaluation of the efficacy of different portal-hypotensive pharmacologic therapies.

The most used method to assess portal pressure is the catheterization of the hepatic vein with determination, via a balloon catheter, of the hepatic vein pressure gradient (HVPG), which is the difference between the wedged (or occluded) hepatic venous pressure and the free hepatic venous pressure.[11] Normal HVPG is 3 to 5 mm Hg. In patients with compensated cirrhosis, an HVPG greater than or equal to 10 mm Hg predicts the development, not only of varices, but of complications that mark the transition from compensated to decompensated cirrhosis.[1,2]

Changes in HVPG during pharmacologic therapy have also been shown to be predictive of clinical outcomes. In patients with a history of variceal hemorrhage, a decrease in HVPG to less than 12 mm Hg or a decrease greater than 20% from baseline significantly reduces the risk of recurrent hemorrhage, ascites, encephalopathy, and death.[12–14] In patients with compensated cirrhosis, even lower reductions in HVPG (>10% from baseline) have been associated with a reduction in the development of varices,[1] first variceal hemorrhage,[15] and ascites.[15] Recent studies show that separate HVPG procedures to assess response to therapy can be obviated by assessing the acute hemodynamic response to intravenous (IV) propranolol (0.15 mg/kg) during a single procedure.[15,16]

Pharmacologic therapies should thus be ideally tailored to a target decrease in HVPG. Even though the HVPG procedure is simple and safe, its use is not widespread in the United States because it is invasive and because it has not been appropriately standardized.[17]

PHARMACOLOGIC THERAPY FOR PORTAL HYPERTENSION
Drugs that Act by Reducing Portal Flow

Increased portal venous inflow secondary to splanchnic vasodilatation can be corrected pharmacologically through the use of splanchnic vasoconstrictors. These drugs have been shown to decrease portal pressure in experimental and proof-of-concept hemodynamic studies. Vasoconstrictors effective in the chronic treatment of portal hypertension are nonselective β-adrenergic blockers (NSBB) (Table 1). Vasoconstrictors effective in the acute therapy for variceal hemorrhage are vasopressin and somatostatin and their respective synthetic analogues.

Table 1
Hemodynamic responders to long-term administration of different pharmacologic therapies in studies including at least 10 patients

First Author (Year)	Setting (Type of Prophylactic Study)	β-Blockers		β-Blockers + Nitrates		No Drugs	
		N treated	N responders (%)	N treated	N responders (%)	N treated	N responders (%)
Groszmann 1990[a,22]	Primary	45	14 (31)			39	7 (18)
Merkel 2000[23]	Primary	29	16 (55)	20	12 (60)	–	–
Banares 2002[24]	Primary	22	5 (23)				
Turnes 2006[25]	Primary	50	19 (38)	21	6 (28)	–	–
Villanueva 2009[15]	Primary	73	25 (34)				
Sharma 2009[26]	Primary	56	21 (38)				
Merkel 2010[27]	Primary	37	13 (35)				
Feu 1995[28]	Secondary	69	25 (36)	–	–	–	–
Villanueva 1996[a,29]	Secondary	–	–	31	14 (45)	31	5 (16)
McCormick 1998[30]	Secondary	14	9 (64)	30	19 (63)	–	–
Villanueva 2001[a,31]	Secondary	–	–	49	25 (51)	46	7 (15)
Patch 2002[a,32]	Secondary	–	–	18	9 (50)		
Abraldes 2003[13]	Secondary	29	11 (33)	44	17 (39)	–	–
Villanueva 2004[33]	Secondary	–	–	132	64 (48)	–	–
Garcia-Pagan 2009[a,34]	Secondary	–	–	135	48 (36)		
Villanueva 2009[a,35]	Secondary	22	7 (32)	27	10 (37)		
Escorsell 2000[36]	Mixed	47	19 (40)	–	–	–	–
Bureau 2002[37]	Mixed	34	13 (38)	21	7 (33)	–	–
Total		527	197 (37)[b]	528	231 (44)[b]	116	19 (16)

Hemodynamic response defined as a decrease in HVPG less than 12 mm Hg and/or a decrease in HVPG greater than 20% from baseline.
[a] Randomized controlled trial.
[b] Difference between NSBB and NSBB+ISMN: $P = .039$.

Recent studies in a rat model of prehepatic portal hypertension show that vascular endothelial growth factor blockade decreases portal pressure and concomitantly decreases the development of portosystemic collaterals and the hyperdynamic splanchnic circulatory state.[18] Although no clinical studies are available, inhibition of angiogenesis may be a future target in the treatment of portal hypertension.

NSBB

These are the most widely evaluated and used drugs in the chronic treatment of portal hypertension (ie, in the prevention of variceal hemorrhage). Their mechanism of action is through both β-1 and β-2 blockade. Although β-1 blockade decreases portal flow through a decrease in cardiac output, β-2 blockade decreases portal flow through splanchnic vasoconstriction via unopposed α-adrenergic activity. As expected, NSBB (propranolol, nadolol, timolol) decrease HVPG to a greater extent compared with selective β-1 adrenergic blockers (atenolol, metoprolol) and are the preferred therapy.[19] The lack of correlation between the postpropranolol decrease in heart rate (β-1 effect) and the decrease in HVPG is further evidence that the β-2 effect plays a more important role.[20]

The most widely used NSBB are propranolol and nadolol. NSBB use is associated with a median reduction in HVPG of approximately 15%,[21] with 37% of the patients being hemodynamic responders (ie, achieving a reduction in HVPG to less than 12 mm Hg and/or a reduction >20% from baseline) (see **Table 1**).[13,15,22–37] The reduction in portal pressure induced by NSBB is lower than the β-blocker–induced reduction in portal blood inflow.[38] This is because of a concomitant increase in collateral resistance secondary to a decrease in collateral flow and diameter.[38] This effect represents an added benefit of NSBB (not assessable by a reduction in portal pressure), which can explain their efficacy in randomized clinical trials (RCT) with only a modest portal pressure–reducing effect.

Although the recommended dosing of propranolol for the treatment of arterial hypertension in patients who are not cirrhotic is 4 times a day, in cirrhosis, because of a slower drug metabolism, twice a day dosing is sufficient. The starting dosage is 20 to 40 mg orally twice a day and this is gradually increased to a maximum of 160 mg twice a day. The lower starting dose (20 mg) is reserved for patients with a baseline low mean arterial pressure. In many RCT, the dose was adjusted to obtain a 25% decrease in heart rate; however, because a change in heart rate is not predictive of a decrease in portal pressure,[20] recent guidelines have recommended the adjustment of NSBB to the highest tolerated dose or to a heart rate of 50 to 55 beats/min.[39] Nadolol has a longer half-life and can be used once daily, which may increase patient adherence. The initial dosage is 20 to 40 mg orally once daily, and this is adjusted to a maximum of 240 mg once daily in the same manner as described for propranolol. Nadolol may have fewer side effects than propranolol because it does not cross the blood-brain barrier, although head-to-head comparisons have not been performed.

The most frequent side effects related to NSBB reported in cirrhosis are lightheadedness, fatigue, and shortness of breath. Some of them disappear with time or after dose reduction. In clinical trials, side effects have led to the discontinuation of NSBB in approximately 15% of the patients. In a study comparing patient preferences between NSBB and band ligation (an endoscopic therapy), more than half the patients favored band ligation because of NSBB-related side effects.[40] In addition, up to 15% of the patients may have relative (sinus bradycardia, insulin-dependent diabetes) or absolute contraindications to NSBB, such as obstructive pulmonary disease, heart failure, aortic valve disease, second- and third-degree atrioventricular heart block, and peripheral arterial insufficiency.

Vasopressin and analogues

Vasopressin is the most potent splanchnic vasoconstrictor available, but it has been abandoned in the therapy for portal hypertension because of its numerous side effects. It is an endogenous nanopeptide that causes vasoconstriction (splanchnic and systemic) by acting on the V1 receptors within the arterial smooth muscle. Having a short half-life, vasopressin can only be administered as a continuous intravenous infusion, and therefore it is only used in an acute setting (ie, in the management of acute variceal hemorrhage). Its continuous intravenous infusion is usually initiated at a dosage of 0.4 units/min that can be titrated up, based on the therapeutic response (cessation of bleeding) and, depending on the development of side effects, to a maximum of 0.8 to 1.0 units/min. Side effects can lead to drug withdrawal in up to 25% of patients, and can include arterial hypertension, myocardial ischemia, arrhythmias, ischemic abdominal pain, and limb gangrene.[41] Vasopressin should be used in combination with nitrates (see later discussion) to reduce side effects.

Terlipressin is a synthetic vasopressin analogue that releases its active form, lysine vasopressin, after 3 glycyl residues are cleaved by endogenous proteases. Because this is a gradual process, the hormone is released slowly, in a sustained manner, minimizing the rate and severity of side effects. It has a longer half-life than vasopressin and can thus be administered in intravenous boluses. Terlipressin is administered by intravenous boluses at a dosage of 2 mg IV every 4 hours for the first 48 hours and can be maintained for up to 5 days at a dosage of 1 mg IV every 4 hours to prevent early rebleeding.[42] The most common side effect of terlipressin is abdominal pain. Serious side effects, including peripheral and myocardial ischemia, occur in less than 3% patients.[42] Although terlipressin is preferred to vasopressin, it is currently not approved for use in the United States.

Somatostatin and analogues

Somatostatin and analogues (octreotide, vapreotide) cause splanchnic vasoconstriction not only through an inhibitory effect on the release of the vasodilator glucagon but also by a local mesenteric vasoconstrictive effect.[43] Intravenous boluses of somatostatin and octreotide cause significant transient reductions in portal pressure.[44,45] However, although a mild reduction in portal pressure is maintained with the continuous infusion of somatostatin,[44] the continuous infusion of octreotide does not result in a sustained reduction in portal pressure.[45] One of the most important effects of somatostatin and analogues is a blunting of postprandial hyperemia,[46] which is useful in the setting of gastrointestinal bleeding when blood has the same effect as food. These drugs have a short half-life and are used in a continuous intravenous infusion in the setting of acute variceal hemorrhage. However, a recent placebo-controlled small study in 18 patients showed that the monthly subcutaneous administration of long-acting octreotide was associated with a significant (26%) decrease in HVPG at 3 months,[47] suggesting that this drug could be used in the chronic treatment of portal hypertension.

Somatostatin is initiated with a single intravenous bolus dose of 250 μg IV followed by a continuous intravenous infusion of 250 μg/h, which is maintained for 5 days. Higher dosages of somatostatin (500 μg/h) have been shown to further decrease HVPG and lower mortality in a subset of patients with bleeding at endoscopy that is difficult to control.[48] Both octreotide and vapreotide are used at an initial bolus of 50 μg intravenously followed by a continuous infusion of 50 μg per hour. As with somatostatin, therapy can be maintained for 2 to 5 days.

The absence of major side effects of somatostatin and analogues represents an important advantage compared with other vasoconstrictive agents. Minor side effects include nausea, vomiting, and hyperglycemia and can occur in up to 30% of patients.[48,49] Octreotide is the only vasoconstrictor available in the United States for control of acute variceal hemorrhage, although its use in this setting is off-label.

Drugs that Act by Reducing Resistance to Blood Flow

Vasodilators such as nitrates, prazosin, clonidine, angiotensin receptor blockers (ARBs) and angiotensin-converting enzyme inhibitors have resulted in significant reductions in HVPG.[21] In studies in which these agents have been administered for 7 days or more, the median reduction in HVPG is around 17%.[21] However, these drugs not only act on the intrahepatic circulation, they also exert a vasodilatory effect on the systemic circulation, leading to arterial hypotension that is frequently symptomatic.[50,51] In several of these studies, a direct correlation has been shown between the decrease in arterial pressure and the decrease in HVPG.[50] This suggests that vasodilators decrease portal pressure mainly through a decrease in portal blood flow secondary to reflex splanchnic vasoconstriction that occurs in response to arterial hypotension. Worsening vasodilatation can also lead to a further decrease in effective arterial blood volume, with consequent aggravation of sodium retention and renal vasoconstriction. Chronic administration of prazosin has been associated with the development of salt retention, ascites, and edema,[52,53] and administration of the ARB irbesartan has been associated with a decrease in creatinine clearance.[51] Furthermore, a trial of isosorbide mononitrate (ISMN) versus placebo in the prevention of first variceal hemorrhage showed a tendency for higher rates of bleeding and late mortality in patients randomized to ISMN.[54]

The use of vasodilators alone is currently not recommended. Nevertheless, a recent meta-analysis of individual patient data from studies that used ARBs and angiotensin-converting enzyme inhibitors shows that, in patients with Child A cirrhosis, these drugs reduce portal pressure with minimal side effects; whereas deleterious effects are mostly observed in patients with decompensated cirrhosis.[55] Future studies should determine the potential of these drugs as alternatives or adjuncts to NSBB in patients with compensated cirrhosis.

Other therapies have been shown, in experimental animals, to improve nitric oxide bioavailability in the liver and to reduce portal pressure. Of these, 2 have been translated to proof-of-concept hemodynamic studies in humans with cirrhosis. One of them is NCX-1000, a nitric oxide-releasing derivative of ursodeoxycholic acid that was found to have no effect on HVPG.[56] The other is simvastatin, which leads to the post-translational upregulation of endothelial nitric oxide synthase. In a small placebo-controlled study of 20 patients, simvastatin was associated with a significant reduction in HVPG, with 32% of hemodynamic responders.[57] Simvastatin was not associated with changes in blood flow, suggesting that it decreased hepatic vascular resistance by acting as a hepatic vasodilator.

Drugs that Act by Reducing Flow and Resistance

The combination of intrahepatic vasodilators and splanchnic vasoconstrictors results in an additive portal pressure–reducing effect (see **Table 1**). This effect was first shown in a hemodynamic study performed in patients with cirrhosis in whom the addition of nitroglycerin to vasopressin led to a further reduction in HVPG, not associated with a further decrease in portal flow[58] This observation suggested that the additional reduction in HVPG induced by nitrates resulted from a decrease in intrahepatic resistance.

This effect has also been observed when ISMN or prazosin are combined with NSBB, with an HVPG reduction of around 20% to 24% with combination therapy, compared with 15% with NSBB alone.[21,59] The rate of HVPG responders with NSBB+ISMN is 44%,[13,23,25,29–35,37] a rate that is significantly higher than that observed with NSBB alone (37%) (see **Table 1**). However, these combinations are associated with more side effects, specifically fluid retention and/or symptomatic hypotension.

Carvedilol is a nonselective β-blocker with weak anti-α_1 adrenergic (vasodilator) activity and therefore acts as a combination of NSBB and vasodilator. When used at a dosage of 25 to 30 mg/d, it has been associated with a significant reduction in HVPG (16%–19%), with 46% being HVPG responders (**Table 2**), which is similar to the response rate of a combination of NSBB and ISMN.[24,60,61] However, as for other combinations of vasoconstrictors and vasodilators, carvedilol at this dosage has been associated with a decrease in mean arterial pressure, fluid retention, and a high rate of patient withdrawal.[60,62]

NATURAL HISTORY OF VARICES AND VARICEAL HEMORRHAGE

Gastroesophageal varices are present in approximately 50% of patients with cirrhosis, with a rate dependent on the severity of liver disease (42% of patients who are Child A vs 72% in Child B/C).[63] Varices develop at a rate of 7% to 8% per year[1] and the transition from small to large varices occurs at the same rate, more commonly among patients with Child B/C cirrhosis.[64] Variceal hemorrhage occurs at a rate of 5% to 15% per year depending on the presence of risk factors, with variceal size, red wale marks on varices, and advanced liver disease (Child B or C) identifying patients at a high risk of variceal hemorrhage.[65] Six-week mortality with each episode of variceal hemorrhage is still around 15% to 25% and also depends on the severity of liver disease.[66,67] Late rebleeding occurs in approximately 60% to 70% of untreated patients, usually within 1 to 2 years of the initial hemorrhage.[68]

The pharmacologic therapy for portal hypertension has been evaluated at each of the stages in the natural history of varices/variceal hemorrhage.

Preprimary Prophylaxis (Prevention of Varices)

A large multicenter RCT of timolol, a NSBB, versus placebo performed in patients with cirrhosis and portal hypertension but without varices, showed a similar rate of development of varices in both treatment groups, with a higher rate of adverse events in the timolol group.[1] Therefore, NSBB are not recommended for the prevention of varices.

Table 2
Long-term effect of carvedilol on portal pressure in studies including at least 10 patients

Study	Setting	n	Mean Dosage (mg/d)	Mean Decrease in HVPG (%)	Hemodynamic Responders (%)
Stanley 1999[60]	Mixed	10	25	16	4 (40)
Banares 2002[a,24]	Primary	24	31	19	13 (54)
Bruha 2006[61]	Mixed	36	25	⁀16	15 (42)
Total		70			32 (46)

[a] Only comparative study with propranolol using a homogenous population of patients without a history of variceal hemorrhage and a baseline HVPG of 12 mm Hg or more. Mean decrease in HVPG with propranolol was 12% and rate of responders was 23% (see **Table 1**).

Primary Prophylaxis (Prevention of First Variceal Hemorrhage)

Patients with medium/large varices are at a high risk of variceal hemorrhage and are the main subgroup of patients with cirrhosis without a previous episode of hemorrhage in whom prophylactic therapy is recommended. In this setting, NSBB have been shown to significantly reduce the risk of first variceal hemorrhage, from 24% to 15% in a median follow-up of 2 years.[41] Adding ISMN does not have an added beneficial effect in this setting, as shown in a double-blind, placebo-controlled trial.[69]

Although meta-analyses of studies comparing NSBB versus endoscopic variceal ligation (EVL) have shown a benefit for EVL, the evidence is weak, because subgroup meta-analysis of trials with adequate design and an acceptable sample size show no differences in the rate of first variceal hemorrhage between groups.[70,71] As these therapies seem equal, choice should depend on local resources, patient preferences, and co-morbidities. It is reasonable to start with NSBB (which should be administered indefinitely) because they have other advantages, such as prevention of bleeding from other portal hypertension sources (portal hypertensive gastropathy and gastric varices) and prevention of ascites (**Table 3**).[15] In patients intolerant of, or with contraindications to, NSBB, EVL should be performed.

A recent single-center RCT showed a significantly lower rate of first variceal hemorrhage with carvedilol compared with EVL (10% vs 23%),[72] without differences in mortality. The dosage of carvedilol used (12.5 mg/d) was lower than that associated with an HVPG reduction (see **Table 2**) and with complications. Larger studies are necessary to evaluate its efficacy compared with NSBB and to determine its mechanism of action.

Patients with small varices with red signs or with advanced liver disease (Child C) are at a similar risk of first hemorrhage compared to those with moderate/large varices and should be treated with NSBB, because banding may be technically more challenging in these patients (see **Table 3**).

Acute Variceal Hemorrhage

A meta-analysis of RCTs for the specific management of acute variceal hemorrhage shows that a combination of endoscopic and pharmacologic therapy is significantly better than endoscopic therapy alone.[73] There are no apparent differences among vasoconstrictors. Notably, the most frequent pharmacologic agent used in these studies was octreotide, the only vasoconstrictor currently available in the United States. Terlipressin is the only vasoconstrictor that has been shown to improve

Table 3 Pharmacologic therapy in the prevention of first variceal hemorrhage (primary prophylaxis)		
Medication	**Dosage**	**Goals**
Propranolol	Initial: 20–40 mg by mouth twice a day Maximum: 160 mg by mouth twice a day	(1) Increase until maximum tolerated OR heart rate of 50–55 beats per minute (2) Continue indefinitely. No need for follow-up EGD
Nadolol	Initial: 20–40 mg once daily Maximum: 240 mg once daily	(1) Increase until maximum OR heart rate of 50–55 beats per minute (2) Continue indefinitely. No need for follow-up EGD

EGD, esophagogastroduodenoscopy.

survival[74] and, if confirmed in RCTs using current standard therapy, it would be the preferred vasoconstrictor. Vasoconstrictor therapy should be initiated as soon as possible, even before diagnostic endoscopy, because this has been shown to improve outcomes (**Table 4**).[75] General recommendations are to maintain vasoconstrictors for 3 to 5 days because this is the time period of highest risk for rebleeding, but this has not been well validated.

Another form of pharmacologic therapy recommended in patients with variceal hemorrhage is antibiotic prophylaxis. In a meta-analysis of 5 trials, antibiotics were associated not only with a decreased risk of infection but also a decreased mortality.[76] Their effect could be related in part to a decrease in the rate of early rebleeding.[77] The preferred antibiotic is oral norfloxacin at a dosage of 400 mg twice a day for 7 days, although IV ceftriaxone at a dosage of 1 g/d is preferable in patients with severe liver disease, particularly in settings of high prevalence of quinolone-resistant organisms.[78]

Other pharmacologic therapies, such as recombinant factor VIIa, have not been shown in RCTs to be of benefit in the management of acute variceal hemorrhage.[79,80]

Secondary Prophylaxis (Prevention of Recurrent Variceal Hemorrhage)

A recent meta-analysis shows that the combination of endoscopic plus pharmacologic therapy reduces overall gastrointestinal and recurrent variceal hemorrhage in patients with cirrhosis who have recovered from an episode of variceal hemorrhage, more than either therapy alone.[81] However, the long-term (82-month) follow-up of one of these studies showed that combination pharmacologic therapy (NSBB plus ISMN) is associated with a better survival compared with EVL.[82] However, this trial did not explore a combination of EVL+NSBB. A review of data obtained from

Table 4
Pharmacologic therapy in the management of acute variceal hemorrhage

Medication	Dosage	Comments
Vasopressin + Nitroglycerin	0.4 units/min continuous IV infusion Intravenously (40 μg/min) or transdermally (10 mg in 24 h)	(1) Should always be used with nitroglycerin to avoid ischemic complications (2) Maximum duration should be 24 h at lowest effective dosage (3) Rarely used
Terlipressin	Initial 48 h: 2 mg IV every 4 h until control of bleeding Maintenance: 1 mg IV every 4 h for up to 5 d to prevent rebleeding	Unavailable in the United States
Somatostatin	Initial IV bolus: 250 μg (can be repeated in the first hour if ongoing bleeding) Maintenance: continuous IV infusion of 250–500 μg/h for 5 d	Unavailable in the United States
Octreotide	Bolus: 50 μg (can be repeated in the first hour if ongoing bleeding) Maintenance: continuous IV infusion of 50 μg/h for 5 d	Available in the United States (off-label use)
Vapreotide	Bolus: 50 μg Maintenance: continuous IV infusion of 50 μg/h for 5 d	Unavailable in the United States

Table 5		
Pharmacologic therapy in the prevention of recurrent variceal hemorrhage (secondary prophylaxis)		
Medication	Dosage	Comments
Propranolol or nadolol	Same as **Table 3**	Same as **Table 3**
Isosorbide mononitrate	Initial: 10 mg by mouth every night Maximum: 20 mg twice a day	(1) Used only in combination with an NSBB (2) Increase until maximum tolerated dose and SBP>95 mm Hg

Abbreviation: SBP, systolic blood pressure.

published secondary prophylaxis randomized trials comparing EVL alone versus EVL+NSBB,[83,84] EVL alone versus NSBB+ISMN,[31,32,85,86] as well as 3 recent studies of EVL plus combination pharmacologic therapy (NSBB+ISMN) versus combination pharmacologic therapy[34,87] or versus EVL alone[88] shows that, at equivalent follow-up times, the combination of EVL plus drugs is associated with the lowest rates of recurrent variceal hemorrhage (14%), overall gastrointestinal hemorrhage (23%), and death (17%). Therefore, the current standard of care for secondary prevention is a combination of EVL and NSBB. In patients who are not candidates or who refuse EVL, the combination of NSBB plus ISMN should be attempted, although this combination is poorly tolerated (**Table 5**).

As mentioned earlier, the lowest rates of recurrent variceal hemorrhage (approximately 10%) are observed in patients who have a hemodynamic response to pharmacologic therapy, defined as a decrease in HVPG to less than 12 mm Hg or a decrease of greater than 20% from baseline levels.[14,68] The more rational approach would be to guide therapy based on the hemodynamic response. A recent RCT compared patients with HVPG-guided pharmacotherapy (nadolol plus ISMN or prazosin) with patients on nadolol+EVL.[35] As expected, patients in the HVPG-guided pharmacotherapy arm showed higher rates of hemodynamic response; however, the rates of recurrent hemorrhage were similar between groups (26% vs 23%). Additional data from larger studies are needed to more clearly define the role of HVPG in the secondary prophylaxis of variceal hemorrhage.

REFERENCES

1. Groszmann RJ, Garcia-Tsao G, Bosch J, et al. Beta-blockers to prevent gastroesophageal varices in patients with cirrhosis. N Engl J Med 2005;353:2254–61.
2. Ripoll C, Groszmann R, Garcia-Tsao G, et al. Hepatic venous pressure gradient predicts clinical decompensation in patients with compensated cirrhosis. Gastroenterology 2007;133:481–8.
3. Bruix J, Castells A, Bosch J, et al. Surgical resection of hepatocellular carcinoma in cirrhotic patients. Prognostic value of preoperative portal pressure. Gastroenterology 1996;111:1018–22.
4. Ripoll C, Groszmann RJ, Garcia-Tsao G, et al. Hepatic venous pressure gradient predicts development of hepatocellular carcinoma independently of severity of cirrhosis. J Hepatol 2009;50:923–8.
5. Bhathal PS, Grossman HJ. Reduction of the increased portal vascular resistance of the isolated perfused cirrhotic rat liver by vasodilators. J Hepatol 1985;1:325–37.

6. Pinzani M, Gentilini P. Biology of hepatic stellate cells and their possible relevance in the pathogenesis of portal hypertension in cirrhosis. Semin Liver Dis 1999;19:397–410.

7. Wiest R, Groszmann RJ. The paradox of nitric oxide in cirrhosis and portal hypertension: too much, not enough. Hepatology 2002;35:478–91.

8. Iwakiri Y, Groszmann RJ. Vascular endothelial dysfunction in cirrhosis. J Hepatol 2007;46:927–34.

9. Sikuler E, Groszmann RJ. Interaction of flow and resistance in maintenance of portal hypertension in a rat model. Am J Physiol 1986;250:G205–12.

10. Fernandez M, Vizzutti F, Garcia-Pagan JC, et al. Anti-VEGF receptor-2 monoclonal antibody prevents portal-systemic collateral vessel formation in portal hypertensive mice. Gastroenterology 2004;126:886–94.

11. Groszmann RJ, Wongcharatrawee S. The hepatic venous pressure gradient: anything worth doing should be done right. Hepatology 2004;39:280–3.

12. Feu F, Bordas JM, Luca A, et al. Reduction of variceal pressure by propranolol: comparison of the effects on portal pressure and azygos blood flow in patients with cirrhosis. Hepatology 1993;18:1082–9.

13. Abraldes JG, Tarantino I, Turnes J, et al. Hemodynamic response to pharmacological treatment of portal hypertension and long-term prognosis of cirrhosis. Hepatology 2003;37:902–8.

14. D'Amico G, Garcia-Pagan JC, Luca A, et al. HVPG reduction and prevention of variceal bleeding in cirrhosis: a systematic review. Gastroenterology 2006;131:1611–24.

15. Villanueva C, Aracil C, Colomo A, et al. Acute hemodynamic response to beta-blockers and prediction of long-term outcome in primary prophylaxis of variceal bleeding. Gastroenterology 2009;137:119–28.

16. La Mura V, Abraldes JG, Raffa S, et al. Prognostic value of acute hemodynamic response to i.v. propranolol in patients with cirrhosis and portal hypertension. J Hepatol 2009;51:279–87.

17. Garcia-Tsao G, Bosch J, Groszmann RJ. Portal hypertension and variceal bleeding–unresolved issues. Summary of an American Association for the Study of Liver Diseases and European Association for the Study of the Liver single-topic conference. Hepatology 2008;47:1764–72.

18. Fernandez M, Mejias M, Angermayr B, et al. Inhibition of VEGF receptor-2 decreases the development of hyperdynamic splanchnic circulation and portal-systemic collateral vessels in portal hypertensive rats. J Hepatol 2005;43:98–103.

19. Mills PR, Rae AP, Farah DA, et al. Comparison of three adrenoceptor blocking agents in patients with cirrhosis and portal hypertension. Gut 1984;25:73–8.

20. Garcia-Tsao G, Grace N, Groszmann RJ, et al. Short term effects of propranolol on portal venous pressure. Hepatology 1986;6:101–6.

21. Garcia-Tsao G. Current management of the complications of cirrhosis and portal hypertension: varices and variceal hemorrhage, ascites and spontaneous bacterial peritonitis. Gastroenterology 2001;120:726–48.

22. Groszmann RJ, Bosch J, Grace N, et al. Hemodynamic events in a prospective randomized trial of propranolol vs placebo in the prevention of the first variceal hemorrhage. Gastroenterology 1990;99(5):1401–7.

23. Merkel C, Marin R, Sacerdoti D, et al. Long-term results of a clinical trial of nadolol with or without isosorbide mononitrate for primary prophylaxis of variceal bleeding in cirrhosis. Hepatology 2000;31:324–9.

24. Banares R, Moitinho E, Matilla A, et al. Randomized comparison of long-term carvedilol and propranolol administration in the treatment of portal hypertension in cirrhosis. Hepatology 2002;36:1367–73.

25. Turnes J, Garcia-Pagan JC, Abraldes JG, et al. Pharmacological reduction of portal pressure and long-term risk of first variceal bleeding in patients with cirrhosis. Am J Gastroenterol 2006;101:506–12.

26. Sharma P, Kumar A, Sharma BC, et al. Early identification of haemodynamic response to pharmacotherapy is essential for primary prophylaxis of variceal bleeding in patients with 'high-risk' varices. Aliment Pharmacol Ther 2009;30: 48–60.

27. Merkel C, Bolognesi M, Berzigotti A, et al. Clinical significance of worsening portal hypertension during long-term medical treatment in patients with cirrhosis who had been classified as early good-responders on haemodynamic criteria. J Hepatol 2010;52:45–53.

28. Feu F, Garcia-Pagan JC, Bosch J, et al. Relation between portal pressure response to pharmacotherapy and risk of recurrent variceal haemorrhage in patients with cirrhosis. Lancet 1995;346:1056–9.

29. Villanueva C, Balanzo J, Novella MT, et al. Nadolol plus isosorbide mononitrate compared with sclerotherapy for the prevention of variceal rebleeding. N Engl J Med 1996;334:1624–9.

30. McCormick PA, Patch D, Greenslade L, et al. Clinical vs hemodynamic response to drugs in portal hypertension. J Hepatol 1998;28:1015–9.

31. Villanueva C, Minana J, Ortiz J, et al. Endoscopic ligation compared with combined treatment with nadolol and isosorbide mononitrate to prevent recurrent variceal bleeding. N Engl J Med 2001;345:647–55.

32. Patch D, Goulis J, Gerunda G, et al. A randomized controlled trial of medical therapy versus endoscopic ligation for the prevention of variceal rebleeding in patients with cirrhosis. Gastroenterology 2002;123:1013–9.

33. Villanueva C, Lopez-Balaguer JM, Aracil C, et al. Maintenance of hemodynamic response to treatment for portal hypertension and influence on complications of cirrhosis. J Hepatol 2004;40:757–65.

34. Garcia-Pagan JC, Villanueva C, Albillos A, et al. Nadolol plus isosorbide mononitrate alone or associated with band ligation in the prevention of variceal rebleeding: a multicenter randomized controlled trial. Gut 2009;58: 1144–50.

35. Villanueva C, Aracil C, Colomo A, et al. Clinical trial: a randomized controlled study on prevention of variceal rebleeding comparing nadolol + ligation vs. hepatic venous pressure gradient-guided pharmacological therapy. Aliment Pharmacol Ther 2009;29:397–408.

36. Escorsell A, Bordas JM, Castaneda B, et al. Predictive value of the variceal pressure response to continued pharmacological therapy in patients with cirrhosis and portal hypertension. Hepatology 2000;31:1061–7.

37. Bureau C, Peron JM, Alric L, et al. "A La Carte" treatment of portal hypertension: adapting medical therapy to hemodynamic response for the prevention of bleeding. Hepatology 2002;36:1361–6.

38. Kroeger RJ, Groszmann RJ. Increased portal venous resistance hinders portal pressure reduction during the administration of beta-adrenergic blocking agents in a portal hypertensive model. Hepatology 1985;5:97–101.

39. Garcia-Tsao G, Sanyal AJ, Grace ND, et al. Prevention and management of gastroesophageal varices and variceal hemorrhage in cirrhosis. Hepatology 2007;46:922–38.

40. Longacre AV, Imaeda A, Garcia-Tsao G, et al. A pilot project examining the predicted preferences of patients and physicians in the primary prophylaxis of variceal hemorrhage. Hepatology 2008;47:169–76.
41. D'Amico G, Pagliaro L, Bosch J. Pharmacological treatment of portal hypertension: an evidence-based approach. Semin Liver Dis 1999;19:475–505.
42. Escorsell A, Ruiz del Arbol L, Planas R, et al. Multicenter randomized controlled trial of terlipressin versus sclerotherapy in the treatment of acute variceal bleeding: the TEST study. Hepatology 2000;32:471–6.
43. Wiest R, Tsai MH, Groszmann RJ. Octreotide potentiates PKC-dependent vasoconstrictors in portal-hypertensive and control rats. Gastroenterology 2000;120: 975–83.
44. Cirera I, Feu F, Luca A, et al. Effects of bolus injections and continuous infusions of somatostatin and placebo in patients with cirrhosis and portal hypertension. A double-blind hemodynamic investigation. Hepatology 1995;22:106–11.
45. Escorsell A, Bandi JC, Andreu V, et al. Desensitization to the effects of intravenous octreotide in cirrhotic patients with portal hypertension. Gastroenterology 2001;120:161–9.
46. Buonamico P, Sabba C, Garcia-Tsao G, et al. Octreotide blunts post-prandial splanchnic hyperemia in cirrhotic patients: a double-blind randomized echo-Doppler study. Hepatology 1995;21:134–9.
47. Spahr L, Giostra E, Frossard JL, et al. A 3-month course of long-acting repeatable octreotide (sandostatin LAR) improves portal hypertension in patients with cirrhosis: a randomized controlled study. Am J Gastroenterol 2007;102: 1397–405.
48. Moitinho E, Planas R, Banares R, et al. Multicenter randomized controlled trial comparing different schedules of somatostatin in the treatment of acute variceal bleeding. J Hepatol 2001;35:712–8.
49. Escorsell A, Bordas JM, Ruiz-del-Arbol L, et al. Randomized controlled trial of sclerotherapy versus somatostatin infusion in the prevention of early rebleeding following acute variceal hemorrhage in patients with cirrhosis. J Hepatol 1998; 29:779–88.
50. Blei AT, Garcia-Tsao G, Groszmann RJ, et al. Hemodynamic evaluation of isosorbide dinitrate in alcoholic cirrhosis: pharmacokinetic-hemodynamic interactions. Gastroenterology 1987;93:576–83.
51. Schepke M, Werner E, Biecker E, et al. Hemodynamic effects of the angiotensin II receptor antagonist irbesartan in patients with cirrhosis and portal hypertension. Gastroenterology 2001;121:389–95.
52. Albillos A, Lledo JL, Banares R, et al. Hemodynamic effects of a-adrenergic blockade with prazosin in cirrhotic patients with portal hypertension. Hepatology 1994;20:611–7.
53. Albillos A, Lledo JL, Rossi I, et al. Continuous prazosin administration in cirrhotic patients: effects on portal hemodynamics and on liver and renal function. Gastroenterology 1995;109:1257–65.
54. Garcia-Pagan JC, Villanueva C, Vila MC, et al. Isosorbide mononitrate in the prevention of first variceal bleed in patients who cannot receive beta-blockers. Gastroenterology 2001;121:908–14.
55. Tandon P, Abraldes JG, Berzigotti A, et al. Renin-angiotensin-aldosterone inhibitors in the reduction of portal pressure: a systematic review and meta-analysis. J Hepatol 2010;53:273–82.
56. Berzigotti A, Bellot P, De Gottardi A, et al. NCX-1000, a nitric oxide-releasing derivative of UDCA, does not decrease portal pressure in patients with cirrhosis: results

of a randomized, double-blind, dose-escalating study. Am J Gastroenterol 2010; 105:1094–101.

57. Abraldes JG, Albillos A, Banares R, et al. Simvastatin lowers portal pressure in patients with cirrhosis and portal hypertension: a randomized controlled trial. Gastroenterology 2009;136:1651–8.

58. Groszmann RJ, Kravetz D, Bosch J, et al. Nitroglycerin improves the hemodynamic response to vasopressin in portal hypertension. Hepatology 1982;2:757–62.

59. Albillos A, Garcia-Pagan JC, Iborra J, et al. Propranolol plus prazosin compared with propranolol plus isosorbide-5-mononitrate in the treatment of portal hypertension. Gastroenterology 1998;115:116–23.

60. Stanley AJ, Therapondos G, Helmy A, et al. Acute and chronic haemodynamic and renal effects of carvedilol in patients with cirrhosis. J Hepatol 1999;30: 479–84.

61. Bruha R, Vitek L, Petrtyl J, et al. Effect of carvedilol on portal hypertension depends on the degree of endothelial activation and inflammatory changes. Scand J Gastroenterol 2006;41:1454–63.

62. Bañares R, Moitinho E, Piqueras B, et al. Carvedilol, a new nonselective beta-blocker with intrinsic anti-alpha$_1$-adrenergic activity, has a greater portal hypotensive effect than propranolol in patients with cirrhosis. Hepatology 1999;30:79–83.

63. Kovalak M, Lake J, Mattek N, et al. Endoscopic screening for varices in cirrhotic patients: data from a national endoscopic database. Gastrointest Endosc 2007; 65:82–8.

64. Merli M, Nicolini G, Angeloni S, et al. Incidence and natural history of small esophageal varices in cirrhotic patients. J Hepatol 2003;38:266–72.

65. North Italian Endoscopic Club for the Study and Treatment of Esophageal Varices. Prediction of the first variceal hemorrhage in patients with cirrhosis of the liver and esophageal varices. A prospective multicenter study. N Engl J Med 1988;319:983–9.

66. Abraldes JG, Villanueva C, Banares R, et al. Hepatic venous pressure gradient and prognosis in patients with acute variceal bleeding treated with pharmacologic and endoscopic therapy. J Hepatol 2008;48:229–36.

67. Augustin S, Muntaner L, Altamirano JT, et al. Predicting early mortality after acute variceal hemorrhage based on classification and regression tree analysis. Clin Gastroenterol Hepatol 2009;7:1347–54.

68. Bosch J, Garcia-Pagan JC. Prevention of variceal rebleeding. Lancet 2003;361: 952–4.

69. Garcia-Pagan JC, Morillas R, Banares R, et al. Propranolol plus placebo versus propranolol plus isosorbide-5-mononitrate in the prevention of a first variceal bleed: a double-blind RCT. Hepatology 2003;37:1260–6.

70. Gluud LL, Klingenberg S, Nikolova D, et al. Banding ligation versus beta-blockers as primary prophylaxis in esophageal varices: systematic review of randomized trials. Am J Gastroenterol 2007;102:2842–8.

71. Bosch J, Berzigotti A, Garcia-Pagan JC, et al. The management of portal hypertension: rational basis, available treatments and future options. J Hepatol 2008; 48(Suppl 1):S68–92.

72. Tripathi D, Ferguson JW, Kochar N, et al. Randomized controlled trial of carvedilol versus variceal band ligation for the prevention of the first variceal bleed. Hepatology 2009;50:825–33.

73. Banares R, Albillos A, Rincon D, et al. Endoscopic treatment versus endoscopic plus pharmacologic treatment for acute variceal bleeding: a meta-analysis. Hepatology 2002;35:609–15.

74. Ioannou G, Doust J, Rockey DC. Terlipressin for acute esophageal variceal hemorrhage. Cochrane Database Syst Rev 2001;(1):CD002147.
75. Levacher S, Letoumelin P, Pateron D, et al. Early administration of terlipressin plus glyceryl trinitrate to control active upper gastrointestinal bleeding in cirrhotic patients. Lancet 1995;346:865–8.
76. Bernard B, Grange JD, Khac EN, et al. Antibiotic prophylaxis for the prevention of bacterial infections in cirrhotic patients with gastrointestinal bleeding: a meta-analysis. Hepatology 1999;29:1655–61.
77. Hou MC, Lin HC, Liu TT, et al. Antibiotic prophylaxis after endoscopic therapy prevents rebleeding in acute variceal hemorrhage: a randomized trial. Hepatology 2004;39:746–53.
78. Fernandez J, Ruiz d A, Gomez C, et al. Norfloxacin vs ceftriaxone in the prophylaxis of infections in patients with advanced cirrhosis and hemorrhage. Gastroenterology 2006;131:1049–56.
79. Bosch J, Thabut D, Bendtsen F, et al. Recombinant factor VIIa for upper gastrointestinal bleeding in patients with cirrhosis: a randomized, double-blind trial. Gastroenterology 2004;127:1123–30.
80. Bosch J, Thabut D, Albillos A, et al. Recombinant factor VIIa for variceal bleeding in patients with advanced cirrhosis: a randomized, controlled trial. Hepatology 2008;47:1604–14.
81. Gonzalez R, Zamora J, Gomez-Camarero J, et al. Meta-analysis: combination endoscopic and drug therapy to prevent variceal rebleeding in cirrhosis. Ann Intern Med 2008;149:109–22.
82. Lo GH, Chen WC, Lin CK, et al. Improved survival in patients receiving medical therapy as compared with banding ligation for the prevention of esophageal variceal rebleeding. Hepatology 2008;48:580–7.
83. Lo GH, Lai KH, Cheng JS, et al. Endoscopic variceal ligation plus nadolol and sucralfate compared with ligation alone for the prevention of variceal rebleeding: a prospective, randomized trial. Hepatology 2000;32:461–5.
84. de la Pena J, Brullet E, Sanchez-Hernandez E, et al. Variceal ligation plus nadolol compared with ligation for prophylaxis of variceal rebleeding: a multicenter trial. Hepatology 2005;41:572–8.
85. Lo GH, Chen WC, Chen MH, et al. A prospective, randomized trial of endoscopic variceal ligation versus nadolol and isosorbide mononitrate for the prevention of esophageal variceal rebleeding. Gastroenterology 2002;123:728–34.
86. Romero G, Kravetz D, Argonz J, et al. Comparative study between nadolol and 5-isosorbide mononitrate vs. endoscopic band ligation plus sclerotherapy in the prevention of variceal rebleeding in cirrhotic patients: a randomized controlled trial. Aliment Pharmacol Ther 2006;24:601–11.
87. Lo GH, Chen WC, Chan HH, et al. A randomized, controlled trial of banding ligation plus drug therapy versus drug therapy alone in the prevention of esophageal variceal rebleeding. J Gastroenterol Hepatol 2009;24:982–7.
88. Kumar A, Jha SK, Sharma P, et al. Addition of propranolol and isosorbide mononitrate to endoscopic variceal ligation does not reduce variceal rebleeding incidence. Gastroenterology 2009;137:892–901.

Therapeutic Potential of Peroxisome Proliferator-Activated Receptors in Chronic Inflammation and Colorectal Cancer

Dingzhi Wang, PhD[a], Raymond N. DuBois, MD, PhD[b],*

KEYWORDS

- Peroxisome proliferator–activated receptor
- Chronic inflammation • Inflammatory bowel disease
- Colorectal cancer

The recognition of chronic inflammation caused by infections or autoimmune diseases as the seventh trait of cancer has highlighted the contribution of inflamed stroma to tumor initiation, growth, and metastasis. Epidemiologic studies indicate that chronic inflammation is clearly associated with increased risk of cancers in several instances, including esophageal, gastric, hepatic, pancreatic, and colorectal cancers (CRC). For example, it has been long known that patients with persistent hepatitis B infection, *Helicobacter pylori* infection, or an immune disorder, such as inflammatory bowel disease (IBD), have a higher risk for developing liver or gastrointestinal tract cancer. It has been estimated that chronic inflammation contributes to the development of approximately 15% of malignancies worldwide.[1] The best evidence for the link between inflammation and tumor progression comes from recent epidemiologic studies and clinical trials that have shown that long-term use of nonsteroidal antiinflammatory drugs (NSAIDs) reduce the relative risk of developing CRC by 40% to 50%.[2]

This work is supported, in part, by the National Institutes of Health Grants RO1DK 62112, P01-CA-77839, R37-DK47297, and P30 CA068485 (R.N.D.). R.N.D. (R37-DK47297) is the recipient of an NIH MERIT award. The authors also thank the National Colorectal Cancer Research Alliance (NCCRA) for their generous support (R.N.D.).
Financial disclosures and conflicts of interest: The authors have nothing to disclose.

[a] Department of Cancer Biology, The University of Texas MD Anderson Cancer Center, Unit 1014; S7.8316A, 6767 Bertner Avenue, Houston, TX 77030, USA
[b] Department of Gastrointestinal Medical Oncology and Cancer Biology, The University of Texas MD Anderson Cancer Center, Unit 118; 1515 Holcombe Boulevard, Houston, TX 77030-4009, USA
* Corresponding author.
E-mail address: rdubois@mdanderson.org

Gastroenterol Clin N Am 39 (2010) 697–707
doi:10.1016/j.gtc.2010.08.014
0889-8553/10/$ – see front matter © 2010 Elsevier Inc. All rights reserved.

The gastrointestinal mucosa forms a complex semipermeable barrier between the host and the largest source of foreign antigens. The mucosal barrier consists of epithelial cell junctions and the underlying stromal elements including immune cells. An abnormal mucosal immune response to bacteria, which make up the intestinal flora, is thought to result in chronic inflammation and the development of IBD. IBD, with its two clinical manifestations of Crohn disease (CD) and ulcerative colitis (UC), is a chronic inflammatory disorder of the gastrointestinal tract. Chronic IBD (especially pancolitis) significantly increases the risk of developing CRC.[3] The observation that 5-aminosalicylic acid (5-ASA), currently used in the treatment of UC, suppresses the development of colitis-associated cancer in an animal model supports this notion.[4]

A large body of evidence indicates that genetic mutations, epigenetic changes, chronic inflammation, diet, and lifestyle are risk factors for cancer.[5–7] Similar to other solid tumors, CRC is a heterogeneous disease with at least 3 major forms: hereditary, sporadic, and colitis-associated CRCs. Patients with familial adenomatous polyposis (FAP), caused by a germline mutation in 1 allele of the tumor suppressor gene *adenomatous polyposis coli* (*APC*), have a near 100% risk of developing CRC by the age of 40 years, if untreated. Somatic loss of *APC* function occurs in about 85% of sporadic colorectal adenomas and carcinomas.[8–10] Hereditary nonpolyposis CRC, which is caused by inherited mutations in genes for DNA mismatch repair, such as *MLH1*, *MSH2*, and *MSH6*, is responsible for approximately 2% to 7% of all diagnosed cases of CRC. The average age at which patients with this syndrome develop cancer is around 44 years as compared with 64 years in the general population. Together with FAP and hereditary nonpolyposis CRC, IBD is among the top 3 high-risk conditions for CRC; therefore, patients with IBD face an increased lifetime risk for developing CRC. Compared with sporadic CRC, colitis-associated CRC affects individuals at a younger age.

Peroxisome proliferator–activated receptors (PPARs), which were initially identified as mediators of the peroxisome proliferators in the early 1990s,[11] belong to the nuclear hormone receptor superfamily and are also ligand-dependent transcription factors. PPARs play a central role in regulating the storage and catabolism of dietary fats via complex metabolic pathways, including fatty acid oxidation and lipogenesis.[12] To date, 3 mammalian PPARs have been identified and are referred to as PPARα (NR1C1), PPARδ/β (NR1C2), and PPARγ (NR1C3). Each PPAR isotype displays a tissue-selective expression pattern. PPARα and PPARγ are predominantly present in the liver and adipose tissue, respectively, whereas PPARδ is expressed in diverse tissues,[13] and its expression in the gastrointestinal tract is very high compared with that in other tissues.[14] As ligand-dependent transcription factors, transcriptional activation by PPARs depends on ligand binding and the interaction of coregulators. PPAR ligands are chemically unrelated molecules, including a variety of fatty acids, fatty acid derivatives, and steroids as well as synthetic compounds. Polyunsaturated fatty acids activate all 3 PPAR isotypes with relatively low affinity.[15] The endogenous fatty acid derivatives, which are mainly converted by cyclooxygenase (COX) and lipoxygenase enzymes, selectively bind and activate each PPAR isotype. For example, 15-deoxy-Δ^{12},Δ^{14}prostaglandin (PG) J_2 (15dPGJ$_2$), a dehydration product of PGD$_2$, is a natural ligand for PPARγ,[16,17] whereas PGI$_2$ can transactivate PPARδ.[18,19]

It is well established that modulation of PPAR activity maintains cellular and whole-body glucose and lipid homeostasis. Hence, great efforts have been made to develop drugs targeting these receptors. For example, PPARγ synthetic agonists, such as troglitazone, rosiglitazone, and pioglitazone, are clinically used for the therapy for non–insulin-dependent diabetes mellitus. The antiatherosclerotic and hypolipidemic agents including fenofibrate and gemfibrozil are PPARα synthetic agonists that induce hepatic lipid uptake and catabolism. Genetic and pharmacologic studies have also revealed that PPARδ agonists are potential drugs for use in the treatment of dyslipidemias, obesity, and insulin resistance.[20–23] Therefore, at present, the PPARδ agonist (GW501516) is in phase 3 clinical trials for the evaluation of the treatment of patients with hyperlipidemias and obesity. In addition to modulation of lipid homeostasis and energy balance, PPARs have emerged as essential molecules in the pathogenesis of IBD and CRC.

PPARS AND IBD

The currently available therapies for IBD include 5-ASA, corticosteroids, antibiotics, immune modulators, and immunosuppressive agents such as azathioprine, 6-mercaptopurine, and cyclosporine. Corticosteroids and immunosuppressive agents are associated with significant risks of unwanted side effects, and not all patients respond to these medications. 5-ASA agents are generally safe but induce remission only in approximately 50% of patients with UC.[24] It is, therefore, essential to develop newer therapeutic interventions for patients with IBD. A growing body of evidence indicates that PPARα and PPARγ have an antiinflammatory effect on IBD, and the agonists of these 2 receptors might serve as a new class of effective therapeutic agents for IBD. The role of PPARδ in IBD remains ambiguous and deserves significant attention, and future research must be directed to better understand the role of PPARs in regulating chronic inflammation in IBD.

PPARα

PPARα is highly expressed in mouse colonic epithelial cells facing the intestinal lumen,[25] and its expression is induced by glucocorticoids (GCs).[26] Subsequent studies have further demonstrated that PPARα mediates the antiinflammatory effects of GC in a mouse model of chemically induced colitis.[27] In this study, treatment with dexamethasone, a potent synthetic member of the GC class of steroid drugs, suppressed the formation of dinitrobenzene sulfuric acid (DNBS)–induced colitis in wild-type mice but not in PPARα knockout mice. Consistent with these results, the deletion of PPARα promoted the severity of colitis in DNBS-treated mice, whereas activation of PPARα by its agonist significantly reduced colonic inflammation in this mouse model.[28] However, there is no report thus far on the precise role of PPARα in genetic models of IBD (transgenic and knockout models).

PPARγ

Although PPARγ is predominantly present in the liver and adipose tissue, it is also expressed in the intestinal epithelium, immune cells, and adipocytes. However, patients with UC, but not those with CD, show decreased PPARγ levels in colonic epithelial cells compared with normal controls.[29] This observation raises the hypothesis that microbe-host interactions, chronic inflammation, and/or genetic predisposition may lead to low PPARγ levels in colonic epithelial cells, which in turn may result in unrestrained inflammation. Several lines of evidence support the notion that PPARγ may serve as a new therapeutic target in IBD. In mouse models of chemically induced colitis, 5-ASA treatment had a beneficial effect on colitis only in wild-type mice and not in heterozygous PPARγ$^{+/-}$ mice, demonstrating that PPARγ mediates the antiinflammatory effect of 5-ASA.[30] Furthermore, treatment with a PPARγ ligand, thiazolidinedione, markedly reduced colonic inflammation in mouse models of chemically induced colitis[31,32] and interleukin (IL)-10 deficient mice (a genetic model of colitis),[33] suggesting that activation of PPARγ suppresses inflammation in IBD.

Because PPARγ is expressed in intestinal epithelial cells, macrophages, and T and B lymphocytes, it is critical to understand the contribution of PPARγ present in each of these cell types to this protection. The results from 2 studies showed that the disruption of PPARγ in colonic epithelial cells worsened colonic inflammatory lesions in dextran sulfate sodium (DSS)–treated mice, indicating that PPARγ expression in epithelial cells is required for the prevention of experimental IBD.[34,35] Similarly, mice with deficiency of PPARγ in CD4 T lymphocytes are more sensitive to trinitrobenzene sulfonic acid–induced colitis because the deficiency of PPARγ in regulatory T cells impaired their ability to prevent effector CD4 T lymphocyte–induced colitis.[36] Moreover, mice with a targeted disruption of PPARγ in macrophages displayed an increased susceptibility to DSS-induced colitis compared with wild-type littermates, demonstrating that PPARγ is required for macrophage-mediated protection against colitis.[37] Consistent with these results, an increase in PPARγ expression by adenovirus-mediated gene transfer attenuated colonic inflammation induced by DSS in mice.[38] In addition, a recent study showed that the antiinflammatory effects of PPARγ on IBD are via maintenance of innate antimicrobial immunity in the mouse colon.[39] The results from 1 randomized placebo-controlled trial and 1 open-label trial showed that a PPARγ agonist, rosiglitazone, has therapeutic efficacy in humans with UC.[40,41] Collectively, all of these studies support a rationale to develop PPARγ agonists as potential therapeutic and prophylactic agents against IBD.

PPARδ

Little is known about the role of PPARδ in IBD, and the results from 2 mouse models of IBD are controversial. Deletion of PPARδ significantly exacerbated colitis, whereas treatment with a PPARδ agonist did not affect the clinical symptoms in the DSS-treated mouse model.[42] This study implies that PPARδ, like PPARγ, exerts antiinflammatory effects in IBD via a ligand-independent mechanism. In contrast with this observation, administration of a PPARδ agonist caused enhanced colitis in IL-10–deficient mice (a genetic model of colitis), suggesting that PPARδ has a proinflammatory effect.[43] Therefore, further studies are necessary to clarify the biologic functions of PPARδ in the modulation of IBD.

PPARS AND CRC

In addition to these metabolic and inflammatory properties, the roles of PPARs in CRC progression have been extensively investigated. PPARs can function as either tumor suppressors or accelerators, suggesting that these receptors are potential candidates as drug targets for cancer prevention and treatment.

PPARα

Less is known about the role of PPARα in human cancer, although long-term administration of a PPARα agonist induces the development of hepatocarcinomas in mice but not in PPARα-null animals, conclusively demonstrating that PPARα mediates these effects in promoting liver cancer.[44] In spite of the fact that activation of PPARα by exogenous agonists generally causes inhibition of tumor cell growth in cell lines derived from CRC, melanoma, and glial brain tumors,[45–47] the physiologic significance of PPARα in the regulation of CRC progression is also less well characterized than that of PPARγ and PPARδ.

PPARγ

Because of the elevated expression of PPARγ in CRC[48] and its involvement in regulating cellular differentiation, PPARγ has become a point of interest in CRC studies. However, studies of PPARγ mutation in human colon tumor samples and CRC cell lines have produced controversial results. One study has shown that 8% of the patients with primary human CRCs had a loss-of-function mutation in 1 allele of the PPARγ gene.[49] Recent data revealed that a Pro12Ala polymorphism in the *PPARγ* gene is associated with an increased risk of CRC.[50,51] These results suggest a putative role for this receptor as a tumor suppressor. In contrast, another study showed that the mutant PPARγ gene was not detected in human colon carcinoma samples or CRC cell lines, suggesting that PPARγ mutations in human CRC may be a rare event.[52]

It is well established in numerous in vitro studies that activation of PPARγ results in growth arrest of colon carcinoma cells through induction of cell cycle arrest or/and apoptosis. However, the effect of PPARγ on CRC progression in vivo is controversial because of conflicting results from different mouse models of colon cancer. Although PPARγ agonists inhibit colorectal carcinogenesis in xenograft models and azoxymethane (AOM)-induced colon cancer model,[53,54] these drugs are reported to have either tumor-promoting or tumor-inhibiting effects in a mouse model of FAP, the *Apc^Min/+* mouse. Multiple studies showed that administration of PPARγ agonists significantly increases the number of colon adenomas in the *Apc^Min/+* [55–57] and even in wild-type C57BL/6 mice.[58] However, other studies showed that treatment of 2 different *Apc* mutant models (*Apc^Min/+* and *Apc^Δ1309*) with a PPARγ agonist pioglitazone reduced the polyp number in small and large intestines in a dose-dependent manner.[59,60] These divergent effects of PPARγ might be related to drug doses and bioavailability and/or the animal models that are used. These paradoxic observations seem to have been resolved by genetic studies, showing that the heterozygous disruption of PPARγ is sufficient to increase tumor numbers in AOM-treated mice and that intestinal-specific PPARγ knockout promotes tumor growth in *Apc^Min/+* mice.[61,62] Thus, genetic evidence supports the hypothesis that PPARγ serves as a tumor suppressor in CRC. In addition, a combined treatment of mice with a selective COX-2 inhibitor and a PPARγ agonist significantly inhibited the incidence and multiplicity of inflammation-associated colonic adenocarcinoma induced by AOM or DSS.[63] A retrospective cohort study revealed that treatment of diabetic patients with a PPARγ agonist (thiazolidinedione) exhibited a mild trend toward risk reduction of CRC, although this difference did not reach statistical significance.[64] Collectively, these findings further support the rationale of developing PPARγ agonists as antitumor agents.

PPARδ

The role of PPARδ in colorectal carcinogenesis is more controversial than that of PPARγ. The first evidence linking PPARδ to carcinogenesis actually came from studies on gastrointestinal cancer. PPARδ was identified as a direct transcriptional target of APC/β-catenin/Tcf pathway and as a repression target of NSAIDs.[65,66] A large case-control study showed that the protective effect of NSAIDs against colorectal adenomas was modulated by a polymorphism in the *PPAR* gene.[67] Moreover, COX-2-derived PGI_2 directly transactivates PPARδ,[18] and COX-2-derived PGE_2 indirectly induces PPARδ activation in CRC, hepatocellular carcinoma, and cholangiocarcinoma cells.[68–70] In addition, PPARδ expression and activity are also induced by oncogenic K-Ras.[71] These studies indicate that PPARδ is a focal point of crosstalk between oncogenic signaling pathways.

Similar to PPARγ, investigation of PPARδ expression in human and mouse colonic tumor samples and CRC cell lines generated controversial results. Some reports showed that PPARδ is elevated in most human CRCs and in tumors arising in the $Apc^{Min/+}$ mice and AOM-treated rats,[18,65] in agreement with the observations that activation of the β-catenin/Tcf pathway by APC mutation or K-Ras upregulates PPARδ expression. PPARδ proteins are accumulated only in human CRC cells with highly malignant morphology.[72] Downregulation of PPARδ is correlated with antitumor effects of dietary fish oil and pectin in rats treated with radiation and AOM.[73] However, other reports showed that PPARδ expression is lower in human cancer tissues and adenomas from the $Apc^{Min/+}$ mice than in normal control tissues.[74,75]

In a murine xenograft cancer model, the disruption of both PPARδ alleles by deletion of its exons 4 and 6 in human HCT116 colon carcinoma cells decreased tumorigenicity, suggesting that activation of PPARδ promotes tumor growth.[76] To further determine whether PPARδ attenuates or promotes intestinal tumor growth, 3 mouse models of CRC were used, including AOM-treated, $Apc^{Min/+}$, and Mlh-null mice. Mlh is a DNA mismatch repair gene that is involved in hereditary nonpolyposis CRC. Conflicting data were obtained from studies in AOM-treated and $Apc^{Min/+}$ mice. For example, activation of PPARδ by a selective synthetic PPARδ agonist (GW501516) or a PPARδ endogenous activator (PGE_2) accelerated intestinal adenoma growth in $Apc^{Min/+}$ mice by promoting tumor cell survival.[68,77] In contrast, another PPARδ ligand (GW0742) inhibited colon carcinogenesis in AOM-treated mice but promoted small intestinal polyp growth in $Apc^{Min/+}$ mice.[78] It is not clear whether PPARδ mediates the effects of GW0742 in $Apc^{Min/+}$ mice in this study. A genetic study showed that loss of PPARδ by deletion of its exons 4 and 5 attenuated small and large intestinal adenoma growth and demonstrated that PPARδ mediated the tumor-promoting effects of the PPARδ ligand (GW501516) and PGE_2 in $Apc^{Min/+}$ mice.[68,79] In a recent study with a tissue-specific deletion of PPARδ exon 4 in the colon, loss of PPARd inhibited colonic carcinogenesis in AOM-treated mice,[80] further confirming the notion that PPARδ serves as a tumor accelerator. On the other hand, several other studies have shown different results when using PPARδ mutant mice generated by germline deletion of PPARδ exon 8. Deletion of PPARδ exon 8 enhances polyp growth in $Apc^{Min/+}$ and AOM-treated mice in the absence of exogenous PPARδ stimulation.[75,81] In Mlh-null mice, no significant differences are evident in the number and size of intestinal adenomas between wild-type and PPARδ mutant mice (deletion of PPARδ exon 8).[75] The conflicting results regarding the effect of PPARδ on intestinal tumorigenesis in $Apc^{Min/+}$ and AOM-treated mice could be attributed to differences in the specific targeting strategy used to delete PPARδ. Deletion of PPARδ exon 4 and/or 5, which encode an essential portion of the DNA binding domain, is thought to disrupt PPARδ's function as a nuclear transcription factor and inhibit tumorigenesis. The deletion of exon 8, the last PPARδ exon, is postulated to generate a hypomorphic allele, which retains some aporeceptor function. Indeed, the observation that the high rates of embryonic mortality and abnormal placental development occurred in mice in which PPARδ exons 4 and 5 were deleted but not in mice in which PPARδ exon 8 was deleted supports this hypothesis.[82,83] Taken together, not enough evidence is available to establish whether PPARδ has pro- or anti-tumorigenic effect on CRC progression, and the role of PPARδ in cancer biology remains unclear.

SUMMARY

Emerging evidence indicates that PPARγ suppresses inflammation in IBD and tumor growth in CRC. In contrast to PPARγ, conflicting results have emerged regarding the role of PPARδ in IBD and colon carcinogenesis. Therefore, further investigation is warranted before considering modulation of PPARδ as an effective therapy for chemoprevention and treatment of IBD and CRC.

REFERENCES

1. Kuper H, Adami HO, Trichopoulos D. Infections as a major preventable cause of human cancer. J Intern Med 2000;248(3):171–83.
2. Smalley WE, DuBois RN. Colorectal cancer and nonsteroidal anti-inflammatory drugs. Adv Pharmacol 1997;39:1–20.
3. Lewis JD, Deren JJ, Lichtenstein GR. Cancer risk in patients with inflammatory bowel disease. Gastroenterol Clin North Am 1999;28(2):459–77, x.
4. Ikeda I, Tomimoto A, Wada K, et al. 5-aminosalicylic acid given in the remission stage of colitis suppresses colitis-associated cancer in a mouse colitis model. Clin Cancer Res 2007;13(21):6527–31.
5. Vogelstein B, Kinzler KW. Cancer genes and the pathways they control. Nat Med 2004;10(8):789–99.
6. Ting AH, McGarvey KM, Baylin SB. The cancer epigenome–components and functional correlates. Genes Dev 2006;20(23):3215–31.
7. Woutersen RA, Appel MJ, van Garderen-Hoetmer A, et al. Dietary fat and carcinogenesis. Mutat Res 1999;443(1–2):111–27.
8. Powell SM, Zilz N, Beazer-Barclay Y, et al. APC mutations occur early during colorectal tumorigenesis. Nature 1992;359(6392):235–7.
9. Jen J, Powell SM, Papadopoulos N, et al. Molecular determinants of dysplasia in colorectal lesions. Cancer Res 1994;54(21):5523–6.
10. Smith AJ, Stern HS, Penner M, et al. Somatic APC and K-ras codon 12 mutations in aberrant crypt foci from human colons. Cancer Res 1994;54(21):5527–30.
11. Issemann I, Green S. Activation of a member of the steroid hormone receptor superfamily by peroxisome proliferators. Nature 1990;347(6294):645–50.
12. Berger JP, Akiyama TE, Meinke PT. PPARs: therapeutic targets for metabolic disease. Trends Pharmacol Sci 2005;26(5):244–51.
13. Michalik L, Desvergne B, Wahli W. Peroxisome-proliferator-activated receptors and cancers: complex stories. Nat Rev Cancer 2004;4(1):61–70.
14. Higashiyama H, Billin AN, Okamoto Y, et al. Expression profiling of peroxisome proliferator-activated receptor-delta (PPAR-delta) in mouse tissues using tissue microarray. Histochem Cell Biol 2007;127(5):485–94.
15. Kersten S, Wahli W. Peroxisome proliferator activated receptor agonists. EXS 2000;89:141–51.
16. Forman BM, Tontonoz P, Chen J, et al. 15-Deoxy-delta 12, 14-prostaglandin J2 is a ligand for the adipocyte determination factor PPAR gamma. Cell 1995;83(5):803–12.
17. Kliewer SA, Lenhard JM, Willson TM, et al. A prostaglandin J2 metabolite binds peroxisome proliferator-activated receptor gamma and promotes adipocyte differentiation. Cell 1995;83(5):813–9.
18. Gupta RA, Tan J, Krause WF, et al. Prostacyclin-mediated activation of peroxisome proliferator-activated receptor delta in colorectal cancer. Proc Natl Acad Sci U S A 2000;97(24):13275–80.
19. Forman BM, Chen J, Evans RM. Hypolipidemic drugs, polyunsaturated fatty acids, and eicosanoids are ligands for peroxisome proliferator-activated receptors alpha and delta. Proc Natl Acad Sci U S A 1997;94(9):4312–7.

20. Wang YX, Lee CH, Tiep S, et al. Peroxisome-proliferator-activated receptor delta activates fat metabolism to prevent obesity. Cell 2003;113(2):159–70.

21. Tanaka T, Yamamoto J, Iwasaki S, et al. Activation of peroxisome proliferator-activated receptor delta induces fatty acid beta-oxidation in skeletal muscle and attenuates metabolic syndrome. Proc Natl Acad Sci U S A 2003;100(26): 15924–9.

22. Oliver WR Jr, Shenk JL, Snaith MR, et al. A selective peroxisome proliferator-activated receptor delta agonist promotes reverse cholesterol transport. Proc Natl Acad Sci U S A 2001;98(9):5306–11.

23. Evans RM, Barish GD, Wang YX. PPARs and the complex journey to obesity. Nat Med 2004;10(4):355–61.

24. Sutherland LR, May GR, Shaffer EA. Sulfasalazine revisited: a meta-analysis of 5-aminosalicylic acid in the treatment of ulcerative colitis. Ann Intern Med 1993; 118(7):540–9.

25. Mansen A, Guardiola-Diaz H, Rafter J, et al. Expression of the peroxisome proliferator-activated receptor (PPAR) in the mouse colonic mucosa. Biochem Biophys Res Commun 1996;222(3):844–51.

26. Bernal-Mizrachi C, Xiaozhong L, Yin L, et al. An afferent vagal nerve pathway links hepatic PPARalpha activation to glucocorticoid-induced insulin resistance and hypertension. Cell Metab 2007;5(2):91–102.

27. Riccardi L, Mazzon E, Bruscoli S, et al. Peroxisome proliferator-activated receptor-alpha modulates the anti-inflammatory effect of glucocorticoids in a model of inflammatory bowel disease in mice. Shock 2009;31(3):308–16.

28. Cuzzocrea S, Di Paola R, Mazzon E, et al. Role of endogenous and exogenous ligands for the peroxisome proliferators activated receptors alpha (PPAR-alpha) in the development of inflammatory bowel disease in mice. Lab Invest 2004; 84(12):1643–54.

29. Dubuquoy L, Jansson EA, Deeb S, et al. Impaired expression of peroxisome proliferator-activated receptor gamma in ulcerative colitis. Gastroenterology 2003; 124(5):1265–76.

30. Rousseaux C, Lefebvre B, Dubuquoy L, et al. Intestinal antiinflammatory effect of 5-aminosalicylic acid is dependent on peroxisome proliferator-activated receptor-gamma. J Exp Med 2005;201(8):1205–15.

31. Su CG, Wen X, Bailey ST, et al. A novel therapy for colitis utilizing PPAR-gamma ligands to inhibit the epithelial inflammatory response. J Clin Invest 1999;104(4): 383–9.

32. Dubuquoy L, Bourdon C, Peuchmaur M, et al. [Peroxisome proliferator-activated receptor (PPAR) gamma: a new target for the treatment of inflammatory bowel disease]. Gastroenterol Clin Biol 2000;24(8–9):719–24 [in French].

33. Lytle C, Tod TJ, Vo KT, et al. The peroxisome proliferator-activated receptor gamma ligand rosiglitazone delays the onset of inflammatory bowel disease in mice with interleukin 10 deficiency. Inflamm Bowel Dis 2005;11(3):231–43.

34. Adachi M, Kurotani R, Morimura K, et al. Peroxisome proliferator activated receptor gamma in colonic epithelial cells protects against experimental inflammatory bowel disease. Gut 2006;55(8):1104–13.

35. Mohapatra SK, Guri AJ, Climent M, et al. Immunoregulatory actions of epithelial cell PPAR gamma at the colonic mucosa of mice with experimental inflammatory bowel disease. PLoS One 2010;5(4):e10215.

36. Hontecillas R, Bassaganya-Riera J. Peroxisome proliferator-activated receptor gamma is required for regulatory CD4 + T cell-mediated protection against colitis. J Immunol 2007;178(5):2940–9.

37. Shah YM, Morimura K, Gonzalez FJ. Expression of peroxisome proliferator-activated receptor-gamma in macrophage suppresses experimentally induced colitis. Am J Physiol Gastrointest Liver Physiol 2007;292(2):G657–66.
38. Katayama K, Wada K, Nakajima A, et al. A novel PPAR gamma gene therapy to control inflammation associated with inflammatory bowel disease in a murine model. Gastroenterology 2003;124(5):1315–24.
39. Peyrin-Biroulet L, Beisner J, Wang G, et al. Peroxisome proliferator-activated receptor gamma activation is required for maintenance of innate antimicrobial immunity in the colon. Proc Natl Acad Sci U S A 2010;107(19):8772–7.
40. Lewis JD, Lichtenstein GR, Deren JJ, et al. Rosiglitazone for active ulcerative colitis: a randomized placebo-controlled trial. Gastroenterology 2008;134(3): 688–95.
41. Lewis JD, Lichtenstein GR, Stein RB, et al. An open-label trial of the PPAR-gamma ligand rosiglitazone for active ulcerative colitis. Am J Gastroenterol 2001;96(12): 3323–8.
42. Hollingshead HE, Morimura K, Adachi M, et al. PPARbeta/delta protects against experimental colitis through a ligand-independent mechanism. Dig Dis Sci 2007; 52(11):2912–9.
43. Lee JW, Bajwa PJ, Carson MJ, et al. Fenofibrate represses interleukin-17 and interferon-gamma expression and improves colitis in interleukin-10-deficient mice. Gastroenterology 2007;133(1):108–23.
44. Peters JM, Cattley RC, Gonzalez FJ. Role of PPAR alpha in the mechanism of action of the nongenotoxic carcinogen and peroxisome proliferator Wy-14,643. Carcinogenesis 1997;18(11):2029–33.
45. Grabacka M, Plonka PM, Urbanska K, et al. Peroxisome proliferator-activated receptor alpha activation decreases metastatic potential of melanoma cells in vitro via down-regulation of Akt. Clin Cancer Res 2006;12(10):3028–36.
46. Strakova N, Ehrmann J, Bartos J, et al. Peroxisome proliferator-activated receptors (PPAR) agonists affect cell viability, apoptosis and expression of cell cycle related proteins in cell lines of glial brain tumors. Neoplasma 2005;52(2):126–36.
47. Grau R, Punzon C, Fresno M, et al. Peroxisome-proliferator-activated receptor alpha agonists inhibit cyclo-oxygenase 2 and vascular endothelial growth factor transcriptional activation in human colorectal carcinoma cells via inhibition of activator protein-1. Biochem J 2006;395(1):81–8.
48. DuBois RN, Gupta R, Brockman J, et al. The nuclear eicosanoid receptor, PPAR-gamma, is aberrantly expressed in colonic cancers. Carcinogenesis 1998;19(1): 49–53.
49. Sarraf P, Mueller E, Smith WM, et al. Loss-of-function mutations in PPAR gamma associated with human colon cancer. Mol Cell 1999;3(6):799–804.
50. Slattery ML, Curtin K, Wolff R, et al. PPARgamma and colon and rectal cancer: associations with specific tumor mutations, aspirin, ibuprofen and insulin-related genes (United States). Cancer Causes Control 2006;17(3):239–49.
51. Landi S, Moreno V, Gioia-Patricola L, et al. Association of common polymorphisms in inflammatory genes interleukin (IL)6, IL8, tumor necrosis factor alpha, NFKB1, and peroxisome proliferator-activated receptor gamma with colorectal cancer. Cancer Res 2003;63(13):3560–6.
52. Ikezoe T, Miller CW, Kawano S, et al. Mutational analysis of the peroxisome proliferator-activated receptor gamma gene in human malignancies. Cancer Res 2001;61(13):5307–10.
53. Sarraf P, Mueller E, Jones D, et al. Differentiation and reversal of malignant changes in colon cancer through PPARgamma. Nat Med 1998;4(9):1046–52.

54. Osawa E, Nakajima A, Wada K, et al. Peroxisome proliferator-activated receptor gamma ligands suppress colon carcinogenesis induced by azoxymethane in mice. Gastroenterology 2003;124(2):361–7.
55. Lefebvre AM, Chen I, Desreumaux P, et al. Activation of the peroxisome proliferator-activated receptor gamma promotes the development of colon tumors in C57BL/6J-APCMin/+ mice. Nat Med 1998;4(9):1053–7.
56. Saez E, Tontonoz P, Nelson MC, et al. Activators of the nuclear receptor PPARgamma enhance colon polyp formation. Nat Med 1998;4(9):1058–61.
57. Pino MV, Kelley MF, Jayyosi Z. Promotion of colon tumors in C57BL/6J-APC(min)/+ mice by thiazolidinedione PPARgamma agonists and a structurally unrelated PPARgamma agonist. Toxicol Pathol 2004;32(1):58–63.
58. Yang K, Fan KH, Lamprecht SA, et al. Peroxisome proliferator-activated receptor gamma agonist troglitazone induces colon tumors in normal C57BL/6J mice and enhances colonic carcinogenesis in Apc(1638 N/+) Mlh1(+/-) double mutant mice. Int J Cancer 2005;116(4):495–9.
59. Niho N, Takahashi M, Kitamura T, et al. Concomitant suppression of hyperlipidemia and intestinal polyp formation in Apc-deficient mice by peroxisome proliferator-activated receptor ligands. Cancer Res 2003;63(18):6090–5.
60. Niho N, Takahashi M, Shoji Y, et al. Dose-dependent suppression of hyperlipidemia and intestinal polyp formation in Min mice by pioglitazone, a PPAR gamma ligand. Cancer Sci 2003;94(11):960–4.
61. Girnun GD, Smith WM, Drori S, et al. APC-dependent suppression of colon carcinogenesis by PPARgamma. Proc Natl Acad Sci U S A 2002;99(21):13771–6.
62. McAlpine CA, Barak Y, Matise I, et al. Intestinal-specific PPARgamma deficiency enhances tumorigenesis in ApcMin/+ mice. Int J Cancer 2006; 119(10):2339–46.
63. Kohno H, Suzuki R, Sugie S, et al. Suppression of colitis-related mouse colon carcinogenesis by a COX-2 inhibitor and PPAR ligands. BMC Cancer 2005;5:46.
64. Govindarajan R, Ratnasinghe L, Simmons DL, et al. Thiazolidinediones and the risk of lung, prostate, and colon cancer in patients with diabetes. J Clin Oncol 2007;25(12):1476–81.
65. He TC, Chan TA, Vogelstein B, et al. PPARdelta is an APC-regulated target of nonsteroidal anti-inflammatory drugs. Cell 1999;99(3):335–45.
66. Ouyang N, Williams JL, Rigas B. NO-donating aspirin isomers downregulate peroxisome proliferator-activated receptor (PPAR)delta expression in APC(min/+) mice proportionally to their tumor inhibitory effect: Implications for the role of PPARdelta in carcinogenesis. Carcinogenesis 2006;27(2):232–9.
67. Siezen CL, Tijhuis MJ, Kram NR, et al. Protective effect of nonsteroidal anti-inflammatory drugs on colorectal adenomas is modified by a polymorphism in peroxisome proliferator-activated receptor delta. Pharmacogenet Genomics 2006; 16(1):43–50.
68. Wang D, Wang H, Shi Q, et al. Prostaglandin E(2) promotes colorectal adenoma growth via transactivation of the nuclear peroxisome proliferator-activated receptor delta. Cancer Cell 2004;6(3):285–95.
69. Xu L, Han C, Wu T. A novel positive feedback loop between peroxisome proliferator-activated receptor-delta and prostaglandin E2 signaling pathways for human cholangiocarcinoma cell growth. J Biol Chem 2006;281(45):33982–96.
70. Xu L, Han C, Lim K, et al. Cross-talk between peroxisome proliferator-activated receptor delta and cytosolic phospholipase A(2)alpha/cyclooxygenase-2/prostaglandin E(2) signaling pathways in human hepatocellular carcinoma cells. Cancer Res 2006;66(24):11859–68.

71. Shao J, Sheng H, DuBois RN. Peroxisome proliferator-activated receptors modulate K-Ras-mediated transformation of intestinal epithelial cells. Cancer Res 2002; 62(11):3282–8.

72. Takayama O, Yamamoto H, Damdinsuren B, et al. Expression of PPARdelta in multistage carcinogenesis of the colorectum: implications of malignant cancer morphology. Br J Cancer 2006;95(7):889–95.

73. Vanamala J, Glagolenko A, Yang P, et al. Dietary fish oil and pectin enhance colonocyte apoptosis in part through suppression of PPAR{delta}/PGE2 and elevation of PGE3. Carcinogenesis 2007;29(4):790–6.

74. Chen LC, Hao CY, Chiu YS, et al. Alteration of gene expression in normal-appearing colon mucosa of APC(min) mice and human cancer patients. Cancer Res 2004;64(10):3694–700.

75. Reed KR, Sansom OJ, Hayes AJ, et al. PPARdelta status and Apc-mediated tumourigenesis in the mouse intestine. Oncogene 2004;23(55):8992–6.

76. Park BH, Vogelstein B, Kinzler KW. Genetic disruption of PPARdelta decreases the tumorigenicity of human colon cancer cells. Proc Natl Acad Sci U S A 2001;98(5):2598–603.

77. Gupta RA, Wang D, Katkuri S, et al. Activation of nuclear hormone receptor peroxisome proliferator-activated receptor-delta accelerates intestinal adenoma growth. Nat Med 2004;10(3):245–7.

78. Marin HE, Peraza MA, Billin AN, et al. Ligand activation of peroxisome proliferator-activated receptor beta inhibits colon carcinogenesis. Cancer Res 2006; 66(8):4394–401.

79. Wang D, Wang H, Guo Y, et al. Crosstalk between peroxisome proliferator-activated receptor delta and VEGF stimulates cancer progression. Proc Natl Acad Sci U S A 2006;103(50):19069–74.

80. Zuo X, Peng Z, Moussalli MJ, et al. Targeted genetic disruption of peroxisome proliferator-activated receptor-delta and colonic tumorigenesis. J Natl Cancer Inst 2009;101(10):762–7.

81. Harman FS, Nicol CJ, Marin HE, et al. Peroxisome proliferator-activated receptor-delta attenuates colon carcinogenesis. Nat Med 2004;10(5):481–3.

82. Peters JM, Lee SS, Li W, et al. Growth, adipose, brain, and skin alterations resulting from targeted disruption of the mouse peroxisome proliferator-activated receptor beta(delta). Mol Cell Biol 2000;20(14):5119–28.

83. Nadra K, Anghel SI, Joye E, et al. Differentiation of trophoblast giant cells and their metabolic functions are dependent on peroxisome proliferator-activated receptor beta/delta. Mol Cell Biol 2006;26(8):3266–81.

New Pharmacologic Therapies in Gastrointestinal Disease

John L. Wallace, PhD, MBA[a],*, Jose G.P. Ferraz, MD, PhD[b]

KEYWORDS

- Ulcer • Acid • Inflammation • Irritable bowel
- Nonsteroidal anti-inflammatory drug

Many gastrointestinal (GI) diseases remain poorly responsive to therapies, and even in the cases of conditions for which there are many effective drugs, there is still considerable room for improvement. This article is focused on drugs for digestive disorders that have entered the marketplace recently, or are expected to reach the marketplace within the next 1 to 2 years. For indications in which there are few treatment options (eg, nonsteroidal anti-Inflammatory drug [NSAID]-gastropathy), discussion of drugs that are earlier in development is provided. Some of these drugs have been discussed in preceding articles of this issue, and for some classes of drugs and indications (eg, inflammatory bowel disease) there are articles elsewhere in this issue that review new and emerging therapies.

ACID SUPPRESSION
Novel Proton Pump Inhibitors

Proton pump inhibitors (PPIs) are the most effective drugs for treatment of acid-related disorders, such as peptic ulcer disease, ulceration caused by NSAIDs, gastroesophageal reflux disease (GERD), dyspepsia, and stress-mediated ulceration (ie, that occurring in the intensive care setting). These drugs act by specifically inhibiting the activity of proton pumps in the canalicular membrane of gastric parietal cells, which are responsible for secretion of acid in the stomach. For inhibition to occur, the proton pumps must be expressed by the parietal cells, and this expression only occurs when they are actively secreting acid, such as with a meal. Thus, one limitation of PPIs is that they need to be given just before a meal to be maximally effective. This limitation has

This work was supported by a research grant from the Canadian Institutes of Health Research.
Disclosure: Dr Wallace is one of the founders of NicOx S.A. and Antibe Therapeutics Inc.
[a] Farncombe Family Digestive Health Research Institute, McMaster University, 1200 Main Street West, Hamilton, Ontario L8N 3Z5, Canada
[b] Inflammation Research Network, University of Calgary, 3330 Hospital Drive NW, Calgary, Alberta T2N 4N1, Canada
* Corresponding author.
E-mail address: jwalla@mcmaster.ca

a significant effect on patient compliance, and limits the on-demand use of the drug for symptomatic relief.[1]

Despite the enormous commercial success of PPIs, there remains a significant unmet need in providing adequate suppression of gastric acid secretion, particularly for patients with GERD. Indeed, as many as 25% of GERD patients are not satisfied with their therapy.[2] These needs can be divided into 2 categories: rapid onset of symptom relief and sustained activity (particularly through the night). The lack of a rapid onset of activity of PPIs is largely attributable to the fact that they are acid-labile, so PPIs have to be administered in formulations that protect the drug until it enters the duodenum. The lack of sustained activity is mainly manifest as nocturnal acid breakthrough (NAB). NAB occurs in a significant percentage of regular PPI users (GERD and non-GERD).[3] It is largely related to the earlier-mentioned need to take PPIs in conjunction with a meal, along with the relatively short plasma half-lives of most PPIs. In short, taking a PPI with the last meal consumed before a patient goes to bed does not provide acid suppression for long enough to control nocturnal acidification and maintain a sufficiently elevated intragastric pH until the patient wakes in the morning. A further complication is that GERD patients are often instructed not to ingest food for at least 3 hours before going to sleep.

Several new PPIs have been designed to address the 2 key issues presently limiting the effectiveness/use of these drugs: the need for a faster relief of symptoms and the need for prevention of NAB. **Table 1** lists some of the new PPIs (recently launched or in late stage of development). Those developed to have a faster onset of symptom relief include Zegerid and VECAM. Zegerid is a formulation containing omeprazole and sodium bicarbonate. The sodium bicarbonate raises intragastric pH to provide rapid relief of symptoms during the lag-time between ingestion of the omeprazole and its onset of activity. VECAM is a formulation containing omeprazole with a "meal-mimicking agent." The rationale of this approach is to overcome the meal-dependence of omeprazole by way of the meal-mimicking agent, which stimulates gastric acid secretion and thereby facilitates omeprazole's interaction with the proton pumps in parietal cells.

As shown in **Table 1**, solving the NAB problem is the focus of more drug development than the need for faster onset of activity. Dexlansoprazole is a delayed-release formulation of the R-enantiomer of lansoprazole. The patients should be able to take dexlansoprazole with their final meal of the day, several hours before bedtime. The delayed release of the active ingredient several hours later would then provide significant suppression of acid secretion through the night. A somewhat similar approach was taken in the design of DM-3458. DM-3458 remains in the stomach for 4 to 6 hours before releasing omeprazole. AGN-201904-Z is an acid-stable prodrug of omeprazole that exhibits a prolonged half-life compared with conventional omeprazole; therefore AGN-201904-Z should provide better nighttime suppression of acid secretion. There are also some new PPIs that may also offer a solution to NAB. Tenatoprazole and Ilaprazole are both reported to exhibit prolonged acid secretion as compared with older PPIs.

Potassium-Competitive Acid Inhibitors

The next generation of acid suppressors will likely be the potassium-competitive acid inhibitors (P-CAI).[1] The drugs act by competitively inhibiting the potassium-binding region of the H^+,K^+-ATPase on activated parietal cells. These drugs also accumulate within the parietal acid compartment to a much greater extent than do PPIs, and this accumulation contributes to their enhanced antisecretory activity. An additional enhancement of activity is achieved as a result of more favorable pharmacokinetic

Table 1
Novel PPIs in development

Drug	Company	Description	Objective
AGN-201904-Z	Alevium	Sodium salt of acid, stable prodrug of omeprazole	Continued metered absorption, resulting in prolonged plasma half-life
DM-3458	Depomed	"Gastroretentive" omeprazole	Delayed release of omeprazole provides better nighttime suppression of acid secretion
Ilaprazole	Takeda	Novel PPI	Increased acid suppression and duration of action compared with omeprazole
Tenatoprazole	Mitsubishi	Novel PPI (sodium salt of S-enantiomer)	Prolonged acid suppression compared with other PPIs
VECAM	Vecta	Omeprazole + "meal-mimicking agent"	Faster absorption; more effective acid suppression
Zegerid	Santarus	Sodium bicarbonate + omeprazole	Faster onset of activity, increased absorption and bioavailability of omeprazole

Abbreviation: PPI, proton pump inhibitor.

properties of P-CAIs versus PPIs.[4,5] Unlike PPIs, the duration of activity of P-CAIs is directly related to their plasma half-life. Also, a full effect is observed after a single dose of a P-CAI, as compared with the need for several doses of a PPI before achieving a full effect.

Combination Histamine H₂-Receptor Antagonists–PPIs

Although the introduction of PPIs has largely supplanted the use of histamine H$_2$-receptor antagonists (H$_2$-RAs), there remains a significant niche for these drugs, such as in the treatment of nocturnal symptoms of GERD.[6] A proof-of-concept of the utility of combination H$_2$-RAs and PPIs was provided by the study of Fandriks and colleagues.[7] Coadministration of omeprazole (20 mg) and famotidine (10 mg daily) led to a significantly faster onset of antisecretory activity (ie, raising intragastric pH >4) as compared with omeprazole alone, as well as improving the duration of acid suppression.

Prokinetics

Serotonin (5-HT) is an important mediator of normal secretory and motor function in the GI tract.[8] The enterochromaffin cell is the major source of serotonin in the gut, and the gut accounts for more than 90% of serotonin in the human body. Serotonin plays a role in triggering peristaltic reflexes and can modulate the release of other mediators that influence smooth muscle contraction. The effects of serotonin are complex, with different receptors sometimes producing opposing effects on contractility (eg, 5-HT$_3$ vs 5-HT$_4$).[8]

Serotonergic prokinetic agents have been in use for many years, but serious adverse cardiac events (fatal cardiac arrhythmias) led to the withdrawal of cisapride and tegaserod. Cisapride remains available in some countries under very strict conditions (restricted investigational drug protocol) for treatment of certain conditions, including pseudo-obstruction, gastroparesis, and GERD. Thus, its use is limited and there is a considerable gap left for the treatment of conditions characterized by disturbed GI motility. Recently, a new 5-HT$_4$ agonist, prucalopride, was approved in Europe for symptomatic treatment of chronic constipation in women who have not obtained adequate relief from treatment with laxatives.

Prucalopride acts throughout the intestine. Although not affecting gastric emptying, prucalopride increases oral-cecal and colonic transit in healthy volunteers.[9] These effects are attributed to enhancement, via activation of 5-HT$_4$ receptors, of cholinergic neurotransmission. Prucalopride has been shown to promote normalization of bowel habits (improved stool consistency and frequency) in patients with chronic idiopathic constipation.[10] Prucalopride has also been shown to be effective in patients who are dissatisfied with conventional laxatives.[11] Like some other prokinetics, prucalopride blocks a potassium channel called the HERG channel, and thereby has the potential to trigger cardiac arrhythmias, but only at concentrations well above those likely to be achieved with clinically relevant doses.[12]

CONSTIPATION

Drugs that enhance fluid secretion, and thereby facilitate intestinal transit, represent a new area of drug development for motility disorders. Generally speaking, this broad class of drugs works via modulation of ion channels on intestinal or colonic enterocytes. Lubiprostone is one such drug that was recently introduced for the treatment of chronic constipation and in constipation-predominant irritable bowel syndrome (IBS-C). Lubiprostone is a prostaglandin E$_1$ derivative that stimulates chloride secretion by colonocytes, resulting in increased passive movement of water into the lumen. This process acts to improve stool consistency, facilitating normalization of bowel movements. Lubiprostone is poorly absorbed, producing its actions locally at the lumen-colonocyte interface. Lubiprostone, therefore, has a low incidence of serious adverse effects, which could result in more widespread applications in the future. Lubiprostone is presently approved for the treatment of chronic constipation in adults, and of IBS-C in women. Two pivotal clinical trials established the safety and efficacy of lubiprostone.[13] These trials involved more than 1100 patients diagnosed with IBS-C, more than 90% of whom were women. More patients treated with lubiprostone reported moderate or significant relief of symptoms of IBS-C over a 12-week treatment period than the patients who received a placebo. Efficacy of lubiprostone for treating men with IBS-C has not been conclusively demonstrated. In addition to being approved for treating women with IBS-C, a higher dose of lubiprostone has been approved by the US Food and Drug Administration (USFDA) for treatment of chronic idiopathic constipation.[13]

Linaclotide is a minimally absorbed peptide agonist of the guanylate cyclase C receptor. By increasing levels of cyclic guanosine monophosphate within enterocytes, linaclotide stimulates secretion and motility. In clinical trials, linaclotide has shown considerable promise for the treatment of chronic constipation and IBS-C, with a very good safety profile.[10] Studies in laboratory animals also point to antinociceptive effects of linaclotide, which if reproduced in humans would increase the utility of linaclotide for treating pain-predominant conditions such as IBS-C. In late 2009, Ironwood Pharmaceuticals and Forest Laboratories, who are codeveloping linaclotide for chronic constipation and IBS-C, reported the results of 2 phase 3 clinical trials. These trials evaluated the effectiveness of once-daily dosing with linaclotide in patients with chronic constipation. In both trials, statistical significance was achieved for the primary end point (complete spontaneous bowel movements) and all prespecified secondary end points (including measures of abdominal discomfort and bloating) were met. One of these studies was recently described in a full publication.[14] As shown in **Fig. 1**, linaclotide markedly and dose-dependently improved spontaneous

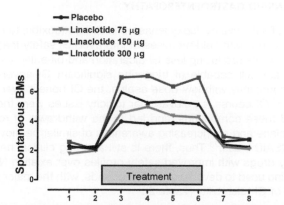

Fig. 1. Dose-dependent improvement of spontaneous bowel movements (BMs) with linaclotide in patients with chronic constipation. A significant ($P<.05$) improvement was observed with all doses of linaclotide as compared with the placebo group. Data were also collected for 2 weeks before and 2 weeks after the treatment period. (*Adapted from* Lembo AJ, Kurtz CB, MacDougall JE, et al. Efficacy of linaclotide for patients with chronic constipation. Gastroenterology 2010;138:886–95; with permission.)

bowel movements. Indeed, linaclotide "was associated with few adverse effects and produced rapid and sustained improvements of bowel habits, abdominal symptoms, global relief, and quality of life in patients with chronic constipation."[14]

Opioid-Induced Constipation

Opioids relax intestinal smooth muscle, interfering with propulsive contractions. The actions are mediated via μ-opioid receptors. Many patients taking opioids for pain relief, such as after surgery, experience significant impairment of intestinal motility (itself a significant source of discomfort). Alvimopan is a peripherally acting μ-opioid receptor antagonist. Alvimopan has very limited ability to cross the blood-brain barrier, and therefore can block the peripheral actions of opiates that are mediated through the μ-receptor without affecting other, desirable actions of opiates. Thus, the constipation normally associated with opiate use can be minimized, without affecting the analgesic effects of the opiate. As a result, greater compliance can also be achieved.

The USFDA has approved alvimopan for acceleration of the restoration of normal bowel function in adults after intestinal resection surgery. The goal of intestinal resection surgery is to accelerate the postoperative recovery and improve bowel function, allowing the patient to reestablish a normal diet more quickly. It is hoped that postoperative ileus (a temporary impairment of GI motility that is often seen when opioid analgesics are used postoperatively) can be alleviated through the use of alvimopan. In 5 randomized, double-blind, placebo-controlled clinical trials (phase 3), alvimopan significantly accelerated the time to recovery of GI function and to hospital discharge after bowel resection.[15]

Methylnaltrexone bromide was approved by the USFDA in April 2008 for restoration of bowel function in patients with late-stage, advanced illnesses who require continuous opioids to relieve pain. Clinical trials demonstrated efficacy of methylnaltrexone bromide in initiating bowel movements in end-stage patients with cancer. In one trial, methylnaltrexone bromide given every other day for 2 weeks was found to produce bowel movements in half of the patients, compared with only 8% to 15% of patients treated with placebo.[16]

PREVENTION OF NSAID GASTROENTEROPATHY

The introduction of selective cyclooxygenase-2 inhibitors (coxibs) to the marketplace in the mid-1990s came with bold promises of improved GI safety that have not been fully realized.[17,18] While producing less GI ulceration and bleeding than conventional NSAIDs, coxibs are still capable of triggering significant GI adverse events, and when given concomitantly with low-dose aspirin, the GI benefit over a conventional NSAID is lost.[19–22] Of course, cardiovascular toxicity issues were the main focus of concerns around these compounds, and led to the withdrawal of rofecoxib (Vioxx) from the marketplace and an increasing awareness of similar cardiovascular toxicity with the entire NSAID class.[23] Thus, there is still a strong clinical need for effective anti-inflammatory drugs with improved safety profiles over existing NSAIDs. Several strategies are being used to develop such compounds, with the major focus still being on improvement of GI tolerability (**Table 2**).

Concomitant Acid Suppression

One of the most active areas for development of GI-sparing NSAIDs is that involving coadministration of an NSAID with an inhibitor of gastric acid secretion. It should be noted that, although there is good evidence for beneficial effects of substantive acid suppression in reducing gastric damage caused by NSAIDs,[24] there are little if any

Table 2
Drugs in development for reducing NSAID gastroenteropathy

Company	Product Name	Composition	Principle for GI Safety	Phase
AstraZeneca	Axanum	Aspirin + esomeprazole	Acid inhibition	Filed
AstraZeneca/Pozen	Vimovo	Naproxen + esomeprazole	Acid inhibition	Filed
Covidien	Pennsaid	Diclofenac in dimethyl sulfoxide	Reduced GI exposure (dermal administration)	Filed
NicOx	Beprana	NO-releasing naproxen	Mucosal protection	Filed
AstraZeneca	PN 200	Naproxen + esomeprazole	Acid inhibition	Phase 3
Covidien	Pennsaid Plus	Diclofenac in dimethyl sulfoxide	Reduced GI exposure (dermal administration)	Phase 3
Horizon	HZT 501	Famotidine + ibuprofen	Acid inhibition	Phase 3
PLx Pharma	Ibuprofen-PC	Ibuprofen + phosphatidylcholine	Reduced topical irritancy on gastric mucosa	Phase 3
AstraZeneca	PN 100	Lansoprazole + naproxen	Acid inhibition	Phase 1
Pozen	PN 100	Naproxen + lansoprazole	Acid inhibition	Phase 1
Horizon	HZT 502	Famotidine + ibuprofen	Acid inhibition	Phase 1
Antibe Therapeutics	ATB-346	H_2S-releasing naproxen	Mucosal protection	Preclinical

data demonstrating protective effects against the small intestinal damage and bleeding caused by NSAIDs. As outlined in **Table 2**, several companies are developing drugs that corelease an NSAID (naproxen, aspirin, or ibuprofen) and a PPI (omeprazole, esomeprazole, or lansoprazole) and many of these compounds are already filed with the USFDA or in very late stages of development. Others are combining the NSAID with a high dose H_2-RA (eg, famotidine), which has been shown to reduce the incidence of NSAID gastropathy.[25]

Reduced Topical Irritancy

Based on the premise that a significant component of the mechanism of GI injury by NSAIDs is related to their topical irritancy (as opposed to systemic effects, such as suppression of prostaglandin synthesis),[18] some companies are developing NSAIDs that have reduced irritant effects either through a novel mechanism of action or through reduced GI exposure. The latter involves formulation of a conventional NSAID (diclofenac) in dimethyl sulfoxide for dermal administration. The dimethyl sulfoxide (45% w/w) facilitates absorption of the diclofenac across the skin. When applied to an inflamed joint, these compounds are reported to produce significant symptomatic relief, but with lower systemic levels of the NSAID they produce less GI injury than when the drug is given orally.[26]

Another strategy to reduce the topical irritant properties of NSAIDs is that taken by PLx Pharma, who has developed NSAIDs that are preassociated with phosphatidylcholine. Extensive preclinical work has demonstrated that these compounds are less likely to damage the gastric epithelium in rodents, and produce less severe mucosal injury while retaining the anti-inflammatory effects of the parent NSAID.[27] However, in a 6-week, randomized, double-blind endoscopy study (125 patients), there was no significant difference in GI damage between PL-1100 (ibuprofen preassociated with phosphatidylcholine) and an equivalent dose of ibuprofen, except in the subgroup of patients older than 55 years.[28]

Mucosal Protection

The discovery that nitric oxide (NO) was a potent gastroprotective substance that modulates many aspects of GI mucosal defense led to the development of NO-releasing NSAIDs,[29] which are also referred to as CINODs (cyclooxygenase-inhibiting NO donors).[30,31] NicOx's lead CINOD, naproxcinod (Beprana), has recently been filed with regulatory agencies in the United States and Europe. The compound has shown improved GI tolerability in some, but not all clinical trials.[31] However, naproxcinod has also been shown to have significantly less detrimental effects on systemic blood pressure than naproxen and rofecoxib.[32,33] Thus, it is likely that improved cardiovascular toxicity is the major differentiating factor between naproxcinod and existing NSAIDs, at least in the short term.

Like NO, hydrogen sulfide (H_2S) has been shown to exert protective effects in the GI tract and to accelerate the healing of preexisting ulcers.[34,35] Antibe Therapeutics is developing several H_2S-releasing drugs, including H_2S-releasing NSAIDs. Derivatives of naproxen, diclofenac, and indomethacin have been reported,[36–38] with ATB-346 (naproxen) being the most advanced in preclinical characterization. When tested in models of compromised gastric mucosal defense, ATB-346 produced negligible damage (approximately one-hundredth that of comparable doses of naproxen) despite exhibiting comparable anti-inflammatory activity to the parent drug.[38] Moreover, as shown in **Fig. 2**, when administered to mice with preexisting gastric ulcers, ATB-346 significantly accelerated ulcer healing.[38] This accelerated ulcer healing

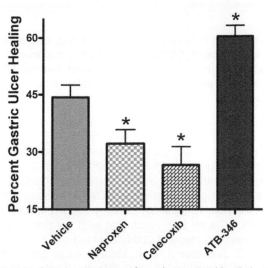

Fig. 2. Healing of gastric ulcers in rats is significantly impaired by daily treatment with anti-inflammatory doses of naproxen or celecoxib, but is accelerated by treatment with a comparable dose of a hydrogen sulfide-releasing naproxen derivative (ATB-346). *$P<.05$ versus the vehicle-treated group. (*Data from* Wallace JL, Caliendo G, Santagada V, et al. Markedly reduced toxicity of a hydrogen sulfide-releasing derivative of naproxen (ATB-346). Br J Pharmacol 2010;159:1236–46; with permission.)

was in contrast to the impairment of ulcer healing observed with comparable anti-inflammatory doses of naproxen or celecoxib.

SHORT BOWEL SYNDROME

Short bowel syndrome (SBS) is a disabling, often life-threatening condition that typically occurs after extensive bowel resection most commonly after repeated bowel resections for the treatment of Crohn disease. Owing to the reduced absorptive capacity after extensive bowel resection, patients are unable to sufficiently absorb nutrients, and consequently suffer from malnutrition and dehydration, which may be complicated by severe diarrhea and osteopenia. Patients usually depend on parenteral nutrition as a means of restoring fluid, electrolyte, and nutrient balance. Of course, deficiencies of key nutrients and vitamins are associated with several degenerative changes, and systemic infections are a significant risk associated with prolonged use of parenteral nutrition. The discovery of the ability of glucagon-like peptide-2 (GLP-2) to promote the growth of intestinal tissue[39] has led to the development of teduglutide, an analogue of GLP-2, as a potential therapy for SBS. The goal of teduglutide therapy is to restore the absorptive capacity of the intestine and thereby reduce the dependence of the patient on parenteral nutrition. Teduglutide is being developed by NPS Pharmaceuticals and Nycomed for both SBS and inflammatory bowel disease. The drug is presently in phase 3 clinical trials for both adults and children with SBS. Early studies of teduglutide in SBS patients have demonstrated that 21 days of treatment resulted in an intestinotrophic effect, improved nutrient absorption, and was well tolerated.[40] Teduglutide has been granted orphan drug status in both the United States and Europe for treatment of SBS.

SUMMARY

Despite significant advances in the past few decades (eg, acid suppression, biologic agents for inflammatory bowel disease), GI disease represents an underserved market. Although advances have been made in understanding GI motility, visceral pain, mucosal inflammation, and tissue repair, the major GI diseases remain as significant therapeutic challenges.

REFERENCES

1. Scarpignato C, Hunt RH. Proton pump inhibitors: the beginning of the end or the end of the beginning. Curr Opin Pharmacol 2008;8:677–84.
2. Chey WD, Mody R, Kothari S, et al. Are proton pump inhibitors (PPIs) sufficient in controlling symptoms of gastro-esophageal reflux disease (GERD)? a community-based US survey study. Gastroenterology 2008;124(Suppl 1):A325.
3. Tutuian R, Katz PO, Castell DO. Nocturnal acid breakthrough: pH, drugs and bugs. Eur J Gastroenterol Hepatol 2004;16:441–3.
4. Gedda K, Briving C, Svensson K, et al. Mechanism of action of AZD0865, a K^+-competitive inhibitor of gastric H+, K+-ATPase. Biochem Pharmacol 2007;73: 198–205.
5. Simon WA, Hermann M, Klein T, et al. Soprazan: setting new standards in inhibition of gastric acid secretion. J Pharmacol Exp Ther 2007;321:866–74.
6. Rackoff A, Agrawal A, Hila A, et al. Histamine-2 receptor antagonists at night improve gastroesophageal reflux disease symptoms for patients on proton pump inhibitor therapy. Dis Esophagus 2005;18:370–3.
7. Fandriks L, Lonroth H, Pettersen A, et al. Can famotidine and omeprazole be combined on a once-daily basis? Scand J Gastroenterol 2007;42:689–94.
8. Gershon MD, Tack J. The serotonin signaling system: from basic understanding to drug development for functional GI disorders. Gastroenterology 2007;132: 397–414.
9. Bouras EP, Camilleri M, Burton DD, et al. Selective stimulation of colonic transit by the benzofuran 5HT4 agonist, prucalopride, in healthy humans. Gut 1999;44: 682–6.
10. Gale JD. The use of novel promotility and prosecretory agents for the treatment of chronic idiopathic constipation and irritable bowel syndrome with constipation. Adv Ther 2009;26:519–30.
11. Tack J, Van Outryve M, Beyens G, et al. Prucalopride (resolor(R)) in the treatment of severe chronic constipation in patients dissatisfied with laxatives. Gut 2009;58: 357–65.
12. Chapman H, Pasternack M. The action of the novel gastrointestinal prokinetic prucalopride on the HERG K^+ channel and the common T897 polymorph. Eur J Pharmacol 2007;554:98–105.
13. Carter NJ, Scott LJ. Lubiprostone. In constipation-predominant irritable bowel syndrome. Drugs 2009;69:1229–37.
14. Lembo AJ, Kurtz CB, MacDougall JE, et al. Efficacy of linaclotide for patients with chronic constipation. Gastroenterology 2010;138:886–95.
15. Kraft M, MacLaren R, Du W, et al. Alvimopan (Entereg) for the management of postoperative ileus in patients undergoing bowel resection. Pharmacol Ther 2010;35:44–9.
16. Holzer P. Opioid receptors in the gastrointestinal tract. Regul Pept 2009;155:11–7.
17. Wallace JL. Selective COX-2 inhibitors: is the water becoming muddy? Trends Pharmacol Sci 1999;20:4–6.

18. Wallace JL. Prostaglandins, NSAIDs, and gastric mucosal protection: why doesn't the stomach digest itself? Physiol Rev 2008;88:1547–65.

19. Fiorucci S, de Lima OM, Mencarelli A, et al. Cyclooxygenase-2-derived lipoxin A_4 increases gastric resistance to aspirin-induced damage. Gastroenterology 2002; 123:1598–606.

20. Fiorucci S, Santucci L, Wallace JL, et al. Interaction of a selective cyclooxygenase-2 inhibitor with aspirin and NO-releasing aspirin in the human gastric mucosa. Proc Natl Acad Sci U S A 2003;100:10937–41.

21. Lanas A, Baron JA, Sandler RS, et al. Peptic ulcer and bleeding events associated with rofecoxib in a 3-year colorectal adenoma chemoprevention trial. Gastroenterology 2007;132:490–7.

22. Laine L, Maller ES, Yu C, et al. Ulcer formation with low-dose enteric-coated aspirin and the effect of COX-2 selective inhibition: a double-blind trial. Gastroenterology 2004;127:395–402.

23. Kearney PM, Baigent C, Godwin J, et al. Do selective cyclo-oxygenase-2 inhibitors and traditional non-steroidal anti-inflammatory drugs increase the risk of atherothrombosis? Meta-analysis of randomised trials. BMJ 2006;332:1302–8.

24. Chan FK, Wong VW, Suen BY, et al. Combination of a cyclo-oxygenase-2 inhibitor and a proton-pump inhibitor for prevention of recurrent ulcer bleeding in patients at very high risk: a double-blind, randomised trial. Lancet 2007;12(369):1621–6.

25. Taha AS, Hudson N, Hawkey CJ, et al. Famotidine for the prevention of gastric and duodenal ulcers caused by nonsteroidal antiinflammatory drugs. N Engl J Med 1996;334:1435–9.

26. Moen MD. Topical diclofenac solution. Drugs 2009;69:2621–32.

27. Lichtenberger LM, Barron M, Marathi U. Association of phosphatidylcholine and NSAIDs as a novel strategy to reduce gastrointestinal toxicity. Drugs Today (Barc) 2009;45:877–90.

28. Lanza FL, Marathi UK, Anand BS, et al. Clinical trial: comparison of ibuprofen-phosphatidylcholine and ibuprofen on the gastrointestinal safety and analgesic efficacy in osteoarthritic patients. Aliment Pharmacol Ther 2008;28:431–42.

29. Wallace JL. The 1994 Merck Frosst Award. Mechanisms of nonsteroidal anti-inflammatory drug (NSAID) induced gastrointestinal damage—potential for development of gastrointestinal tract safe NSAIDs. Can J Physiol Pharmacol 1994;72:1493–8.

30. Wallace JL, Del Soldato P. The therapeutic potential of NO-NSAIDs. Fundam Clin Pharmacol 2003;17:11–20.

31. Wallace JL, Viappiani S, Bolla M. Cyclooxygenase-inhibiting nitric oxide donators for osteoarthritis. Trends Pharmacol Sci 2009;30:112–7.

32. Karlsson J, Pivodic A, Aguirre D, et al. Efficacy, safety, and tolerability of the cyclooxygenase-inhibiting nitric oxide donator naproxcinod in treating osteoarthritis of the hip or knee. J Rheumatol 2009;36:1290–7.

33. White WB, Schnitzer TJ, Fleming R, et al. Effects of the cyclooxygenase inhibiting nitric oxide donator naproxcinod versus naproxen on systemic blood pressure in patients with osteoarthritis. Am J Cardiol 2009;109:840–5.

34. Fiorucci S, Distrutti E, Cirino G, et al. The emerging roles of hydrogen sulfide in the gastrointestinal tract and liver. Gastroenterology 2006;131:259–71.

35. Wallace JL, Dicay M, McKnight W, et al. Hydrogen sulfide enhances ulcer healing in rats. FASEB J 2007;21:4070–6.

36. Wallace JL, Caliendo G, Santagada V, et al. Gastrointestinal safety and anti-inflammatory effects of a hydrogen sulfide-releasing diclofenac derivative in the rat. Gastroenterology 2007;132:1261–71.

37. Wallace JL. Hydrogen sulfide-releasing anti-inflammatory drugs. Trends Pharmacol Sci 2007;28:501–5.

38. Wallace JL, Caliendo G, Santagada V, et al. Markedly reduced toxicity of a hydrogen sulphide-releasing derivative of naproxen (ATB-346). Br J Pharmacol 2010;159:1236–46.

39. Drucker DJ. Biologic actions and therapeutic potential of the proglucagon-derived peptides. Nat Clin Pract Endocrinol Metab 2005;1:22–31.

40. Jeppesen PB, Sanguinetti EL, Buchman A, et al. Teduglutide (ALX-0600), a dipeptidyl peptidase IV resistant glucagon-like peptide 2 analogue, improves intestinal function in short bowel syndrome patients. Gut 2005;54:1224–31.

Pharmabiotic Manipulation of the Microbiota in Gastrointestinal Disorders, from Rationale to Reality

Fergus Shanahan, MD[a],*, Stephen M. Collins, MD[b]

KEYWORDS

• Pharmabiotic • Probiotic • Gut microbiota
• Inflammatory bowel disease

An inescapable truism is that the human genome does not encode sufficient information for full development. For optimal maturation, particularly of mucosal tissues and sensory organs, including the immunosensory system, stimulation from the environment is required. In the gut, this is derived from the microbiome. The microbiota colonizing the neonate exerts trophic, metabolic, and protective effects on developing intestinal and extraintestinal organs and is critical for homeostasis throughout life.[1,2] This inner biomass is an asset for health, protective against disease, and yet, depending on the context, some of its components may become a risk factor for disease.[3] Therein is the rationale for exploring the potential benefit of managing or manipulating the human microbiota.

The most striking example in the developed world of successfully targeting a component of gut microbiota in the treatment of disease has been the story of *Helicobacter pylori* with peptic ulcer disease and gastric cancer. The real lesson of

---

FS is supported in part by Science Foundation Ireland (SFI) and SMC by the Canadian Institutes of Health Research (CIHR). FS is a shareholder in Alimentary Health Limited (Cork, Ireland), and has consulted and/or received research grants from Procter and Gamble Company (Cincinatti, USA) and GlaxoSmithKline Limited (Stevenage, UK). SMC receives an unrestricted grant in aid from the Nestlé Research Institute (Lausanne, Switzerland).

[a] Department of Medicine, Alimentary Pharmabiotic Centre, University College Cork, National University of Ireland, Ireland
[b] Farncombe Family Digestive Health Institute, McMaster University Medical Centre, Hamilton, Ontario, Canada
* Corresponding author. Department of Medicine, Alimentary Pharmabiotic Centre, c/o Clinical Science Building, Cork University Hospital Ireland, Ireland
E-mail address: F.Shanahan@ucc.ie

Gastroenterol Clin N Am 39 (2010) 721–726
doi:10.1016/j.gtc.2010.08.006
0889-8553/10/$ – see front matter © 2010 Elsevier Inc. All rights reserved.

that story was that some chronic human diseases can never be solved by research and therapeutics focused exclusively on the host, without due regard for interactions with environmental microbiota. Despite this, most current therapeutic strategies for many disorders including inflammatory bowel disease (IBD) still focus on modifying the host response, while the microbiota, an essential contributor to the pathogenesis, receives limited attention. The significance of this therapeutic omission is striking when considered in light of increasing evidence suggesting that elements of a modern lifestyle represent environmental risk factors for IBD, which act by modifying the alimentary microbiota and thence, the developing immune system.[4] Thus, modern lifestyle factors may link two of the main contributory factors to the pathogenesis of IBD (immunity and microbiota) and, in effect, represent proxy markers of microbial exposure during mucosal immune maturation.

Although antibiotics have served for targeting specific organisms, a bigger challenge is the manipulation of the broader microbial community and whether its composition might even be controlled in neonates at the time of colonization, to confer maximal biodiversity for optimal host–microbe interactions during development. Whether it be practicable, naïve, or futuristic, boosting natural microbial defenses is conceptually appealing to patients and represents a commercial growth area. Clinicians, therefore, need to be equipped with an essential understanding of the current status of the science to give an authoritative response to questions from informed and misinformed patients. The intent here is to present a brief overview of the potential scope for therapeutic manipulation of the microbiota.

TYRANNY OF TERMINOLOGY

Current strategies for manipulating the microbiota involve probiotics, prebiotics, and combinations (synbiotics), although phage viruses or topically active, narrow-spectrum antibiotics might in the future have a role in certain circumstances. Unfortunately, words and labels often outlive their usefulness or are rendered inaccurate by new discoveries. Recall that the term antibiotic, as originally defined, was a secondary metabolite of microbial origin, but in modern usage, it now covers naturally occurring compounds of nonmicrobial origin, such as sulfonamides, in addition to various synthetic and semisynthetic agents. Similarly, accepted definitions of probiotics are probably too restrictive, because they do not reflect usage of dead organisms, bacterial constituents including cell proteins, cell wall polysaccharides, and probiotic DNA or genetically modified organisms. To portray the wider scope of beneficial microbes and their products, the authors have adopted the umbrella term alimentary pharmabiotics. In the current context, an alimentary pharmabiotic is any material with potential health benefit that can be mined from host-microbe-dietary interactions in the gut. In practice, most pharmabiotics (and probiotics) are live whole organisms, usually lactobacilli or bifidobacteria, but other components of the commensal microbiota can be harnessed for their beneficial impact on the host.

ACTION IN VIVO—SEEING IS BELIEVING

Almost every component of probiotics from DNA to cytosolic protein and cell wall has been shown to influence mucosal immune or epithelial cells in vitro.[5] This is hardly surprising, and there is no shortage of reports of such phenomena. However, exposure of cultured host cell lines or isolates to bacteria with which the responding cell has never seen or encountered before is hardly proof of a probiotic mechanism of action. Experiments demonstrating probiotic action in vivo are more convincing. Perhaps the best mechanistic demonstration of probiotic action has been in protection against infection. For example, in a murine model of infection with *Listeria monocytogenes*, the protective effect of the probiotic *L salivarius* UCC118 was shown conclusively to be due to production of an antimicrobial bacteriocin.[6] More importantly, by using a luciferase-based reporter system and bioluminescence imaging, it was possible to track translocated *Listeria* infection in vivo and to visualize the protective influence of the probiotic in vivo. However, the same probiotic also protects against *Salmonella* infection. This is not due to the antimicrobial bacteriocin, however, because an engineered knockout of the bacteriocin was equally protective. To account for this aspect of probiotic action against pathogens, one has to look elsewhere: competitive inhibition and stimulation of innate and acquired immunity.

Not surprisingly, probiotics mimic the indigenous commensals, which are engaged in continual dialog with the host, particularly with enterocytes and dendritic cells. Remarkably, probiotics use a language that is similar to that used by pathogens when engaging with the host. They express microorganism-associated molecular patterns (MAMPs) that engage with the same pattern recognition receptors (PRRs) as do pathogens. This provides the molecular basis of protection by competitive exclusion.[5] For other probiotics, protection against pathogen-induced tissue damage is conferred by stimulation of innate and acquired immunity and in particular, the generation of regulatory T cells. Once again, this aspect of probiotic action has been demonstrated elegantly in vivo. In a murine model of *Salmonella* infection, it was possible to image NF-κB activation in vivo and its attenuation by the probiotic *Bifidobacterium infantis*.[7] The response was not specific to *Salmonella* and was also seen when injected lipopolysaccharide (LPS) was the inflammatory stimulus. It was associated with upregulation of enteric and systemic regulatory T cells, confirmation of which was shown in vivo by transferring the cells to naive recipients in whom LPS-induced activation of NF-κB was suppressed when the cells were derived from probiotic-fed, but not from placebo-fed, mice.

Skeptics of probiotic mechanism have argued that the average daily dose of most probiotics (10^9–10^{12} organisms) is such a tiny fraction of the total resident bacteria, that a meaningful impact on the intestinal ecosystem must be unlikely. Elegant studies with gnotobiotic mice, however, have shown that the resident bacteria adapt to the introduction of a probiotic species and to host dietary changes with alterations in gene expression.[8]

Regrettably, in contrast to the consistent efficacy of probiotics in experimental animals, evidence for clinical efficacy of probiotics in people is relatively sparse, and confounded by a failure by many to appreciate that probiotics are not created equal. The complexity of host–flora interactions needs to be taken into account and tailored to suit the challenges of human disease. Despite this, there are success stories with probiotics in people.

TRANSLATION TO CLINICAL GASTROENTEROLOGY

The circumvention of a historic dependency on culture-based methods to study the microbiota has accelerated interest in the composition of the normal commensal population and manipulation or enhancement thereof. Molecular (nonculture-based) techniques, notably metagenomics, have shown the biodiversity of the enteric microbiota with compositional alterations that may be risk factors for disease.[2] In particular, reduced microbial biodiversity is tantamount to reduced environmental stimulation of the developing immune and digestive systems, with reduced competitive capacity against pathogen invasion.[9]

Those most vulnerable to any disturbance of the enteric microbiota and perhaps most suited to probiotic supplementation are at the extremes of life. It is, therefore, not surprising that the most compelling evidence for probiotic efficacy in people is in premature or low birth weight neonates who are at increased risk of necrotizing enterocolitis (NEC). Meta-analyses of various controlled trials using different probiotics have shown that probiotics not only reduce the risk of NEC but also reduce risk of all causes of mortality.[10] This has prompted pediatricians to ask whether the stage has been reached where it may be inappropriate to deny these vulnerable babies the protection of probiotics. It seems likely that future trials will focus on comparative studies and optimal probiotic regimens.[11,12]

Probiotics also appear to have modest but consistent efficacy in people, where there is loss of biodiversity or significant disruption to the indigenous microbiota, such as that following antibiotic exposure or with acute enteric infections. Despite impressive rationale for their use, however, evidence for efficacy of probiotics in IBD is inconsistent and at variance with what has been observed with many murine models by different research groups.[13] Results of controlled trials in Crohn disease provide no encouragement.[14,15] Experience with probiotics in ulcerative colitis is somewhat better. In particular, the efficacy of E coli (Nissle 1917) has been reported to be equivalent to that of mesalamine for maintenance of remission.[16,17] The best reported results have been in the treatment or prevention of pouchitis. However, after two encouraging controlled trials with a cocktail of eight different bacteria (VSL#3), subsequent reports, and clinical anecdotal experience, have been inconsistent or disappointing.[18,19] Since the impact of intestinal bacteria on the developing immune system is greatest at the earliest stages of postnatal life, the notion of manipulating the microbiota in adulthood as a therapeutic strategy for IBD may be futile, too late to achieve substantial efficacy. This may explain the apparent disparity in efficacy of probiotics in attenuating animal models of IBD with the disappointing data to date in people with the same organisms.

Remarkably, the gastrointestinal (GI) disorder for which the efficacy of some but not all probiotics has been best documented is irritable bowel syndrome.[20] It is self-evident that more controlled trials of different agents and dosing regimens are desirable. Studies of probiotics in other GI disorders are too sparse or limited in design to interpret anything conclusively at present.

PROBIOTICS AND THE CLINICIAN

As with many new fields of human scientific endeavor, the concept of therapeutic manipulation of the microbiota by probiotics or otherwise has been distracted by premature or exaggerated claims from certain enthusiasts. Poorly substantiated claims of efficacy are widespread. However, there is science amidst the snake oil. The evidence base for both probiotic mechanisms of action and for strain-specific efficacy in different indications is beginning to catch up with the clinical impetus. Guidelines for future clinical studies are clear.[21,22] For now, there are important principles to steer clinicians on the use of pharmabiotics or probiotics.

First, it is likely that the greatest role for probiotics in the Western world will be at the extremes of life and in those most vulnerable to infection. Second, probiotics are not uniform, and it should not be assumed that efficacy with one strain applies to another. Nor should it be assumed that the same strain will be equally effective in a different indication. Third, probiotics should only be acquired from a reputable vendor with disclosure of contents and documentation of shelf-life. Fourth, as with most naturally occurring remedies, efficacy with probiotics in any indication is likely to be modest.

Probiotics should be considered as supplements not substitutes for conventional therapy. Fifth, more is not always better. The practice of combining probiotics without knowledge of the activities or antagonism of the ingredients is as foolish as combining drugs without understanding adverse interactions. Sixth, dietary–probiotic interactions should be anticipated. Perhaps the greatest environmental influence on the commensal microbiota is dietary. Prebiotics or dietary poly/oligosaccharides represent the most obvious form of dietary influence on the microbiota or consumed probiotics. Less well appreciated is the potential role of dietary fat on microbial metabolism. It has previously been shown that the microbiota is an environmental regulator of fat storage in people, but more recently it has been shown that microbial metabolism of specific dietary fatty acids in the gut has a profound influence on the composition of bioactive fatty acids in the adipose tissue of the host.[23] This, in turn, influences the immunoinflammatory response. Finally, in choosing a nonpharmacologic approach to management, clinicians must remember that the usual principles of evidence-based therapeutics still apply.

BRAVE NEW WORLD–TURBO PHARMABIOTICS

Genetic engineering of microbes can render them therapeutically functional. This strategy has been exploited with commensal and food-grade bacteria for luminal production and mucosal delivery of anti-inflammatory cytokines such as interleukin-10, prohealing trefoil factors, and immunogenic peptides as vaccines. Safety concerns have been assuaged by containment of the transgenic organism whereby the transgene replaces the thymidylate synthase gene, thereby rendering the organism dependent on a local supply of thymidine or thymine in the gut and unable to survive without these factors in the external environment.[24] Preliminary open-label results with such organisms in people with Crohn disease have been encouraging, but controlled clinical trials are still pending.[25]

REFERENCES

1. Round JL, Mazmanian SK. The gut microbiota shapes intestinal immune responses during health and disease. Nat Rev Immunol 2009;9:313–23.
2. Turnbaugh PJ, Ley RE, Hamady M, et al. The human microbiome project. Nature 2007;449:804–10.
3. Garrett WS, Gordon JI, Glimcher LH. Homeostasis and inflammation in the intestine. Cell 2010;140:859–70.
4. Bernstein CN, Shanahan F. Disorders of a modern lifestyle: reconciling the epidemiology of inflammatory bowel diseases. Gut 2008;57:1185–91.
5. Lebeer S, Vanderleyden J, De Keersmaecker SC. Host interactions of probiotic bacterial surface molecules: comparison with commensals and pathogens. Nat Rev Microbiol 2010;8:171–84.
6. Corr SC, Li Y, Riedel CU, et al. Bacteriocin production as a mechanism for the antiinfective activity of Lactobacillus salivarius UCC118. Proc Natl Acad Sci U S A 2007;104:7617–21.
7. O'Mahony C, Scully P, O'Mahony D, et al. Commensal-induced regulatory T cells mediate protection against pathogen-stimulated NF-κB activation. PLoS Pathogens 2008;4(8):e1000112.
8. Sonnenburg JL, Chen CT, Gordon JI. Genomic and metabolic studies of the impact of probiotics on a model gut symbiont and host. PLoS Biol 2006;4:2213–26.

9. Kitano H, Oda K. Robustness trade-offs and host–microbial symbiosis in the immune system. Mol Syst Biol 2006;2:2006:0022

10. Deshpande G, Rao S, Patole S, et al. Updated meta-analysis of probiotics for preventing necrotizing enterocolitis in preterm neonates. Pediatrics 2010;125: 921–30.

11. Tarnow-Mordi WO, Wilkinson D, Trivedi A, et al. Probiotics reduce all-cause mortality and necrotizing enterocolitis: it is time to change practice. Pediatrics 2010;125:1068–70.

12. Soll RF. Probiotics: are we ready for routine use? Pediatrics 2010;125:1071–2.

13. Hedin C, Whelan K, Lindsay JO. Evidence for the use of probiotics and prebiotics in inflammatory bowel disease: a review of clinical trials. Proc Nutr Soc 2007;66: 307–15.

14. Marteau P, Lémann M, Seksik P, et al. Ineffectiveness of Lactobacillus johnsonii LA1 for prophylaxis of postoperative recurrence in Crohn's disease: a randomised, double-blind, placebo-controlled GETAID trial. Gut 2006;55:842–7.

15. Van Gossum A, Dewit O, Louis E, et al. Multicenter randomized–controlled clinical trial of probiotics (Lactobacillus johnsonii, LA1) on early endoscopic recurrence of Crohn's disease after Ileo–caecal resection. Inflamm Bowel Dis 2007;13: 135–42.

16. Kruis W, Fric P, Pokrotnieks J, et al. Maintaining remission of ulcerative colitis with the probiotic Escherichia coli Nissle 1917 is as effective as with standard mesalazine. Gut 2004;53:1617–23.

17. Rembacken BJ, Snelling AM, Hawkey PM, et al. Nonpathogenic Escherichia coli versus mesalazine for the treatment of ulcerative colitis: a randomised trial. Lancet 1999;354:635–9.

18. Gionchetti P, Rizzello F, Venturi A, et al. Oral bacteriotherapy as maintenance treatment in patients with chronic pouchitis: a double-blind, placebo-controlled trial. Gastroenterology 2000;119:305–9.

19. Mimura T, Rizzello F, Helwig U, et al. Once-daily high-dose probiotic therapy (VSL#3) for maintaining remission in recurrent or refractory pouchitis. Gut 2004; 53:108–14.

20. Brenner DM, Moeller MJ, Chey WD, et al. The utility of probiotics in the treatment of irritable bowel syndrome: a systematic review. Am J Gastroenterol 2009;104: 1033–49.

21. Haller D, Antoine JM, Bengmark S, et al. Guidance for substantiating the evidence for beneficial effects of probiotics: probiotics in chronic inflammatory bowel disease and the functional disorder irritable bowel syndrome. J Nutr 2010;140:690S–7.

22. Wolvers D, Antoine JM, Myllyluoma E, et al. Guidance for substantiating the evidence for beneficial effects of probiotics: prevention and management of infections by probiotics. J Nutr 2010;140:698S–712.

23. Wall R, Ross RP, Shanahan F, et al. The metabolic activity of the enteric microbiota influences the fatty acid composition of murine and porcine liver and adipose tissues. Am J Clin Nutr 2009;89:1393–401.

24. Van Huynegem K, Loos M, Steidler L. Immunomodulation by genetically engineered lactic acid bacteria. Front Biosci 2009;14:4825–35.

25. Braat H, Rottiers P, Hommes DW, et al. A phase I trial with transgenic bacteria expressing interleukin-10 in Crohn's disease. Clin Gastroenterol Hepatol 2006; 4:754–9.

Index

Note: Page numbers of article titles are in **boldface** type.

A

ABT-229 (erythromycin derivative), for GERD, 403
Acid suppression therapy
    for GERD, 397–402
    for NSAID injury, 449–451, 714–716
    new therapies for, 709–712
Acyclovir, for esophagitis, 632
Adalimumab. *See* Tumor necrosis factor-α monoclonal antibodies.
Adefovir dipivoxil, for hepatitis B, 667–675
Adrenocorticotrophic hormone, tumors secreting, 622–624
ADX 10059 (glutamate receptor antagonist), for GERD, 405
AGN 201,904-Z
    for acid suppression, 710–711
    for GERD, 401
Allergy, in proton pump inhibitor therapy, 534–535
Alosetron
    for diarrhea, 500
    for functional gastrointestinal disorders, 537
    for irritable bowel syndrome, 488
Alpha-receptor agonists, for diarrhea, 501
Alvimopan, for constipation, 514, 519–520, 522–523, 714
5-Aminosalicylic acid and related compounds, for inflammatory bowel disease, **559–599**
    administration routes for, 559–560, 562–564, 568
    adverse effects of, 590–591
    dosing of, 566–567
    efficacy of, 569–588
    enemas with, 568
    formulations of, 560, 562–568
    mechanisms of action of, 562
    prodrugs, of, 561
Amoxicillin, for *Helicobacter pylori* infection, 468–469, 484
Amphotericin B, for esophagitis, 631
Analgesics, for radiation esophagitis, 633
Anaphylaxis, in proton pump inhibitor therapy, 534–535
Anemia, in NSAID injury, 447–448
Angiogenesis inhibitors
    for carcinoid tumors, 619
    for colorectal cancer, 602–604
Angiotensin receptor blockers, for portal hypertension, 686
Angiotensin-converting enzyme inhibitors, for portal hypertension, 686
Anidulafungin, for esophagitis, 630

Gastroenterol Clin N Am 39 (2010) 727–745
doi:10.1016/S0889-8553(10)00090-7
0889-8553/10/$ – see front matter © 2010 Elsevier Inc. All rights reserved.

gastro.theclinics.com

Antacids, for GERD, 402
Antibiotics
    for diarrhea, 499
    for neutropenic enterocolitis, 637
    for portal hypertension, 689
Anticholinergic agents, for irritable bowel syndrome, 487
Antidepressants
    for dyspepsia, 485–486
    for GERD, 406
    for irritable bowel syndrome, 488–489
Antiemetic agents, for chemotherapy, 642
Antireflux agents, for GERD, 404–406
Antisecretory therapy, for dyspepsia, 484–485
Antispasmodics, for functional gastrointestinal disorders, 537
Antithymocyte globulin, for graft versus host disease, 638
Anxiolytics, for dyspepsia, 485–486
Arbaclofen placarbil, for GERD, 404–405
Asimadoline, for dyspepsia, 486
Assessing the Safety and Clinical Efficacy of New Dose of 5-ASA (ASCEND) trials,
    566–567
Atiprimod, for pancreatic neuroendocrine tumors, 623
Axitinib, for colorectal cancer, 604
Azathioprine
    hepatotoxicity of, 641
    tumor necrosis factor-α monoclonal antibodies with, for inflammatory bowel
        disease, 550
Azithromycin, for GERD, 403

B

Baclofen, for GERD, 404–405
Balsalazide, for inflammatory bowel disease
    adverse effects of, 590–591
    efficacy of, 569–570, 573–576, 580–582, 584
    formulations of, 563, 565
    mechanism of action of, 565
    structure of, 560–561
Beclomethasone, for graft versus host disease, 638
Berberine, for diarrhea, 501
Beta blockers, nonselective, for portal hypertension, 682–684, 688–690
Bethanechol, for GERD, 402
Bevacizumab
    for carcinoid tumors, 619–620
    for colorectal cancer, 602–604, 607–608
Bifidobacterium
    for constipation, 524
    potential uses of, 723
Biopsy, for NSAID injury, 448
Bisacodyl
    for constipation, 510–511
    for irritable bowel syndrome, 488

Bismuth, for diarrhea, 500
Bleeding
    in cancer therapy, 642
    upper non-variceal, **419–432**
        acid suppression, 419–420
        histamine₂-receptors antagonists not efficacious for, 421–422
        proton pump inhibitors for, 422–428
        somatostatin and analogs not recommended for, 421
        tranexamic acid not recommended for, 420
Blood loss, in NSAID injury, 447–448
BRAF oncogene, as biomarker, 606
BRiTE (Bevacizumab Regimens: Investigation of Treatment Effects) study, 604
Brivanib, for colorectal cancer, 604
Bulk laxatives, for constipation, 510–511

C

CAIRO (Capecitabine, Irinotecan, and Oxaliplatin in advanced colorectal cancer) trial, 607
Calcium carbonate, for functional gastrointestinal disorders, 537
Calmodulin antagonists, for diarrhea, 500
Calprotectin, in NSAID injury, 446–447
Cancer
    colorectal
        chemotherapy for, **601–613**
        peroxisome proliferator-activated receptor modulators for, 700–702
    therapy for, complications of, **629–647**
        constipation, 639–640
        diarrhea, 633–637
        esophagitis, 629–633
        graft versus host disease, 637–639
        hepatotoxicity, 640–642
        neutropenic enterocolitis, 637
        radiation proctitis, 639
Candidiasis, esophageal, in cancer therapy, 630–632
Cannabinoid receptor agonists, for GERD, 405–406
Capecitabine
    diarrhea due to, 633
    for colorectal cancer, 602, 607
    for pancreatic neuroendocrine tumors, 623
Capecitabine, Irinotecan, and Oxaliplatin in advanced colorectal cancer (CAIRO) trial, 607
Carcinoid tumors, well-differentiated, 617–622
Carcinomas, poorly differentiated, 624
Carvedilol, for portal hypertension, 687–688
Caspofungin, for esophagitis, 630
Ceftriaxone, for portal hypertension, 689
Certolizumab pegol. *See* Tumor necrosis factor-α monoclonal antibodies.
Cetuximab, for colorectal cancer, 603–604, 606–608
Charcoal, for diarrhea, 634
Chemotherapy
    complications of, 642–643
        constipation, 639–640

Chemotherapy (*continued*)
    diarrhea, 633–637
    esophagitis, 629–633
    graft versus host disease, 637–639
    hepatotoxicity, 640–642
    neutropenic enterocolitis, 637
  for carcinoid tumors, 621
  for colorectal cancer, **601–613**
  for pancreatic neuroendocrine tumors, 623
  for poorly differentiated carcinomas, 624
Chest pain
  in GERD, 396–397
  in NSAID injury, 436
Chloride channel activators, for constipation, 512, 514
Chloride channel antagonists, for diarrhea, 501
Chloride secretion, diarrhea in, 496–497
Chlorpromazine, for diarrhea, 500
Cholestyramine
  for diarrhea, 500
  for irritable bowel syndrome, 488
Cimetidine, for functional gastrointestinal disorders, 535–537
Cirrhosis, portal hypertension in, 681–695
Cisapride
  for constipation, 523
  for dyspepsia, 485
  for GERD, 402–403
Cisplatin, for poorly differentiated carcinomas, 624
Clarithromycin, for *Helicobacter pylori* infection, 469, 484
Clonidine, for portal hypertension, 686
Clopidogrel, proton pump inhibitor use with, 530–531
Clopidogrel and the Optimization of Gastrointestinal Events Trial (COGENT), 531
Clostridium difficile infections
  in cancer therapy, 636–637
  in proton pump inhibitor therapy, 531–532
Clotrimazole, for esophagitis, 631–632
Codeine, for diarrhea, 498–499, 634
COGENT (Clopidogrel and the Optimization of Gastrointestinal Events Trial), 531
Colchicine, for constipation, 524
Colesevelam, for irritable bowel syndrome, 488
Colon, NSAID injury of, 438–439
Colorectal cancer
  chemotherapy for, **601–613**
    adjuvant, 607–608
    systemic, 601–602
    targeted, 602–607
  peroxisome proliferator-activated receptor modulators for, **697–707,** 700–702
Colorectal Oral Novel Therapy for the Inhibition of Angiogenesis and Retarding
  of Metastases (CONFIRM) study, 604
Constipation
  in cancer therapy, 639–640
  treatment of, **509–527**

alvimopan, 514, 519–520, 522–523, 714
bulk laxatives, 510–511
chloride channel activators, 512, 514
colchicine, 524
guanylate cyclase C activators, 513–514
in irritable bowel syndrome, 487–489
linaclotide, 513–514, 517
lubiprostone, 512, 514, 516
methylnaltrexone, 513–514, 519, 522
mixed laxatives, 511
motilin agonists, 524
neurotrophin-3, 521, 524
new products for, 712–714
NKTR-118, 520
opioid antagonists, 513–514, 522
opioid-induced, 714
osmotic laxatives, 510–512
probiotics and prebiotics, 524
prucalopride, 515, 517–518, 523
serotonergic agonists, 515, 523
stimulant laxatives, 510–511
stool softeners, 510–511
TD-5108, 518
Corticosteroids, for graft versus host disease, 638–639
Crohn's disease
5-aminosalicylic acid compounds for, **559–599**
tumor necrosis factor-α monoclonal antibodies for, **543–557**
Cyclooxygenase-inhibiting nitric oxide donors, for NSAID injury, 716
Cyclophosphamide
for graft versus host disease, 638
hepatotoxicity of, 641
Cytarabine, hepatotoxicity of, 641
Cytochrome 450 enzymes
in clarithromycin metabolism, 469
in metronidazole metabolism, 469–470
in proton pump inhibitor metabolism, 466, 472–473, 530–531
Cytomegalovirus infections, of esophagus, 632

D

Dacarbazine, for pancreatic neuroendocrine tumors, 623
Daunorubicin, hepatotoxicity of, 641
Dexlansoprazole, 398–400, 710
Dexrabeprazole, for GERD, 401
Diarrhea, **495–507**
in cancer therapy, 633–637
in irritable bowel syndrome, 487–489
in stem cell transplantation, 635–636
mechanisms of, 495–498
therapy for, 498–502
Diclofenac, in combinations, for NSAID injury, 715–716

Dicyclomine
 for functional gastrointestinal disorders, 537
 for irritable bowel syndrome, 487
Dietary fiber, for irritable bowel syndrome, 487
Dimethyl sulfoxide, in combinations, for NSAID injury, 715–716
Diphenoxylate
 for diarrhea, 498–499, 634
 for irritable bowel syndrome, 487
DM-3458, for acid suppression, 710–711
Docusate, for constipation, 510–511
Domperidone
 for dyspepsia, 485
 for functional gastrointestinal disorders, 538
 for GERD, 402
Doxorubicin
 for pancreatic neuroendocrine tumors, 623
 hepatotoxicity of, 641
Duodenum
 mucosal injury due to, 436–437, 441
 NSAID injury of, 436–437
Dyspepsia, therapy for, 482–487
 evaluation for, 482–484
 functional, 484–487
 proton pump inhibitors, 530–535
 uninvestigated, 484
Dysphagia
 in GERD, 396–397
 in NSAID injury, 436

E

Eastern Cooperative Oncology Group colorectal cancer trial, 604
Echinocandins, for esophagitis, 630–632
Elderly persons, NSAID injury in, 435
Endoscopy
 for dyspepsia, 484
 for NSAID injury, 445, 447–448
Endostatin, for carcinoid tumors, 619, 621
Enemas, for 5-aminosalicylic acid administration, 568
Enkephalinase inhibitors, for diarrhea, 499–500
Entecavir, for hepatitis B, 667–675
Enteric infections, in proton pump inhibitor therapy, 531–532
Enterocolitis, neutropenic, in cancer therapy, 637
Epidermal growth factor inhibitors, for colorectal cancer, 605–607
Erlotinib, for colorectal cancer, 607
Erythromycin, for GERD, 402–404
Esmoprazole
 for GERD, 398, 400–402
 for non-variceal upper gastrointestinal bleeding, 423
 for NSAID injury, 450–451
 in combinations, for NSAID injury, 715

Esophagitis, in cancer therapy, 629–633
Esophagus
    NSAID injury of, 435–436
    reflux into. See Gastroesophageal reflux disease.
Etanercept, ineffective for inflammatory bowel disease, 545
Etoposide, for poorly differentiated carcinomas, 624
Everolimus, for pancreatic neuroendocrine tumors, 622

F

Famciclovir, for esophagitis, 632
Famotidine
    for functional gastrointestinal disorders, 535–537
    in combinations, for NSAID injury, 715
    omeprazole with, 712
Fedotozine, for dyspepsia, 486
Fistula formation, in cancer therapy, 642
Fluconazole, for esophagitis, 630–631
Fluoropyrimidine capecitabine, for colorectal cancer, 602
Fluoroquinolones, for Helicobacter pylori infection, 470–471
5-Fluorouracil
    diarrhea due to, 633
    for colorectal cancer, 601–603, 607
    for pancreatic neuroendocrine tumors, 623
    hepatotoxicity of, 641–642
FOLFIRI regimen, for colorectal cancer, 602, 604
FOLFOX regimen, for colorectal cancer, 602–604, 607
Folinic acid, for colorectal cancer, 601–603, 607
Functional gastrointestinal disorders, therapy for, **529–542**
    histamine$_2$-receptor antagonists, 535–537
    prokinetic agents, 537–538
    proton pump inhibitors, 530–535
    safety of, 537–538
Fungal infections, in cancer therapy, 630–632

G

Gamma-aminobutyric acid-receptor agonists, for GERD, 404–405
Ganciclovir, for esophagitis, 632
Gastrinomas, 622–624
Gastroenteropancreatic neuroendocrine tumors, **615–628**
    classification of, 616–617
    prevalence of, 615–616
    therapy for
        impediments to, 617
        poorly differentiated carcinomas, 624
        well-differentiated carcinoids, 617–622
        well-differentiated pancreatic, 622–624
Gastroesophageal reflux disease, **393–418**
    clinical manifestations of, 396–397

Gastroesophageal (*continued*)
    economic costs of, 394
    pathophysiology of, 394–395
    prevalence of, 393–394
    therapy for
        acid suppression, 397–402
        antireflux agents, 404
        cannabinoid receptor agonists, 405–406
        current recommendations, 406–408
        gamma-aminobutyric acid-receptor agonists, 404–405
        glutamate receptor antagonists, 405
        histamine$_2$-receptor antagonists, 535–537
        motility agents, 402–404
        mucosal protection, 406
        nonacid suppression, 402–406
        proton pump inhibitors, 530–535, 709–711
        visceral pain modulators, 406
Gefitinib
    for carcinoid tumors, 621
    for pancreatic neuroendocrine tumors, 623
GERD. *See* Gastroesophageal reflux disease.
Glucagon-like peptide-2 analogue, for short bowel syndrome, 717
Glucagonomas, 622–624
Glutamate receptor antagonists, for GERD, 405
Graft versus host disease, in cancer therapy, 637–639
Guanilib, for constipation, 513
Guanylate cyclase C activators, for constipation, 513–514

H

Heartburn, in GERD, 396–397
Helicobacter pylori infection
    eradication therapy for, **465–480**
        amoxicillin, 468–469
        antibiotic combinations, 472
        clarithromycin, 469
        fluoroquinolones, 470–471
        metronidazole, 469–470
        pharmacogenetics of, 472–476
        proton pump inhibitors, 466–467, 472–473
        rescue, 473–476
        tetracyclines, 471–472
    in dyspepsia, 484–485
    NSAID injury and, 439–440
Hemorrhage, variceal, portal hypertension and, 687–690
Hepatic vein pressure gradient, in portal hypertension, 682
Hepatitis, drug-induced, 640–642
Hepatitis B
    drug-induced hepatotoxicity with, 640
    therapy for, **659–680**
        interferon, 661–667

    nucleos(t)ide analogues, 667–675
    viral replication cycle and, 659–660
Hepatitis C
  drug-induced hepatotoxicity with, 641
  therapy for, peginterferon alfa with ribavirin, **649–658**
Herpes simplex infections, of esophagus, 632
Histamine₂-receptor antagonists
  for dyspepsia, 484
  for functional gastrointestinal disorders, 535–537
  for GERD, 397
  not effacious for non-variceal upper gastrointestinal bleeding, 421–422
  proton pump inhibitors with, 712
Hydrogen sulfide, for NSAID injury, 716–717
5-Hydroxyamine, diarrhea due to, 497–498
Hyocyamine, for functional gastrointestinal disorders, 537
Hypergastrinemia, in proton pump inhibitor therapy, 533
Hypertension, portal. See Portal hypertension.

I

Ibuprofen, in combinations, for NSAID injury, 715
IDEAL (Individual Dosing Efficacy versus Flat Dosing to Assess Optimal Pegylated
    Interferon Therapy), 653–654
Ifosamide, hepatotoxicity of, 641
Ilaprazole
  for acid suppression, 710–711
  for GERD, 401
Individual Dosing Efficacy versus Flat Dosing to Assess Optimal Pegylated Interferon
    Therapy (IDEAL) study, 653–654
Inflammation, peroxisome proliferator-activated receptor modulators for, **697–707**
Inflammatory bowel disease
  5-aminosalicylic acid compounds for, **559–599**
  peroxisome proliferator-activated receptor modulators for, 699–700
  tumor necrosis factor-α monoclonal antibodies for, **543–557**
Infliximab. See Tumor necrosis factor-α monoclonal antibodies.
  for graft versus host disease, 638
Insulinomas, 622–624
Interferon, pegylated
  for carcinoid tumors, 619
  for hepatitis B, 661–667
    dose of, 664
    duration of, 664
    efficacy of, 664–666
    mechanisms of action of, 661–663
    pharmacokinetics of, 663
    side effects of, 666–667
  with ribavirin, for hepatitis C, **649–658**
Ion secretion, diarrhea in, 496–497
Irinotecan
  diarrhea due to, 633
  for colorectal cancer, 601–602, 607

Irinotecan (*continued*)
    for poorly differentiated carcinomas, 624
    hepatotoxicity of, 641–642
Irritable bowel syndrome, 487–489
Isosorbide dinitrate, for portal hypertension, 686, 690
Itraconazole, for esophagitis, 630–631

K

Kaolin, for diarrhea, 634
Ketamine, for GERD, 406
KRAS oncogene, as biomarker, 606

L

Lactobacillus
    for constipation, 524
    potential uses of, 723
Lamivudine, for hepatitis B, 640, 664–675
Lanreotide, for carcinoid tumors, 618
Lansoprazole, 710
    for functional gastrointestinal disorders, 530
    for GERD, 399–400
    for *Helicobacter pylori* infection, 467
    for non-variceal upper gastrointestinal bleeding, 423–424, 426
    in combinations, for NSAID injury, 715
Lanza score, for NSAID injury, 448
Laser therapy, for radiation proctitis, 639
Laxatives
    for constipation, 510–512, 640
    for irritable bowel syndrome, 487
Lesogaberan, for GERD, 405
Levofloxacin, for *Helicobacter pylori* infection, 471
Lidocaine, for radiation esophagitis, 633
Linaclotide
    for constipation, 513–514, 517, 713–714
    for irritable bowel syndrome, 488
Linaprazan, for GERD, 402
Liver
    disorders of. *See also* Hepatitis B; Hepatitis C.
        portal hypertension in, 681–695
    drug-induced damage of, 640–642
Loperamide
    for diarrhea, 498–499, 634
    for functional gastrointestinal disorders, 537
    for irritable bowel syndrome, 487
Lubiprostone
    for constipation, 512, 514, 516, 640, 712–713
    for functional gastrointestinal disorders, 537

M

Macrolides, for GERD, 402–404

Magaldrate, for functional gastrointestinal disorders, 537

Magnesium salts
  for constipation, 512
  for irritable bowel syndrome, 487

Mebeverine, for irritable bowel syndrome, 487

Mercaptopurine, hepatotoxicity of, 641

Mesalamine. *See* 5-Aminosalicylic acid and related compounds.

Methotrexate
  hepatotoxicity of, 641
  tumor necrosis factor-α monoclonal antibodies with, for inflammatory bowel
    disease, 550

Methylnaltrexone, for constipation, 513–514, 519, 522, 640, 714

Methylprednisolone, for graft versus host disease, 638

Metoclopramide
  for functional gastrointestinal disorders, 537–538
  for GERD, 402

Metronidazole
  for diarrhea, 636
  for *Helicobacter pylori* infection, 469–470

Micafungin, for esophagitis, 630

Miconazole, for esophagitis, 632

Minocyline, for *Helicobacter pylori* infection, 471–472

Misoprostol, for NSAID injury prevention, 451

Mitemcinal, for constipation, 524

Monoclonal antibodies, tumor necrosis factor-α, **543–557**

Morphine, for diarrhea, 498–499

MOSAIC (Multicenter International Study of Oxaliplatin/5-fluorouracil/Leucovorin in the
  Adjuvant Treatment of Colon Cancer) trial, 607

Mosapride, for dyspepsia, 485

Motilin agonists
  for constipation, 524
  for GERD, 403

Motility, disorders of, diarrhea in, 496

Motility agents, for GERD, 402–404

Mucosal injury, from NSAIDs. *See* Nonsteroidal antiinflammatory drugs, mucosal injury
  due to.

Mucosal protection
  for GERD, 406
  for NSAID injury, 449–451, 716–717

Mucositis, oral, in cancer therapy, 642–643

Multicenter International Study of Oxaliplatin/5-fluorouracil/Leucovorin in the Adjuvant
  Treatment of Colon Cancer (MOSAIC) trial, 607

Mycophenolate mofetil, for graft versus host disease, 638

N

Nadolol, for portal hypertension, 684, 688, 690

Naproxcinod, for NSAID injury, 453, 716

Naproxen, for NSAID injury, 715–716
Nausea and vomiting, in chemotherapy, 642
NCX-1000, for portal hypertension, 686
Neuroendocrine tumors. *See* Gastroenteropancreatic neuroendocrine tumors.
Neurotrophin-3, for constipation, 521, 524
Neutropenic enterocolitis, in cancer therapy, 637
Neutrophil gelatinase–associated lipocalin, in inflammatory bowel disease, 547
Nitroglycerin, for portal hypertension, 686, 689
NKTR-118, for constipation, 520
Nonsteroidal antiinflammatory drugs, **433–464**
    mucosal injury due to
        alternatives to, 453
        clinical features of, 435–439
        colonic, 438–439
        epidemiology of, 434–435
        esophageal, 435–436
        evaluation of, 445–448
        gastroduodenal, 436–437, 441
        mechanisms of, 440–445
        prevention of, 448–451, 714–717
        risk factors for, 439
        selective versus nonselective, 451–453
        small intestinal, 437–438
    usage statistics for, 433
Norfloxacin, for portal hypertension, 689
North Central Cancer Treatment Group, colorectal cancer studies of, 608
NSAIDs. *See* Nonsteroidal antiinflammatory drugs.
Nucleos(t)ide analogues, for hepatitis B, 667–675
    dose for, 669–670
    efficacy of, 671, 673–674
    mechanisms of action of, 667–668
    pharmacokinetics of, 668–669
    resistance to, 670–672
    side effects of, 674–675
Nystatin, for esophagitis, 631

O

Octreotide
    for carcinoid tumors, 618
    for diarrhea, 634
    for portal hypertension, 685–686, 688–689
Odynophagia, in NSAID injury, 436
Olsalazine, for inflammatory bowel disease
    adverse effects of, 590–591
    efficacy of, 569, 572–573, 577, 582–583, 586
    formulations of, 563, 565
    mechanism of action of, 565
    structure of, 560–561
Omeprazole
    famotidine with, 712

for functional gastrointestinal disorders, 530–531
for GERD, 399–401
for *Helicobacter pylori* infection, 466–467
for non-variceal upper gastrointestinal bleeding, 422–426
in pregnancy, 535
sodium bicarbonate with, 710
with meal-mimicking agent, 710
Opioid(s)
    constipation due to, 714
    for diarrhea, 498–499
Opioid agonists, for diarrhea, 634
Opioid antagonists, for constipation, 513–514, 522
Oral rehydration therapy, for diarrhea, 498
Osmotic diarrhea, mechanisms of, 496
Osmotic laxatives, for constipation, 510–512
Oxaliplatin
    for colorectal cancer, 601–602, 607
    hepatotoxicity of, 641–642

P

PACCE (Panitumumab Advanced Colorectal Cancer Evaluation), 607
Pain, visceral, modulators of, 406
Palifermin, for mucositis, 642–643
Pancreatic neuroendocrine tumors, well-differentiated, 622–624
Pancreatitis, in cancer therapy, 642
Panitumumab, for colorectal cancer, 603, 605–607
Panitumumab Advanced Colorectal Cancer Evaluation (PACCE), 607
Pantoprazole
    for functional gastrointestinal disorders, 530
    for GERD, 401
    for non-variceal upper gastrointestinal bleeding, 421, 423–424, 426
Parathyroid hormone–related hormone, tumors secreting, 622–624
Pasireotide, for carcinoid tumors, 618
Peptic ulcer bleeding. *See* Bleeding, upper non-variceal.
Perforation, gastrointestinal, in cancer therapy, 642
Peroxisome proliferator-activated receptor modulators, for colorectal cancer, **697–707**
Pharmacology
    of acid-related disorder therapy. *See* Acid suppression therapy.
    of 5-aminosalicylic acid compounds, **559–599**
    of colorectal cancer therapy, **601–613, 697–707**
    of constipation therapy. *See* Constipation.
    of diarrhea therapy. *See* Diarrhea.
    of dyspepsia therapy, 482–487
    of functional disorder therapy, 537–538
    of gastroesophageal reflux disease therapy, **393–418**
    of gastrointestinal bleeding therapy, upper non-variceal, **419–432**
    of *Helicobacter pylori* infection therapy, **465–480**
    of hepatitis B therapy, **659–680**
    of hepatitis C therapy, **649–658**
    of inflammatory bowel disease therapy, **543–557, 559–599**

Pharmacology (*continued*)
   of irritable bowel syndrome therapy, 487–489
   of neuroendocrine tumor therapy, **615–628**
   of new therapies, **709–720**
   of NSAID injury, **433–464**
   of oncologic therapy, **629–647**
   of peginterferon, **649–658**
   of peroxisome proliferator-activated receptors, **697–707**
   of portal hypertension therapy, **681–695**
   of probiotics, **721–726**
   of ribavirin, **649–658**
   of tumor necrosis factor-α monoclonal antibodies, **543–557**
Plums, dried, for constipation, 511–512
Pneumonia, in proton pump inhibitor therapy, 532–533
Polyethylene glycol
   for constipation, 510–512
   for irritable bowel syndrome, 487
Portal hypertension, **681–695**
   classification of, 682
   pathophysiology of, 681–682
   pressure measurement in, 682
   therapy for
      drugs reducing flow and resistance, 686–687
      drugs reducing portal flow, 682, 684
      drugs reducing resistance to blood flow, 686
      in acute variceal hemorrhage, 688–689
      nonselective beta-adrenergic blockers, 682–684, 688–690
      prophylactic, 687–690
      somatostatin and analogues, 685–686
      vasopressin and analogues, 685
Posaconazole, for esophagitis, 630–631
Potassium-competitive acid blockers
   for GERD, 401–402
   novel, 710, 712
Prazosin, for portal hypertension, 686
Prebiotics, for constipation, 524
Pregnancy
   proton pump inhibitors in, 535
   tumor necrosis factor-α monoclonal antibodies in, 551–553
Prevention of Latent Ulceration Treatment Options (PLUTO), 450–451
Probiotics, **721–726**, 723–724
   clinical use of, 723–725
   for constipation, 524
   for irritable bowel syndrome, 489
   genetic engineering of, 725
   mechanism of action of, 722–723
   terminology of, 722
Proctitis, radiation, 639
Prokinetic agents
   for dyspepsia, 485
   for functional gastrointestinal disorders, 537–538

for GERD, 402–404
novel, 712
PROMID study, of neuroendocrine tumors, 618
Propranolol, for portal hypertension, 684, 688, 690
Prostaglandins
    deficiency of, NSAID injury in, 441–444
    diarrhea due to, 497–498
Proton pump inhibitors
    for dyspepsia, 484
    for functional gastrointestinal disorders, 530–535
        allergy due to, 534–535
        Clostridium difficile due to, 531–532
        drug-drug interactions with, 530–531
        in pregnancy, 535
        osteoporosis due to, 533–534
        pneumonia due to, 532–533
        rebound hypersecretion due to, 533
        vitamin B$_{12}$ deficiency due to, 534
    for GERD, 397–402, 406–408
    for *Helicobacter pylori* infection, 466–467, 472–473
    for non-variceal upper gastrointestinal bleeding, 422–428
        after hospital discharge, 427
        in real-life setting, 426–428
        intravenous, 422–425
        mechanism of action of, 422
        oral, 425–426
        randomized trials of, 423–425
    for NSAID injury, 449–450
    histamine$_2$-receptor antagonists with, 712
    novel, 709–711
Prucalopride
    for acid suppression, 712
    for constipation, 515, 517–518, 523
    for irritable bowel syndrome, 488
Prunes, for constipation, 511–512
Psychotherapy, for dyspepsia, 486
Psychotropic agents, for dyspepsia, 485–486

R

R137696, for dyspepsia, 486
Rabeprazole
    for *Helicobacter pylori* infection, 467
    for non-variceal upper gastrointestinal bleeding, 423, 426
Racecadotril, for diarrhea, 500
RAD001 in Advanced Neuroendocrine Tumors study, 622
Radiation therapy, complications of
    diarrhea, 633–637
    esophagitis, 629–633
    proctitis, 639

Ranitidine
    for functional gastrointestinal disorders, 535–537
    not effacious for non-variceal upper gastrointestinal bleeding, 421–422
Rebound hypersecretion, in proton pump inhibitor therapy, 533
Reflux, gastrointestinal. See Gastroesophageal reflux disease.
Registry of Patients with Upper Gastrointestinal Bleeding Undergoing Endoscopy, 426
Regurgitation, in GERD, 396–397
Renzapride
    for constipation, 523
    for functional gastrointestinal disorders, 538
Resistance, to nucleos(t)ide analogues, 670–672
Revaprazan, for GERD, 402
Ribavirin, with peginterferon alfa, for hepatitis C, **649–658**
Rifaximin
    for diarrhea, 637
    for irritable bowel syndrome, 489
Riluzole, for GERD, 405

S

Secretory diarrhea, mechanisms of, 496
Selective cyclooxygenase-2 inhibitors, mucosal injury due to
    epidemiology of, 434–435
    evaluation of, 445–448
    gastroduodenal, 437
    mechanisms of, 440–441, 443, 445
    risk factors for, 439
    versus nonselective COX inhibitors, 451–453
Selective serotonin reuptake inhibitors, for GERD, 406
Senna, for constipation, 510–511
Serotonergic agonists, for constipation, 515, 523
Serotonin, diarrhea due to, 497–498
Short bowel syndrome, 717
Simvastatin, for portal hypertension, 686
Small intestine, NSAID injury of, 437–438
Sodium, absorption of, diarrhea in, 497
Sodium picosulfate, for constipation, 510–511
Somatostatin and analogs
    for carcinoid tumors, 618
    for diarrhea, 499
    for portal hypertension, 685–686, 689
    not recommended for non-variceal upper gastrointestinal bleeding, 421
Somatostatinomas, 622–624
Sorafenib
    for carcinoid tumors, 619
    for pancreatic neuroendocrine tumors, 623
Soraprazan, for GERD, 402
SP-303, for diarrhea, 501
Stem cell transplantation
    diarrhea due to, 635–636
    graft versus host disease in, 637–639

Stimulant laxatives, for constipation, 510–511
Stomach
    mucosal injury due to, 436–437, 441
    NSAID injury of, 436–437
Stool softeners, for constipation, 510
Streptozocin, for pancreatic neuroendocrine tumors, 623
Substance P
    antagonists of, for diarrhea, 504
    diarrhea due to, 498
Sucralfate
    for diarrhea, 634
    for functional gastrointestinal disorders, 537
    for GERD, 406
Sucrose permeability test, for NSAID injury, 445–446
Sulfasalazine, for inflammatory bowel disease
    efficacy of, 564, 569–574, 576–577, 579–580, 583–584
    formulations of, 563
    mechanism of action of, 564
    structure of, 560–561
Sunitinib
    for carcinoid tumors, 619
    for pancreatic neuroendocrine tumors, 622–623

T

Tandospirone, for dyspepsia, 486
TD-5108 (Velusetrag), for constipation, 518, 523
Teduglutide, for short bowel syndrome, 717
Tegaserod
    for constipation, 510–511, 523
    for functional gastrointestinal disorders, 538
    for GERD, 403, 406
Telbivudine, for hepatitis B, 667–675
Temozolomide, for pancreatic neuroendocrine tumors, 623
Temsirolimus, for carcinoid tumors, 621
Tenatoprazole
    for acid suppression, 710–711
    for GERD, 398, 401
Tenofovir, for hepatitis B, 667–675
Terlipressin, for portal hypertension, 685, 688–689
Tetracyclines, for Helicobacter pylori infection, 471–472
Thalidomide, for carcinoid tumors, 619
6-Thioguanine, hepatotoxicity of, 641
Thrombosis, in cancer therapy, 642
Tranexamic acid, not recommended for non-variceal upper gastrointestinal
    bleeding, 420
Transplantation, stem cell
    diarrhea due to, 635–636
    graft versus host disease in, 637–639
Trazodone, for GERD, 406

Trial to Assess Improvement in Therapeutic Outcomes by Optimizing Platelet Inhibition
    with Prasugrel-Thrombolysis in Myocardial Infarction (TRITON-TIMI), 531
Tricyclic antidepressants
    for dyspepsia, 485–486
    for GERD, 406
    for irritable bowel syndrome, 488–489
TRITON-TIMI (Trial to Assess Improvement in Therapeutic Outcomes by Optimizing Platelet
    Inhibition with Prasugrel-Thrombolysis in Myocardial Infarction), 531
TU-199 (tenatoprazole isomer), for GERD, 398, 401
Tumor necrosis factor-α monoclonal antibodies, **543–557**
    combination therapy with, 550
    immunogenicity of, 549–550
    in pregnancy, 551–553
    mechanisms of action of, 545–548
    pharmacokinetics of, 548–549
    safety of, 551
    structures of, 545
    successive therapy with, 550–551
Tumors, neuroendocrine. See Gastroenteropancreatic neuroendocrine tumors.

U

Ulcer(s)
    in NSAID injury, 436–437
    oral, in cancer therapy, 642–643
    peptic. See Bleeding, upper non-variceal.
Ulcerative colitis
    5-aminosalicylic acid compounds for, **559–599**
    tumor necrosis factor-α monoclonal antibodies for, **543–557**

V

Valacyclovir, for esophagitis, 632
Valganciclovir, for esophagitis, 632
Vancomycin, for diarrhea, 636–637
Vapreotide, for portal hypertension, 685–686, 689
Varicella-zoster virus infections, of esophagus, 632
Varices and variceal hemorrhage, portal hypertension and, 687–690
Vascular endothelial growth factor inhibitors, for colorectal cancer, 602–604
Vasoactive intestinal peptide antagonists, for diarrhea, 501–502
Vasodilators, for portal hypertension, 686
Vasopressin and analogues, for portal hypertension, 685, 689
Vatalanib
    for carcinoid tumors, 619
    for colorectal cancer, 604
VECAM, for acid suppression, 710–711
Velusetrag (TD-5108), for constipation, 518, 523
Verification of Esmoprazole for NSAID Ulcers and Symptoms (VENUS) study, 450–451
VIPomas, 622–624
Viral infections, in cancer therapy, 632
Visceral pain modulators, for GERD, 406
Voriconazole, for esophagitis, 630–631

W

WIN 55,212-2 (cannabinoid receptor agonist), for GERD, 405–406
World Health Organization, neuroendocrine tumor classification of, 616–617

X

XELOX regimen, for colorectal cancer, 602–604

Z

Zaldaride maleate, for diarrhea, 500
Zegerid, for acid suppression, 710–711

Moving?

Make sure your subscription moves with you!

To notify us of your new address, find your **Clinics Account Number** (located on your mailing label above your name), and contact customer service at:

Email: journalscustomerservice-usa@elsevier.com

800-654-2452 (subscribers in the U.S. & Canada)
314-447-8871 (subscribers outside of the U.S. & Canada)

Fax number: 314-447-8029

Elsevier Health Sciences Division
Subscription Customer Service
3251 Riverport Lane
Maryland Heights, MO 63043

*To ensure uninterrupted delivery of your subscription,
please notify us at least 4 weeks in advance of move.